The Hatherleigh Guide to Psychopharmacology

The Hatherleigh Guides Series

The
Hatherleigh
Guide to
Psychopharmacology

Hatherleigh Press • New York

The Hatherleigh Guide to Psychopharmacology

Project Editor: Stacy M. Powell
Indexer: Sandi Frank
Cover Design: Gary Szczecina

© 1999 Hatherleigh Press
A Division of The Hatherleigh Company, Ltd.
1114 First Avenue, Suite 500, New York, NY 10021-8325

This book is printed on acid-free paper.

Compiled under the auspices of the editorial boards of *Directions in Psychiatry, Essential Psychopharmacology, Directions in Mental Health Counseling, Directions in Clinical and Counseling Psychology, and Directions in Rehabilitation Counseling*.

Library of Congress Cataloging-in-Publication Data

The Hatherleigh Guide to Psychopharmacology.
      p.   cm. -- (The Hatherleigh guides series; 11)
   Includes bibliographical references and indexes.
   ISBN 1-57826-022-1 (alk. paper)
   1. Psychopharmacology—Handbooks, manuals, etc. I. Title: Guide to psycho-
     pharmacology. II. Title: Psychopharmacology. III. Series.
   RC456.H38   1996 vol. 11
   [RM315]
   616.89 S--dc21
   [615'. 78]   99–11869
                                                                     CIP

March 1999

10 9 8 7 6 5 4 3 2 1
Printed in the USA

The Hatherleigh Guide to Psychopharmacology
was compiled under the auspices of the editorial boards of
Directions in Psychiatry, Essential Psychopharmacology,
Directions in Mental Health Counseling,
Directions in Clinical and Counseling Psychology, and
Directions in Rehabilitation Counseling

v

Table of Contents

Illustrations

Introduction

It always surprises and dismays me that, in spite of the enormous amount of information available to professionals about psychopharmacological agents, these drugs continue to be widely used in ineffective and sometimes even dangerous ways. Only recently, I was asked to consult in the case of a young woman who had been maintained on serotonergic reputake inhibitors for years, and was abruptly taken off them when she had to undergo major surgery and general anesthesia. After her operation, she appeared to be in good spirits for several weeks. In spite of a long history of depression and several previous suicide attempts, her psychiatrist did not restart her on antidepressants. Moreover, when she informed him that she was deeply depressed again, with urges to end her life, he failed to offer the protection she required. Shortly after she left his office, she made a serious, nearly successful suicidal attempt.

On another occasion, I was asked to see a patient who did not respond as expected to antidepressant therapy, although several different drugs had been used in adequate dosages and for sufficient periods of time. A brief, careful history strongly suggested hypothyroidism, and indeed, appropriate testing confirmed the diagnosis. When thyroid hormone was administered in conjunction with the patient's antidepressant medication, her depression steadily abated.

Finally, I recall consulting with a patient, a 47-year-old woman, who developed side-effects to very small doses of several diffierent SSRIs. I'd seen this problem several times before, and I usually end up keeping the patient on very low doses, if there is any effectiveness, or finding another type of antidepressant for the patient. But I also routinely inquire about psychodynamic issues that may relate to the patient's perception of medication usage or her interaction with me, her doctor. In this case I asked her about experiences with doctors throughout the course of her life. Indeed she had experienced several traumas in this context, one as a child when she was severely punished for hiding from a pediatrician when he made a house call, and another when she lilterally leaped off the operating table as she was about to be given anesthesia for a tonsillectomy. While her adverse reaction to medication was quite real, it also had a significant psychological overlay, and I observed moderate improvement in her response to and tolerance of the antidepressant that she was taking at that time.

I cite these three clinical anecdotes to emphasize how important it is to approach the practice of psychopharmacology in a genuinely sophisticated way. Up-to-date information, experience, alertness, thoroughness, careful monitoring, and real understanding of the psychodynamic and psychosocial issues in every patient's situation are essential ingredients of good management. Because many patients receive several different medications, some psychiatric, some related to other medical illnesses, a working knowledge of drug-drug interactions is critical.

The Hatherleigh Guide to Psychopharmacology contains much pertinent data to help us achieve such a standard of practice—antidepressants and mood stabilizers, antipsychotics in schizophrenia, drug-drug interactions in adults, adolescents, and children, cross cultural perspectives, and insights into how patients themselves view pharmacotherapy. As valuable a reference as it is, such data is only one component of informed practice. The rest is up to the determination and conscientiousness of the practitioner.

Frederic Flach, MD
New York Presbyterian Hospital,
New York, NY

1　The Patient's View of Antipsychotic Pharmacotherapy

Klaus Windgassen, MD

Dr. Windgassen is Professor of Psychiatry, University of Münster, Germany, and Director of Remscheid Psychiatric Hospital, Remscheid, Germany.

Editor's Note

In this chapter, the author reminds us that our most difficult patients, those with schizophrenic symptoms, require us to vigorously deploy all of our skills to provide for their well-being. The schizophrenic patient's impaired ability to pinpoint the sources of his or her anguish poses an enormous challenge to the practitioner, and it is a mistake to think that the proliferation of psychopharmacologic treatments has somehow simplified this process. There is no drug that compensates for an inadequate assessment of the patient with schizophrenia.

The patient with schizophrenia counts on us to be patient and persistent, to differentiate between symptoms and medication side effects, to prioritize our treatment approach from our patients' vantage point, to account for variables predictive of outcome which the patients themselves may not be capable of communicating to us in clear and specific terms. The author recommends that we seek to identify the global subjective experience of these patients, as determined by personality, situation, severity of illness, assessment of coping strength, and the presence of psychosocial supports, and then tailor our treatment approach accordingly.

It is key to attend constantly to the symptoms and side effects that pose the patient the most difficulty. Among the useful and fascinating insights in this chapter is the proposal that the patient's experience of a lack of positive drug effects exerts a greater influence on the patient's sense of the value of antipsychotic pharmacotherapy. Thus, it would seem that patients who reject pharmacotherapy see no good reason to take these drugs, as opposed to responding primarily to negative medication side effects, for example. We also learn that patients experiencing acute schizophrenic episodes subjectively report enormous benefits from the alleviation of restlessness and anxiety and the restoration of a balanced emotional state that atypical antipsychotic drugs can make possible. Therefore, it would seem that targeting such symptoms should be a priority in treating this patient population, both from the standpoint of enhancing treatment compliance and of addressing the most disturbing effects of schizphrenia and antipsychotic medication(s).

Contradictory Evaluations

The established efficacy of antipsychotic pharmacotherapy has paved the way for progress in the treatment of patients with schizophrenia. For example, the use of antipsychotics has dramatically reduced hospitalization periods, with far more patients than before reaping the benefits of environmentally-oriented, sociotherapeutic, and psychotherapeutic treatment methods on an outpatient basis. Many patients whose symptoms once would have consigned them to long-term hospitalization can now lead reasonably normal lives as members of outpatient programs for the rehabilitation of persons with chronic and severe mental illness. **Moreover, the relapse-preventing effect of antipsychotics has been substantiated in more than 40 placebo-controlled studies.**

On the other hand, **the media and the general public still evince a deep-rooted skepticism toward antipsychotic medications, not infrequently rejecting them out of hand as "chemical strait-jackets."** However, the same stereotype was used at the turn of the century to reject drugs for treating schizophrenic psychoses.[1] Even without the experience of motor-impairing side effects, the chemical strait-jacket metaphor seems a fitting way of expressing reservations against *any* form of drug therapy for patients with schizophrenia.

In view of these discrepancies, **special attention must be paid to the subjective rating of patients undergoing antipsychotic pharmacother-**

apy. Compliance provides inadequate information in this respect. Although the patient complies with the medical prescription based on his or her experience of the prescribed antipsychotic, the patient's decision to use such an agent over time is also influenced by numerous other factors, e.g., the patient's level of awareness of any symptoms in need of treatment, how strongly the psychotic symptoms affect the patient, and the patient's estimate of the risk of relapse, to name a few. Noncompliance is widespread among patients with schizophrenia—a median of 41% was reported by Young et al.[2] on the basis of 21 studies evaluated; the noncompliance rate among physically ill patients is often on a similar scale.[3] Moreover, changes in medication on the patient's own initiative are by no means confined to reducing the dose or discontinuing antipsychotic drug intake: 27 out of 178 schizophrenic patients (15%) enrolled in a study by Hornung et al.[4] *increased* their medication on their own initiative within a two-year period. The majority of them rated their subjective experience with the increased dose as essentially good, whereas patients with experience in discontinuing antipsychotic intake themselves without the guidance of the psychiatrist reported an essentially poor effect.

Methodological Problems

How schizophrenic patients actually experience and rate their treatment, in particular their antipsychotic therapy, is a matter of considerable therapeutic significance, and one which has long been neglected on the scientific front. Yet, all studies published on this issue conclude that psychotic patients, too, come to grips very seriously not only with their illness but also with their treatment. *To dismiss their experiences and reports out of hand as psychotically distorted assessments of reality is not only therapeutically counterproductive but also scientifically untenable.*

There are several methodological problems involved in gaining useful insights from subjective ratings and experiences. The claims of a patient undergoing antipsychotic pharmacotherapy can be *measured* neither with objective ratings nor even in physical terms. Yet ratings, attitudes, and changes in well-being are at least semiquantitative. Moreover, how the patient experiences the treatment in detail is a matter for qualitative analysis. Irrespective of these methodological problems, generally valid statements about how schizophrenic patients view their antipsychotic therapy are not to be expected from the very outset. The situations in which antipsychotics are used in the treatment of schizophrenia are too varied: acute treatment versus long-term therapy and relapse prevention; an outpatient setting versus hospitalization; so-called positive versus negative symptoms; different antipsychotics with pronounced variations in their action and side effects profile; and patients with versus patients without previous experience with antipsychotics. Although some of these specific variables can be controlled with effort if the sample is carefully selected, this does not apply to a number of others.

The patient's experience of drug therapy presumably depends as well on the extent to which the pharmacotherapy is coordinated with psychotherapeutic and sociotherapeutic measures within the framework of a comprehensive overall treatment plan. In particular, attention should be paid to the impact of the effects of drugs on the therapist-patient relationship. In this context, studies from the early days of the "neuroleptic era" are still of interest today, specifically with regard to the effects of the medications on the patient's psychodynamics. The studies describe a drug-induced change in defense mechanisms as well as the intrapsychic significance of pharmacologic side effects.[5]

The subjective experiences of physical side effects of antipsychotic therapy reported below apply primarily to acute treatment. In maintenance therapy and relapse prevention, unpleasant psychic side effects of the drugs are easily overlooked or underestimated in their significance to the patient.

The Patient's Experience of Antipsychotic Medication

When patients with schizophrenia are questioned systematically on their subjective response to antipsychotics, the majority of effects reported are unpleasant ones. This applies, on the one hand, in purely quantitative terms. On the other hand, patients tend to emphasize negative experiences whereas positive effects of drugs are generally mentioned only in matter-of-fact terms.

In one of my own studies of acute schizophrenics,[6,7] the patients complained primarily of changes in physical experience. Many patients were disturbed, above all, by restricted motor activity and sedation. Closer investigation reveals the following insights.

Physical Side Effects:

The physical side effects of medication are often sensed and felt differently by the patient than the formulations used in everyday language might first suggest. For instance, antipsychotic sedation is often referred to as "drowsiness." **Yet, in response to systematic questioning, four-fifths of the patients enrolled in our study stated that the sort of drowsiness they felt was previously unknown to them. They identified its apparent "unreasonableness."** In contrast to everyday tiredness, it is not the outcome of a previous effort: "I always have to fight to keep my eyes open. It's a *leaden* drowsiness that doesn't come from exhaustion." Here, the patient is expressing not so much a directly sensed difference but rather attempting to designate in retrospect what is sensed as distinctly "different."

Patients also note a localized physical malaise: "It was practically only my head that was involved in the drowsiness. I mean not my whole body .... it wasn't evenly distributed. It was practically in my eyes and in my head."

Patients experience an almost physical restlessness with simultaneous suppression: "I felt as though I were on drugs ... drowsy, and yet really wound up. Then there was a feeling somewhere between drowsiness and being highly stimulated and wound up." Normal drowsiness wasn't there at all at the beginning. The drowsiness was also experienced as resignation: "It isn't a real need for sleep. I think something is switched off."

Initial Dystonia:

One and the same change is experienced subjectively in very different ways. For example, **initial dystonia can be experienced by the patient as inexplicable physical discomfort** ("Well, my mouth, it refused to close. So I just tried to do it mechanically with my own hands. Because then the pain in my upper and lower jaw subsided. I really was afraid because I didn't know how long that would go on. And I especially didn't know why it hurt so much ... I'd really prefer not to talk about it, it was so terrible..."); **his or her body having a will of its own** ("My teeth were grinding hard and uncontrollably." — "My head, it wanted to lean to the right. My eyes, they wanted to look upwards. And my tongue, it just wouldn't do what I wanted any more..."); **stigmatizing** ("Yes, that was embarrassing ... that other people see it. That really did worry me."); and the **embodiment of being mental ill in self-perception** ("Yes, I see in [initial dystonia] that I am ill and that I have to get out of it, out of this illness.").

The patient's experience of physical side effects depends not only on their type and intensity, but also on the frequency and intensity of psychotic symptoms and, perhaps above all, on motivational factors determined by the patient's history. This was clearly expressed in a study *of antipsychotic-induced galactorrhea.*[8] More than half the female patients experienced galactorrhea as closely linked to their own femininity, (e.g., as *a reinforcement of their heretofore undermined feminine identity*). This may explain the unexpected finding that *galactorrhea was given a positive rating* far more often than a negative rating by those concerned.

Subjective Response — Psychological and Behavioral Changes:

Emotional instability, tormenting anxiety, intolerable restlessness, and occasionally the direct experience of impending ego-disintegration or ego-fragmentation are predominant features of the self-experience of many patients during the acute schizophrenic episode. It is not only the therapist's view, but also the experience of the majority of patients, that **the alleviation of restlessness and anxiety and the restoration of a balanced emotional state are the crucial beneficial psychological effects of antipsychotics in acute treatment. However, a number of patients not only experience a reduced intensity of distressing, burdensome feelings, but also suffer from generalized emotional impoverishment and from the loss of their emotional responsiveness. Such a loss is often associated with indifference, a feeling of emptiness, and a lack of ideas.** These disturbances may occur at an early stage of treatment or develop over the course of time.

Unlike the known physical side effects, undesirable psychological effects of antipsychotic therapy are not readily identifiable in many cases. They are often difficult to delineate from morbogenic impairments. However, more attention has been focused on dysphoric responses in recent years, especially with regard to the extent to which subjective response is a predictor of outcome in antipsychotic therapy.

The term *dysphoric response* denotes all emotional and cognitive changes perceived subjectively by the patient using antipsychotics

and experienced as unpleasant. Scientific investigation of possible correlations between subjective response and outcome (or between subjective response and compliance) requires operationalized recording and, if possible, quantification of the patient's subjective response. However, highly differentiated statements regarding the subjective experience of patients treated with antipsychotics makes this very difficult to accomplish. **The operationalized methods used for recording the patient's subjective response are diverse.** They include calculation of selected, differently weighted items from the Brief Psychiatric Rating Scale,[9] a semistructured interview with a quantifying, subjective rating of the current medication,[10] or a *Drug Attitude Inventory.*[11] Additionally, for methodological reasons, a dysphoric response is not always taken to refer to one and the same phenomenon in different studies. Yet this factor alone cannot account for the varying results: whereas some authors reported a correlation between early negative subjective response to antipsychotics with less favorable outcome to treatment,[9,10,12–14] others were unable to confirm this correlation despite their operationalized methods having been partially the same.[15–17] **Whether early subjective response is a direct predictor of responsiveness to psychotic symptoms is quite questionable. However, it may well be a predictor of noncompliance in the further course of treatment**[18,19] **and thus indirectly of the treatment outcome.**

Some authors recorded a correlation between a dysphoric response and the extrapyramidal motoric effects of antipsychotics, especially akathisia and akinesia, whereas others found no differences in the frequency and intensity of side effects between patients with dysphoric and nondysphoric responses.

The studies by Böker et al.[20,21] **suggest that dysphoric responses related to using antipsychotics in acute treatment of patients with schizophrenia are due primarily to negative experiences in the cognitive arena. What is involved is a direct antipsychotic effect on cognitive processes; studies involving healthy probands have shown that such agents may cause reversible cognitive disturbances. However, another factor which seems to play a role is that the patient is once again confronted increasingly with the burdensome aspects of his or her situation as well as a longstanding cognitive impairment, once the antipsychotic effect improves the patient's assessment of reality.** Feelings of powerlessness and helplessness may result. "The therapeutically desired weakening of psychotic symptoms obviously entails disruption of previous, albeit pathological, attempts to cope with reality."[21,p.104] That this also constitutes therapeutic progress is clear.

Morbogenic or Pharmacogenic?

Most physical side effects of antipsychotics can be delineated without difficulty from morbogenic changes (even allowing for exceptions, as illustrated by functional sexual disturbances). In contrast, **it is often impossible to distinguish between morbogenic and pharmacogenic disturbances in antipsychotic-induced psychological impairments referred to as dysphoric responses.** On the one hand, loss of concentration, emotional impoverishment or depressed mood, restlessness or disinterest are also common symptoms of untreated patients with schizophrenia. On the other hand, emotional and cognitive disturbances of this kind also are reported in self-experiments by healthy persons and in studies involving healthy probands (e.g., the self-experiment carried out as early as 1954 by the Swiss psychiatrist couple Ernst).[22-27] They also occur in nonpsychotic patients using antipsychotics (e.g., in Tourette's syndrome).[28,29]

The possibility of there being a correlation between dysphoric response and the dopamine-antagonistic effect of antipsychotics is under discussion. Numerous studies based on animal experiments illustrate the significance of the dopaminergic system in the so-called reward system. Bearing in mind the complexity and multidimensionality of human experience, however, animal models of this kind are certainly incapable of illuminating more than very limited partial aspects of the dysphoric response of patients with schizophrenia treated with antipsychotics.

As we listen to a patient's subjective reactions to medication, the line between side effects and illness becomes increasingly difficult to distinguish.[30] On the level of subjective experience, a dichotomized classification of morbogenic vs. pharmacogenic changes is a dubious practice. Even an unequivocally pharmacogenic event (e.g., initial dystonia) becomes an experience akin to stigmatization or an experienced loss of control over one's body, primarily through the patient's reaction. **This subjective reaction is determined not only by who the patient is but also by his or her situation and illness, and how he or she copes with** these. Conversely, patients are often incapable of recognizing and experiencing illness-induced changes (e.g. what is alien to them in their emotional lives) until the antipsychotic effects of the drug set in.

Patient Ratings of Pharmacotherapy

In view of the predominance of unpleasant or even decidedly burdensome experiences patients on antipsychotics have described in detail, a generally negative **rating of pharmacotherapy** by patients would not be surprising. Yet the results of empirical studies put the matter in a different light: **Positive ratings were in the majority, reaching 50%–60% in most studies**[7,31–33] and a higher level, as expected, in samples of highly compliant patients.[34] **The rating of antipsychotic pharmacotherapy by patients with acute schizophrenia**[6,7] **is not much less positive than that of patients on long-term antipsychotic depot medication.**[25,33] **A predominantly negative rating of antipsychotics by patients is rather the exception.**[36] In general, the rate of "predominantly critical" or "unequivocally rejecting" patient ratings is between 25% and 30%.

Reasons for Approval and Rejection:

Considering both the subjective patient *experiences* and patient *ratings* of antipsychotic pharmacotherapy, Rogers et al.[32] came to the following conclusion after questioning 360 patients treated with antipsychotics: "In the *qualitative* data there were more negative than positive comments about major tranquillizers, despite the fact that, in the statistical results, twice as many people describe the drugs as helpful."[32,p.133] **What accounts for pharmacotherapy being given a positive overall rating while negative experiences predominated when effects were reported in detail?**

In a study of inpatients with acute schizophrenia treated with antipsychotics, all changes registered by the patients themselves and subjectively ascribed to the drug were noted and counted.[7] If the patient's view is to be recorded, those responses considered by the therapist to describe effects which are *not* drug-induced must not be excluded. Conversely, changes considered by the therapist to be pharmacogenic were not taken into account, unless the patient rated them explicitly as drug-induced effects.

"**Drug effects**" **assessed by each patient as positive were compared** with those experienced as unpleasant. On average, the negative effects reported by the patients outnumbered the positive effects by three to one. The difference was most pronounced in those patients rejecting pharmacotherapy but also was recorded in patients rating the drugs as helpful and beneficial to themselves personally. Statistically significant group differences were not found with respect to changes experienced as unpleasant and ascribed to the medication, but were recorded with respect to the number of "effects" subjectively sensed as positive; these were quoted as highly significant more frequently by those patients who believed themselves to be benefiting from the medication. In other words: **it is obviously not the occurrence of undesirable side effects that is fundamentally forming the patient's attitude toward antipsychotic therapy.** The patient's experience of a lack of positive drug effects exerts a far greater influence on the patient's view of antipsychotic drugs. Thus, **it would seem that patients who reject pharmacotherapy saw no good reason to take these drugs.**

In a study on compliance in antipsychotic relapse prevention, Linden also concludes **"that patients are not so much kept from a therapy by negative therapeutic effects but that they endorse a treatment because of positive therapeutic effects."**[37] Bossert et al.[38] investigated the influence of previous therapeutic experiences on the attitude of acute psychotic inpatients to pharmacotherapy. **Patients with schizophrenia who had previous experience with antipsychotics were more content with their therapy and reported significantly fewer subjective undesirable side effects than patients without such experience.** A comparison study showed that **patients with a consenting attitude to pharmacotherapy were able to report previous experiences of positive changes in their subjective state of health significantly more often than those who refused treatment were.**[39]

Therapeutic Consequences

From the patient's view, drugs are expected to alleviate affective symptoms, such as depression, anxiety, or restlessness. Accordingly, those changes described by patients as positive apply primarily to the affective area or to the remission of psychotic thought incoherence and disturbed concentration. **Delusions and hallucinations are experienced** by patients not so much as complaints but rather as incursions from outside or as disturbed relationships. The remission of these psychotic phenomena therefore is linked less directly with drug intake in the unreflected experience of the patient than the alleviation of distressing feelings of anxiety or fear.

The question of patient attribution is of substantial therapeutic significance: even mild physical side effects are tangible to the patient and readily attributable to his or her medication. In contrast, the antipsychotic effects can be only inferred, at least in part, but not directly experienced as an effect of the pharmacotherapy. One patient, for instance, reported that he had "not really anything positive" to say about his medication: "*So it's only the negative side effects that I notice. From what I know, I can only imagine that I might well be far worse off without the tablets.*" Another patient stated: "I didn't know what was really happening and what was just imagined by me. I believe the medicine can help me there—although I don't actually notice it."

In general, a drug is taken to alleviate specific complaints. If this effect is tangible to the patient, he or she is content with the therapy and is willing to continue it, provided no negative side effects diminish its value. For some patients with schizophrenia, however, the situation is seen in another light, giving rise to such statements as: "I don't feel anything negative, so I take it." There is some evidence that more than a small proportion of acute psychotic patients give antipsychotic therapy a positive rating without registering any positive drug effects themselves.[6] These patients, then, must have other crucial motives. For instance, they may expect the antipsychotic to have primarily unpleasant effects, and the absence of the dreaded effects is the reason for their approval of the medication.

The absence of dreaded side effects may initially promote acceptance. However, this will certainly not be sufficient in the long-term to motivate the patient to continue his or her medication, especially as the very discreet, initially almost imperceptible side effects are forced increasingly into the foreground of the patient's experience. Then, the acute symptoms become more remote and their deterrent effect fades. The task confronting the therapist is not only to keep side effects to a minimum but also to help the patient perceive the favorable effects of treatment which, unlike side effects, are not directly perceptible in most cases. This requirement for its part addresses the importance of psychotherapeutic guidance; it is only through this that the prescribing of the antipsychotic becomes medical treatment.

Implications for Practice

Psychotic disorders are not always so disturbing and distressing as to necessitate immediate antipsychotic therapy. If the psychiatrist makes a point in such cases of understanding fully the suffering to which the patient is exposed (and not only of making a diagnosis), the antipsychotic medication subsequently recommended is more likely to be accepted by the patient.

During acute therapy, it is, of course, vital to minimize side effects by prescribing the right antipsychotic in the right dose. For psychological reasons, oral medication is preferable to parenteral medication because it encourages the patient to take an active part in the therapy from the outset.

When treating acute psychotic patients, the psychiatrist must not rely solely on the information on possible side effects given during the briefing to be present in the patient's mind when such effects occur. Rather, he or she must make a point of addressing side effects repeatedly. If patients are aware that the psychiatrist is not playing down or denying the undesirable side effects, many of them are more willing to temporarily endure certain medication-induced restrictions.

Side effects may occasionally have a direct negative impact on the patient's self-healing powers. If the patient feels threatened in his ego activity or ego vitality and attempts to reassure himself through motor activity, his concern may be increased by restricted motor activity or antipsychotic sedation. Instead of suppressing this attempt at self-reassurance, oppurtunities for physical activity should be given to the patient to help him experience autonomous movement. Physical therapy (e.g., sport or kinetotherapy to counter restricted motor activity, hydrotherapy to counter orthostatic dysfunctions and sedation) is often helpful in such cases and has a comforting effect on many patients.

It is important to help the patient at an early stage to recognize the connection between alleviation of symptoms and medication (e.g., "I'm so glad your medication is helping you and that you're beginning to feel better."). However, it is important to the patient that his or her psychiatrist's interest is not confined to the remission of symptoms (or at most to potential side effects). It is only when the patient feels that the psychiatrist is aiming not only at eliminating disorders but also at restoring quality of life that he or she feels in good hands.

Measures aimed at encouraging the patient to be independent and to become an expert on his or her own illness as much as possible should extend to medication. In the course of time, many patients learn in cooperation with their doctor to adapt the dose themselves—within certain agreed limits—according to current stress levels and well-being. However, the doctor must continue to address the need for continued therapy even when the symptoms have receded, with medication being codetermined in relevant cases.

In subsequent treatment stages the doctor should make a point of reminding the patient occasionally of the benefit of continued medication, with reference being made to the different experiences of individual patients (e.g., what situations which used to subject the patient to excessive stress and which triggered a psychotic episode can he or she now cope with under the protection of antipsychotic therapy?). The unpleasant side effects, which should never be denied or played down by the therapist, are thus given a counterweight.

The best possible understanding of the patient is the best precondition for treatment, pharmacotherapy included. The patient-therapist relationship is strongly influenced by the therapist's ability to empathize with the patient, not only in the experiencing of the psychosis but also in the subjective experiences with the therapeutic measures. If the patient senses this empathy, he is more likely to be willing to follow medical advice. Or, as Diamond[30] put it: We must listen to our patients before they will listen to us.

References

1. Wolff. Trionalkur. *Centralbl Nerven Psychiatrie*.1901;12:281–283.

2. Young JL, Zonana HV, Shepler L. Medication noncompliance in schizophrenia: codification and update. *Bul Am Acad Psychiatry Law*. 1986; 14:105–122.

3. Ley P. Improving Patients' understanding, recall, satisfaction, and compliance. In: Broome AK, ed. Health Psychology. New York: Chapman and Hall; 1989. Quoted in: Mayer C, Soyka M. Compliance bei der therapie schizophrener mit neuroleptika-eine ubersicht. *Fortschr Neurol Psychiatr*. 1992;60:212–222.

4. Hornung WP, Buchkremer G, Redbrake M, Klingber S. Patientmodifizierte Medikation. Wie gehen schizophrene Patienten mit ihren Neuroleptika um? *Nervenarzt*. 1993; 64:434–439.

5. Azima H, Sarwer-Foner GJ. Psychoanalytic formulations of the effect of drugs in pharmacotherapy. In: Bordeleau JM, ed. *Extrapyramidal System and Neuroleptics*. Montreal: Editions Psychiatriques; 1961:507—522.

6. Windgassen K. *Schizophreniebehandlung aus der Sicht des Patienten*. Berlin: Springer; 1989.

7. Windgassen K. Treatment with neuroleptics: the patient's perspective. *Acta Psychiatr Scand*. 1992; 86:405–410.

8. Wesselmann U, Windgassen K. Galactorrhea: subjective response by schizophrenic patients. *Acta Psychiatr Scand*. 1995;91:152–155.

9. Singh MM, Smith JM. Kinetics and dynamics of response to Haloperidol in acute schizophrenia—a longitudinal study of the therapeutic process. *Compr Psychiatry*. 1973;14:393–414.

10. Van Putten T, May PRA. Subjective response as a predictor of outcome in pharmacotherapy. *Arch Gen Psychiatry*. 1978;35:477–480.

11. Hogan TP, Awad AG, Eastwood R. A self-report scale predictive of drug compliance in schizophrenics: reliability and discriminative validity. *Psychol Med*. 1983;13:177–183.

12. May PRA, Van Putten T, Yale C, et al. Predicting individual responses to drug treatment in schizophrenia. *J Nerv Ment Dis*. 1976; 126:177–183.

13. Singh MM, Kay RS. Dysphoric response to neuroleptic treatment in schizophrenia: its relationship to autonomic arousal and prognosis. *Biol Psychiatry*. 1979;14:277–294.

14. Awad AG, Hogan TP. Early treatment events and prediction of response to neuroleptics in schizophrenia. *Prog Neuropsychopharmacol Biol Psychiatry*. 1985;9:585–588.

15. White K, Busk J, Eaton E, et al. Dysphoric response to neuroleptics as a predictor of treatment outcome with schizophrenics. *Int Pharmacopsychiatry*. 1981;16:34–38.

16. Ayers T, Liberman RP, Wallace CJ. Subjective response to antipsychotic drugs: failure to replicate predictions of outcome. *J Clin Psychopharmacol*. 1984;4:89–93.

17. Gaebel W, Pietzker A, Ullrich G, Schley J, Müller-Oerlinghausen B. Möglichkeiten der Voraussage des Erfolges einer Akutbehandlung mit Perazin anhand der Reaktion auf eine Perazintestdosis. In: Helmchen H, Hippius H, Tölle R, eds. *Therapie mit Neuroleptika—Perazin*. Stuttgart: Thieme; 1988; 159–172.

18. Van Putten T, May PRA, Marder SR, Wittman LA. Subjective response to antipsychotic drugs. *Arch Gen Psychiatry*. 1981; 38:187–190.

19. Van Putten T, May PRA, Marder SR. Response to antipsychotic medication: the doctor's and the consumer's view. *Am J Psychiatry*. 1984; 141:16–19.

20. Böker W, Brenner HD, Alberti L. Untersuchung subjektiver Neuroleptikawirkung bei Schizophrenen. *Therapiewoche*. 1982; 32:3411–3421.

21. Brenner HD, Böker W, Rui C. Subjektive Neuroleptikawirkung bei Schizophrenen und ihre Bedeutung für die Therapie In: Hinterhuber H, Schubert H, Kulhanek F (Hrsg.). *Seiteneffekte und Störwirkungen der Psychopharmaka S. Stuttgart*: Schattauer; 1986: 97-107.

22. Ernst K. Psychopathologische Wirkungen des Phenothiazinderivates "Largactil" ("Megaphen") in Selbstversuchen und bei Kranken. *Arch Psychiatr Nervenkr*. 1954; 192:573–590.

23. Heimann H, Witt PN. Die Wirkung einer einmaligen Largactilgabe bei Gesunden. *Mschr Psychiatr Neurol*. 1955; 129:104–128.

24. Degkwitz R. Zur Wirkungsweise von Psycholeptica anhand langfristiger Selbstversuche. *Nervenarzt.* 1964; 35:491–496.

25. Kendler KS. A medical student's experience with akathisia. *Am J Psychiatry.* 1976; 133:454–455.

26. Belmaker RH, Wald D. Haloperidol in normals. *Br J Psychiat.* 1977; 131:222–223.

27. Anderson, Reker D. Prolonged adverse effects of haloperidol in normal subjects. *N Engl J Med.* 1981; 305:643–644.

28. Bruun RD. Subtle and underrecognized side effects of neuroleptic treatment in children with Tourette's disorder. *Am J Psychiatry.* 1988; 145:621–624.

29. Caine E, Polinsky R. Haloperidol-induced dysphoria in patients with Tourette syndrome. *Am J Psychiatry.* 1979; 136:1216–1217.

30. Diamond R. Drugs and the quality of life: the patient´s point of view. *J Clin Psychiatry.* 1985; 46(5,2):29–35.

31. Soskis DA. Schizophrenic and medical inpatients as informed drug consumers. *Arch Gen Psychiatr.* 1978; 35:645–647.

32. Rogers A, Pilgrim D, Lacey R. *Experiencing Psychiatry: Users' View of Services.* London: Macmillan, in association with MIND Publications; 1993.

33. Larsen EB, Gerlach J. Subjective experience of treatment, side-effects, mental state and quality of llife in chronic schizophrenic out-patients treated with depot neuroleptics. *Acta Psychiatr Scand.* 1996;93:381–388.

34. Linden M, Chaskel R. Information and consent in schizophrenic patients in long-term treatment. *Schizophr Bull.* 1981;3:132–236.

35. Trenckmann U. Wirkungen und Nebenwirkungen im Erleben der Patienten. *Psychiatr Prax.* 1990; 17:184–187.

36. Davidhizar RE. Beliefs, feelings and insight of patients with schizophrenia about taking medication. *J Adv Nurs.* 1987; 12:177–182.

37. Linden M. Negative vs. positive Therapieerwartungen und Compliance vs. Non Compliance. *Psychiatr Prax.* 1987; 14:132–136.

38. Bossert S, Dose M, Emrich HM, Garcia D, Junker M, Raptis K, Weber MM. Psychologische Wirkungen von Behandlungsvorerfahrungen mit Neuroleptika. *Nervenarzt.* 1990; 61:301–305.

39. Marder SR Mebane A Chien C Winslade WJ Swann E VanPutten T. A comparison of patients who refuse and consent to neuroleptic treatment. *Am J Psychiatry.* 1983; 140:470–472.

2   The Pharmacology and Drug Interactions of the Newer Antidepressants

Robert L. DuPont, MD

Dr. DuPont is Clinical Professor of Psychiatry, Georgetown University,School of Medicine, Washington, DC, and President, Institute for Behavior and Health, Inc., Rockville, MD.

Editor's Note

The newer antidepressants are increasingly well known to patients and physicians alike. The selective serotonin-reuptake inhibitors (fluoxetine [Prozac], sertraline [Serzone], and paroxetine [Paxil]) as well as nefazodone [Serzone], fluvoxamine [Luvox], venlafaxine [Effexor], and bupropion [Wellbutrin] offer efficacy comparable to older agents but lack many of the side effects and toxicities associated with tricylics and monoamine oxidase inhibitors.

As a result, the most common of these agents have been used by an unprecedented number of patients, and are increasingly likely to be prescribed by primary care physicians. "Simpler drugs" should not be confused with "simple," however. The new antidepressants have pharmacokinetic characteristics and drug interactions that require clinical attention.

In this chapter, Dr. DuPont reviews the characteristics and interactions of greatest clinical import. The metabolism and half-lives of several drugs, for example, have implications for appropriate dosing. Switching from one drug to another requires an understanding of potential interactions and the elimination rate of the previous agent.

Interactions between the cytochrome P-450 enzyme system and medications are of considerable importance and an evolving knowledge. Certain drugs inhibit and others induce P-450 enzymes. These effects can alter blood levels of concomitantly taken medications, leading to changes in efficacy and a greater risk of adverse effects. Clinicians should be aware of both specific drug interactions and the pharmacologic principles that underlie them.

Introduction

Most of the newer antidepressants pose a risk of drug interactions because they inhibit clusters of P-450 enzymes involved in the metabolism of other medications. Drug interactions involving these antidepressants can change plasma levels by a factor of three or more, which is most likely to be clinically significant for medications that have low therapeutic indexes. **Drug interactions are of increasing importance because of their perilous impact on our aging patient population, the rising simultaneous use of multiple medications, and the growing concern about the costs of medical care.**

The new generation of antidepressants—beginning in the United States with the introduction of fluoxetine (Prozac) in 1988 and now including a total of four selective serotonin-reuptake inhibitors (SSRIs) plus four novel medications—has transformed the treat-ment of a variety of disorders, including the affective and anxiety disorders. **Compared with the earlier antidepressants, particularly the tricyclic antidepressants (TCAs), these newer antidepressants have a more benign side-effect profile and a wider range of usage. They are relatively safe in overdoses, a major risk with the TCAs. They lack both the minor but often troubling side effects of the TCAs** (i.e., dry mouth, constipation, weight gain) **as well as the more serious adverse events** (i.e., disturbances in cardiac rhythm, dizziness, hypotension).

In the past year, a controversy has developed surrounding the extent to which these medications cause drug interactions. To put this controversy into perspective and to protect patients from both adverse drug interactions, as well as from decisions based on unreasonable fears of drug interactions, requires an understanding of the metabolism of these medications and how they interact with other commonly prescribed medications. The issues involved are evolving rapidly. Because most of the research on drug interactions is based on in vitro studies and because there is great individual variability in the metabolism of medications, there is considerable uncertainty about the clinical significance of many potential interactions. **Concerns about drug interactions have been spurred by QT prolongation and torsades de pointes-type ventricular tachycardia** (sometimes fatal), **which can result from drug interactions involving erythromycin** (E-Mycin) **and ketoconazole** (Nizoral) **with astemizole** (Hismanal), **terfenadine** (Seldane), **and cisapride** (Propulsid). **These medications involve the same hepatic enzymes that are affected by some of the newer antidepressants.**[1] **Concerns about drug interactions involving antidepressants first surfaced when the newer antidepressants were combined with TCAs, sometimes leading to serious adverse events.**

This chapter will review interactions involving the newer antidepressants, and will focus on the needs of practicing physicians. Physicians should stay informed about these issues as new information becomes available; much of it is reflected in package inserts and the *Physicians' Desk Reference* (PDR).[2] A recent article by Nemeroff and associates in the *American Journal of Psychiatry* authoritatively reviews this controversy.[3]

Pharmacodynamics and Pharmacokinetics

Pharmacology is divided into pharmacodynamics and pharmacokinetics.[4] The former describes the effects of medications at their sites of action, which for the antidepressants are the synapses of specific brain neurons, primarily involving serotonin and norepinephrine receptors. **Pharmacodynamic drug interactions occur at the site of action, such as the potentiation of sedation from using an antidepressant along with alcohol or another sedative. In contrast, pharmacokinetics describes the absorption, distribution, protein binding, metabolism, and excretion of medications.** In essence, pharmacodynamics is the study of what drugs do to the body, whereas pharmacokinetics is the study of what the body does to drugs. With respect to the antidepressants, pharmacodynamics is the brain's story, whereas pharmacokinetics is the liver's story.

Because all the antidepressants are highly lipophilic, which is the basis of their ability to penetrate the blood-brain barrier; are rapidly and nearly completely absorbed from the intestines, as well as widely distributed after oral administration; and are bound to plasma proteins, the clinically relevant pharmacokinetic issues primarily relate to their metabolism. Metabolism is divided into phase I, oxidative metabolism, and phase II, conjugation with glucuronide and related reactions. Both phases of metabolism are accomplished primarily in the microsomes of hepatocytes and make the antidepressant molecules more water soluble and, therefore, more efficiently eliminated by the kidneys. With respect to the newer antidepressants, phase I metabolism is the primary step by which drug interactions occur.

The metabolic effects of the antidepressants involve their interactions with the P-450 enzymes, which are the major metabolic pathways for foreign chemicals, including all medications. The P-450 enzymes also metabolize some endogenous substances, including prostaglandins, fatty acids, and steroids.

Table 2.1 presents a pharmacokinetic comparison of the eight new antidepressants plus clomipramine (Anafranil) **and amitriptyline** (Elavil), **highlighting some of their most important pharmacologic features. Introduced in the United States at about the same time as fluoxetine, clomipramine is a TCA with serotonin activity that may explain** its role in the treatment of obsessive-compulsive disorder (OCD). Amitriptyline is included in Table 2.1 because it was one of the first TCAs and because it remains widely used for its sedative properties and for management of chronic pain.

Dosing Issues:

Because some patients respond well to some antidepressants but not to others, these medications are not simply interchangeable. A patient's ability to tolerate the antidepressants—the individual side-effect picture—is a major factor in the selection of specific antidepressants. Because there is great variation in side effects and because clinicians cannot predict individual patient responses in terms of either therapeutic benefits or side effects, selection of particular antidepressants is largely a matter of trial and error, as physicians work with their patients to find the best choices of medications and the best doses. [5,6]

All the drugs listed in Table 2.1 have been approved by the Food and Drug Administration for the treatment of depression except fluvoxamine (Luvox), **which currently has been approved in the United States only for the treatment of OCD.** Fluvoxamine has been approved to treat depression in Europe and in most countries world-

Table 2.1

Pharmacokinetic Comparison of Antidepressants

	Sertraline	Fluoxetine	Paroxetine	Nefazodone	Fluvoxamine
Half-life (h)	26	24–72*/96–144†	21 (mean)	2–4	15.6
Metabolite activity	20%–30%	Equal	Inactive	3 variably active	Questionable
Metabolite half-life (h)	62–104	96–384	—	1.5–18.0	14–16
Steady state (days)	7–10	28–35	≈10	1–5	7
Dose-proportional plasma levels	Yes	No	No	No	No
Protein-binding (%)	98	94.5	93–95	99	80
Dose reduction in elderly patients	No	Yes	Yes	Yes	Yes

	Venlafaxine	Clomipramine	Amitriptyline	Bupropion	Mirtazapine
Half-life (h)	3–7	19–37	9–46	14	20–40
Metabolite activity	Equal	Equal	Equal	4 variably active	10% activity
Metabolite half-life (h)	9–13	54–77	16–88	8–24	20–40
Steady state (days)	3	7–14	4–10	Variable	3–4
Dose-proportional plasma levels	Yes	No	Yes	Yes	Yes
Protein-binding (%)	25–29	97	90–97	80	85
Dose reduction in elderly patients	No	Yes	Yes	Yes	No

* Acute administration, † Chronic administration

Reprinted by permission of the publisher from Ereshefsky L, Overman GP, Karp JK. Current psychotropic dosing and monitoring guidelines. *Prim Psychiatry.* 1996;3:21–45. Copyright 1996 by MBL Communications.

wide. Some of these drugs have other approved indications, as noted in Table 2.2, which also shows typical dose ranges for starting treatment and for maintenance therapy for a wide selection of antidepressants as well as provides information about therapeutic plasma concentrations. Fluoxetine and sertraline (Zoloft) may be used at lower doses for elderly patients, although there is nothing in the package inserts to suggest that a lower dose for elderly patients is necessary.

Although the SSRIs and clomipramine are specifically indicated for the treatment of OCD, the antidepressants as a class have a broad spectrum of clinical uses in both depression and anxiety and are frequently used to treat disorders outside their approved indications. Many of these antidepressants either have been or will soon be approved for use in anxiety disorders, including panic disorder, social phobia, and generalized anxiety disorder.[7] Fluoxetine also has been approved to treat bulimia nervosa.

All the antidepressants have an onset of therapeutic benefit after several weeks of regular dosing and are used every day for months or years. None has been shown in controlled trials to have significantly greater antidepressant efficacy than imipramine (Tofranil) or the other antidepressants. The older TCAs (imipramine, amitriptyline) are tertiary amines, whereas the newer TCAs are secondary amines (desipramine [Norpramin] and nortriptyline [Pamelor]). By the 1980s, the secondary TCAs had all but replaced the tertiary TCAs because they had similar efficacies but fewer side effects.

None of the newer antidepressants is suitable for as-needed use as are the benzodiazepines in the treatment of clinically significant anxiety, except when sedating antidepressants (most often trazodone [Desyrel] and amitriptyline) **are used to treat insomnia.** Food has relatively little effect on the absorption of the newer antidepressants; exceptions include sertraline (food increases absorption of this agent) and nefazodone (Serzone; food decreases absorption of this agent). All of the newer antidepressants are 80% or more protein bound, except venlafaxine (Effexor), which is nearly 27% protein bound. All the eight newer antidepressants have active metabolites, except paroxetine (Paxil) and fluvoxamine. Neither the effect of food on absorption nor protein binding is thought to be clinically important when using these drugs.

In clinical practice, doses of the older and the newer antidepressants

Table 2.2
Antidepressant Pharmacotherapy

Drug Plasma	Typical Starting Dosage(mg)	Typical DosageRange* (mg/dL)	FDA Indication(s)	Proposed Therapeutic Concentration (ng/mL)
Amitriptyline	25 t.i.d. or 50 every night	50–300	Depression	120–250
Amoxapine	50 b.i.d.	508–600	Depression, psychotic depression	—
Bupropion	100 b.i.d.	200–450‡	Depression	<100
Clomipramine	25 to 100 every day in divided doses within first 2 weeks	25–250	OCD	100–250
Desipramine	25 t.i.d.	100–300	Depression	115–180
Doxepin	25 t.i.d.	75–300	Depression	70–250
Fluoxetine	20 every day	20–80	Depression, obsessive-compulsive disorder	—
Fluvoxamine	50 every day	50–300	OCD	—
Imipramine	25 t.i.d.	75–300	Depression, childhood enuresis	200–250 §
Maprotiline	25 t.i.d.	75–225	Depression	—
Mirtazapine	15 every night	15–45	Depression	—
Nefazodone	100 b.i.d.	200–600	Depression	—
Nortriptyline	25 t.i.d.	75–150	Depression	50–150 §
Paroxetine	20 every morning	20–50	Depression, panic disorder	—
Phenelzine	15 t.i.d.	15–90	Depression, atypical depression	—
Protriptyline	5 t.i.d.	15–60	Depression	70–250
Sertraline	50 every morning	50–200	Depression	—
Tranylcypromine	Individualized	30–60	Depression, depression without melancholia	—
Trazodone	50 t.i.d.	150–600	Depression	—
Trimipramine	25 t.i.d.	50–300	Depression	—
Venlafaxine	18.75 b.i.d.	75–375	Depression	—

* In geriatric patients, the appropriate dosage is widely variable but generally is one half the young adult dosage range for TCAs and for compounds with significant cardiovascular toxicity Parent and metabolite; ‡ Not >150 mg/dose, § Therapeutic drug monitoring is well established; **t.i.d.** = three times a day; **b.i.d.** = twice a day; **OCD** = Obsessive-Compulsive Disorder Reprinted by permission of the publisher from Ereshefsky L, Overman GP, Karp JK. Current psychotropic dosing and monitoring guidelines. Prim Psychiatry, 1996;3:21–45. Copyright 1996 by MBL Communications.

are managed according to the clinical response of each patient to determine the best doses over a period of weeks or months. When disturbing side effects occur, dose escalation is slowed, stopped, or reversed. Generally, the dose of an antidepressant is increased slowly as tolerated until therapeutic response is adequate or the maximum recommended dose is achieved. **Benefits may occur within 1 week of starting treatment but may take up to 10 weeks to be fully realized. Therapeutic benefits usually are seen over months, and even years, of continuous therapy. In contrast, side effects usually occur within a few doses of the medication, and many side effects subside gradually at stable dose levels.**

For all the newer and older antidepressants, except nortriptyline, there is a poor correlation between either therapeutic effect or adverse reactions and plasma levels.[4] For this reason, the primary use of determinations of plasma levels with the newer antidepressants is to establish patient compliance. Plasma levels for particular doses of all the antidepressants show wide individual variations in healthy patients and even wider variations in medically compromised patients. For example, the half-life of amitriptyline in a large sample of healthy patients ranged from 9 to 46 hours.[8] This is a fivefold variation for a relatively simple chemical in the absence of hepatic or renal disease. Because of this wide variation, it is useful to have a general sense of the half-lives of these medications.

Half-Lives:

The widely differing elimination half-lives of the eight newer antidepressants (and the active metabolites of six of the agents), unlike the pharmacokinetic parameters previously discussed, are clinically important in some settings. Like the TCAs, most of the newer antidepressants have elimination half-lives of approximately 24 hours for the parent compound and roughly similar half-lives for their major psychoactive metabolites (see Table 2.1). Sertraline, bupropion (Wellbutrin), fluvoxamine, mirtazapine (Remeron), and paroxetine have half-lives of approximately 24 hours. **The half-lives of the parent compounds are only a few hours for both nefazodone and venlafaxine, which explains why these two non-SSRI antidepressants are recommend-ed for twice-a-day dosing to maintain relatively steady plasma levels.** Fluvoxamine has a half-life of approximately 16 hours and no active metabolite, which may explain why the manufacturer recommends twice-a-day dosing. However, the half-life of fluvoxamine is close enough to 24 hours to explain why many experienced clinicians prescribe it once a day, like the other SSRIs.

Bupropion is a special case with its recommended dosing of three times a day despite its half-life, which is similar to that of fluvoxamine. The inconvenient divided dosing for bupropion is suggested in part to limit the peak plasma levels that occur after once-a-day dosing because of the potential for seizures with high plasma levels. A sustained-release form of bupropion was recently introduced and is recommended for twice-a-day dosing. In the future, sustained-release forms of the other two antidepressants now recommended for multiple daily dosing may become available to permit once-a-day dosing, which is an important advantage in terms of patient compliance.

With respect to half-life, fluoxetine is the one outlier among the antidepressants. It has roughly a 6-day half-life for the parent compound and up to a 16-day half-life for its major active metabolite, norfluoxetine. It takes approximately five times the half-life to reach a steady state in the plasma with continuing stable dosing. Similarly, it takes approximately five times the half-life to eliminate 90% of the medication from the body. Given these general pharmacokinetic principles, the time to reach a steady state and the time to reach 90% clearance are both longer for fluoxetine than for any other antidepressant. **For simplicity, consider fluoxetine to require nearly 30 days to reach a steady state** (and to reach elimination once dosing stops). **The equivalent time for the other newer antidepressants is roughly 7 days** (see Table 2.1).

In the treatment of both affective and anxiety disorders, a long half-life has the clear advantage because it reduces the clinical importance of missed doses, which are common in all medical treatments. With a short half-life medication, missed doses can lead to breakthrough depression, panic, and other serious symptoms, as well as to withdrawal symptoms.[5] A poorly maintained clinical response or intermittent withdrawal can lead to discontinuation of treatment.

However, a long half-life can be problematic in the management of side effects because it takes a long time for the medication to be eliminated from a patient's plasma. **Clinical experience has shown that most side effects of the newer antidepressants are reduced or elimi-**

**nated within a few days of stopping the medication, even with fluox-
etine.** This rapid reduction in side effects, even for a long half-life medication, is the result of decreased plasma levels that is correlated with a
reduction in side effects long before 90% of the medication is eliminated from the body. When these two factors are combined (better
maintained clinical effects despite occasionally missed doses and rapid
reduction in side effects even for long half-life antidepressants), the
scale is tipped toward the long half-life of fluoxetine as an important
clinical advantage.

**Another area in which the long half-life of fluoxetine can prove
problematic is when a switch from an SSRI to a monoamine oxidase
inhibitor (MAOI), such as phenelzine (Nardil) or tranylcypromine
(Parnate), is indicated. Inhibition of hepatic enzymes is probably
close to zero nearly 1 week after stopping paroxetine, nearly 1–2
weeks after stopping sertraline, and nearly 6 weeks after stopping
fluoxetine. Thus, when switching from an SSRI to an MAOI, it is
desirable to use a short half-life SSRI. With its 24-hour half-life and
no active metabolite, paroxetine may be the best choice, because it is
undesirable for seriously depressed patients to have to wait 6 weeks
without an antidepressant before starting an MAOI. SSRI–MAOI
combination therapy is contraindicated because it may lead to what
has become known as the serotonin syndrome, a potentially fatal
adverse event.**[9,10]

**Half-lives do not correlate with the speed of onset of therapeutic
effects or the speed of onset of most adverse experiences with the
antidepressants. Thus, nefazodone does not have a more rapid onset
of action than does fluoxetine. In fact, none of the antidepressants,
new or old, has been shown to be superior to the others in terms of
rapid onset.** Because these medications produce prompt changes in
neurotransmitter levels (serotonin and norepinephrine) despite the
clinically undesirable delay in onset of therapeutic benefits, it is clear
that the efficacy of antidepressants involves a slower, more complex
neuroadaptation than a simple shift in neurotransmitter levels at brain
synapses.

The P-450 Enzymes

Absorbed on the spectrophotometer at 450 nm, the hepatic enzymes that metabolize foreign chemicals are contained in the cytochrome P-450 enzyme system. A total of 34 of the P-450 enzymes have been identified in humans. Although they are primarily located in the liver, these enzymes are also located in the brain, the intestines, and other tissues. Each of the individual P-450 enzymes is named using a number, a letter, and then another number. A specific enzyme is identified first by its family (shown as 1 to 4 or sometimes as I to IV), then by its subfamily (shown as a letter), and finally by its specific gene (shown with a number). One of the best studied P-450 enzymes is cytochrome P-450 enzyme system 2D6, sometimes labeled more simply 2D6 or IID6. **When an enzyme is induced, it metabolizes its substrates more effectively. When an enzyme is inhibited, it metabolizes its substrates less effectively.**

Most people have an abundance of a particular P-450 enzyme (a normal state), although some people lack one or more of these enzymes (a genetic deficiency). People who have a specific P-450 enzyme completely inhibited by an antidepressant (or other substance) function like people who are genetically deficient in that enzyme, becoming transformed from normal metabolizers into poor metabolizers while they take the inhibiting substance.

The fact that most people who lack one of the P-450 enzymes on a genetic basis seem to function without problems (including in their use of medications that are normally metabolized by their deficient enzymes) helps to keep these issues in perspective and to explain some of the well-known individual variability in the metabolism of all medications. One explanation for the common observation that clinical outcomes are not more variable (including more adverse events) despite this variability in metabolism is that multiple enzymatic pathways exist in the liver for the metabolism of many drugs.

Poor metabolizers of a particular compound can be distinguished by identifying the ratio of the parent compound to its major metabolite in the plasma. Poor metabolizers have little or no metabolite after administration of a medication that they metabolize poorly. Normal metabolizers have a larger amount of the metabolite than of the parent compound within a few hours of the first dosage. Poor metabolizers eliminate a drug more slowly and primarily or exclusively as the parent compound. Patients who lack a specific P-450 enzyme on a genetic basis show no effect when they take a medication that inhibits this enzyme.

Some medications induce specific P-450 enzymes, whereas others inhibit specific enzymes. All medications are substrates of one or more P-450 enzymes. Although none of the newer antidepressants is known to induce any P-450 enzyme, other psychotropic medications do induce some of these enzymes. Many of the newer antidepressants inhibit clusters of these P-450 enzymes and are themselves metabolized by enzymes that they inhibit. Although it has been suggested that this "autoinhibition" may be important, an abundance of clinical experience indicates it is not a significant problem. For example, both fluoxetine and sertraline inhibit 2D6, an enzyme that metabolizes these two medications. There is no evidence that blood levels of these medications increase once steady-state levels have been achieved in a few weeks of stable dosing, even after years of continuous dosing.

Of the P-450 enzymes, four have been demonstrated to have clinical significance: 1A2, 2C (9 and 19), 2D6, and 3A4. Genetic polymorphism exists for the 2C and 2D6 enzymes and also may exist for the 1A2 enzymes.

1A2:

Fluvoxamine inhibits 1A2, which can raise plasma levels of theophylline (Quibron), **clozapine** (Clozaril), **tacrine** (Cognex), **acetaminophen** (Tylenol). **At high doses, fluoxetine and paroxetine also inhibit 1A2. Caffeine is metabolized by 1A2, so inhibition of this enzyme can produce heightened and prolonged reactions to this common but often overlooked cause of clinically significant anxiety and panic.**

2C:

The 2C system is important with respect to the metabolism of phenytoin (Dilantin). Like the TCAs, phenytoin has a relatively low therapeutic index, with potentially serious adverse events. **The 2C enzymes metabolize diazepam** (Valium), **clomipramine, amitriptyline, and imipramine as well as** omeprazole (Prilosec), **warfarin** (Coumadin), **tolbutamide, and some nonsteroidal anti-inflammatory agents. Paroxetine, fluoxetine, sertraline, and fluvoxamine inhibit the 2C enzymes.**

2D6:

Fluoxetine, sertraline, and paroxetine—but not fluvoxamine—all inhibit 2D6, which can markedly increase plasma levels of TCAs (including desipramine and nortriptyline) **when the TCAs are coadministered with one of the SSRIs. Inhibition of 2D6 is potentially serious with coadministration of type 1C antiarrhythmics, such as encainide** (Enkaid), **flecainide** (Tambocor), **and propafenone** (Rythmol). **These agents have low therapeutic indexes and produce potentially lethal adverse reactions. Inhibition of the 2D6 enzyme is also important with the coadministration of the TCAs because they are primarily metabolized by this enzyme and because they have low therapeutic indexes. Thus, even small increases in plasma levels of TCAs can produce adverse events, including potentially lethal disturbances in cardiac rhythm. Many drugs other than fluoxetine, paroxetine, and sertraline also inhibit the 2D6 enzyme; they include quinidine** (Quinidex), **cimetidine** (Tagamet), **fluphenazine** (Prolixin), **haloperidol** (Haldol), **thioridazine** (Mellaril), **amitriptyline, desipramine, and clomipramine.**

One of the most hotly debated issues involving drug interactions is whether sertraline is significantly different from fluoxetine and paroxetine with respect to inhibition of 2D6 and the metabolism of TCAs. Preskorn and colleagues[11] have taken a strong position: sertraline (50 mg) is significantly less likely to raise plasma levels of desipramine than is fluoxetine (20 mg). Nemeroff[12] has taken an equally strong position: sertraline, paroxetine, and fluoxetine produce similar effects on the 2D6 enzyme. The argument hinges on dose equivalence, to some extent, because both sides agree that all three SSRIs inhibit the 2D6 enzyme. Nemeroff[12] argues that fluoxetine (20 mg) is more reasonably compared with sertraline (150 mg) in the treatment of depression, in which case there is little difference between the effects of sertraline on plasma levels of TCAs and the effects of fluoxetine or paroxetine. **Elevations in plasma concentrations of TCAs over baseline have ranged from 58% to 150% for sertraline** (at a dose of 50 mg) **to 110% to 375% for fluoxetine** (at a dose of 20 mg).

3A4:

Nefazodone and fluvoxamine (and, to a much lesser extent, fluoxetine and sertraline) **inhibit 3A4, which can raise plasma levels of ter-**

fenadine, astemizole, carbamazepine (Tegretol), alprazolam (Xanax), and triazolam (Halcion). Of the P-450 enzymes, 3A4 is the most abundant (60%, whereas all other isoenzymes make up only 40%). The substrates of 3A4 include terfenadine and astemizole as well as midazolam (Versed), diazepam, carbamazepine, sertraline, TCAs, calcium channel blockers, cyclosporine (Neoral), erythromycin, steroids, codeine, quinidine, and lidcaine (Xylocaine). Grapefruit juice is a potent inhibitor of 3A4, although the component of grapefruit juice responsible for these effects has not been identified.[13] The clinical significance of this remarkable in vitro finding remains unclear, but it underscores the fact that in vitro inhibition of P-450 enzymes may be of little or no practical importance.

Summary

In summary, the most common and important drug interactions involving the newer antidepressants are the inhibition of 2D6 by fluoxetine, paroxetine, and sertraline with coadministered TCAs and the inhibition of 3A4 by fluvoxamine, nefazodone, and others as it relates to the simultaneous use of alprazolam, astemizole, terfenadine, and triazolam. In particular, the low-therapeutic indexes of the two nonsedating antihistamines are a cause of concern because of potentially serious toxicity (life-threatening arrhythmias) and because most patients using these medications do not consider them to be medically worrisome. Clinicians should consider the general risk of drug interactions for the class of SSRIs until proven otherwise and treat these three SSRIs similarly regarding possible drug interactions involving the inhibition of both 2D6 and 3A4.

As additional studies are reported, more is understood about drug interactions, including those involving the newer antidepressants. The Food and Drug Administration considers research and clinical data used in the package inserts and in the PDR. The Administration's handling of possible drug interactions changes constantly. For this reason, it is useful to refer to the most recent editions of the PDR and other references to keep abreast of these issues.

Drug Interaction Profiles

Significant clinical problems involving drug interactions with the newer antidepressants can result from the simultaneous use of other drugs that are normally metabolized by specific P-450 enzymes when these enzymes are inhibited. This can lead to higher blood levels and slower elimination of the coadministered medication than would have been expected without the simultaneous use of the antidepressant. **The elevated plasma levels that may result from such drug interactions can lead to toxicity, a problem most often seen with medications that have low therapeutic indexes.**

The prototype for drug interactions involving the antidepressants is the simultaneous use of a TCA (which has a low therapeutic index) with one of the SSRIs. This combination is not rare, and the consequences of drug interactions when the SSRIs are combined with the TCAs can be serious.[3]

When the SSRIs were first introduced, it was relatively common to switch patients from a TCA to an SSRI, usually because of side effects that limited the tolerability of the TCA. Sometimes, the SSRI was simply added to the TCA, which occasionally led to serious adverse events. This problem triggered the investigation of the mechanism underlying this drug interaction and ultimately led to the rapidly growing interest in the effect of the newer antidepressants on the P-450 enzymes.[14,15] Today, the more common pattern of combination occurs when a patient fails to respond adequately to an SSRI, usually the first-line treatment of depression (and many of the anxiety disorders), in which case a TCA augmentation strategy may be employed. An inadequate response to an antidepressant must be considered within the context of alternative ways of handling inadequate clinical responses to the SSRIs (see subsequent discussion of augmentation strategies).

The Role of Enzyme Inhibition:

Venlafaxine, bupropion, and mirtazapine are substrates for the P-450 enzymes, but none is known to be a clinically significant inhibitor of any of these enzymes. Table 2.3 shows the potentially important drug interactions for the newer antidepressants. From a clinical perspective, it is acceptable to consider all drugs in either group as potential causes of enzyme inhibition. Not all the predicted drug

Table 2.3
Antidepressants and Cytochrome P-450 Enzyme Involvement

Cytochrome	Polymorphism	Substrates	Inhibitors	Potentially Significant Interactions Between Inhibitors (and Substrates)
1A2 (P448)	Possible	Phenacetin, caffeine, theophylline, demethylation of TCAs,)(haloperidol,***	Fluvoxamine	Fluvoxamine haloperidophenytoin, teophylline, caffeine)
2C	Yes: 2–3% of whites; 15–25% of Asians	Diazepam, demethylation of TCAs, wariann,|| tolbutamide,|| phenytoin||	Fluvoxamine, fluoxetine,|| sertraline||	Fluvoxamine, fluoxetine (phenytoin) Sertraline (diazepam, tolbutamide)
2D6 (debrisoquin hydroxylase; sparteine hydroxylase)	Yes: 5–8% of whites; lower in Asians and African Americans	Haloperidol,* thioridazine, perphenazine, clozapine,‡ risperidone, hydroxylation of nortriptyline & desipramine; paroxetine, venlafaxine, codeine, beta blockers: timolol, metroprolol, propranolol*; type 1C antiarrhythmics: encainide, flecanide, propaferone	Quinidine, fluphenazine, leyopromazine, fluoxetine, noriluoxetine, paroxetine, sertraline	Fluoxetine, sertraline, paroxetine (TCAs, type 1C antiarrhythmics, some antipsychotics)
3A4	Possible	Demethylation of TCAs, triazoiam, verapamil, midazolam, alprazolam, carpamazepine,|| cyclosporin, [terfenadine], [astemizole], quinidine, erythromycin, lidocaine [cisapride]	Ketoconazole, sertraline,|| fluoxetine,|| fluvoxamine, nefazodone§	Fluoxetine, sertraline (carbamazepine) Nefazodone (alprazolam, triazolam)

* Catalyzes a minor pathway of reversible metabolism
** Evidence based on significant elevation of haloperidol concentrations during concomitant fluvoxamine administration Additional name for the same enzyme
‡ At least partially oxidized through this enzyme
§ Evidence based on significant inhibition of alprazolam/triazolam metabolism
|| Suspected but not confirmed
Material in italics has been added since original publication.
[NB material in brackets has been associated with cardiac irregularities.]
Reprinted by permission of the publisher from DeVane CL. Antidepressants and cytochrome P450 enzyme involvement. *Am J Med.* 1994: 97(suppl 6A);19S. Copyright 1994 by Excerpta Medica Inc.

interactions will occur because of individual variations and because multiple metabolic pathways often exist. Table 2.3 shows the substrates for the most important P-450 enzymes, making it a helpful checklist when coadministering other medications with the antidepressants. For example, if a patient is taking fluvoxamine, Table 2.3 shows it to be a potent inhibitor of enzymes 1A2, 2C, and 3A4. Because the list of substrates for the P-450 enzymes is long, it is not likely to be remembered by prescribing physicians. However, it is not difficult to review this list or the PDR when using the antidepressants and other medications because drug interactions are not limited to either the antidepressants or to other psychotropic medications.

A growing body of experience has shown that drug interactions involving the newer antidepressants, with the exception of the well-known interaction of the SSRIs with the TCAs and the MAOIs, are uncommon in practice. Table 2.4 offers a simplified summary of the most important pharmacokinetic interactions of the newer antidepressants. (Since the data in Table 2.4 were compiled, new studies suggest that there is little clinical risk in the coadministration of fluoxetine and terfenadine.)

Fluoxetine and paroxetine were widely studied in clinical trials prior to the identification of the potential for these drug interactions. **In these clinical trials, 5,500 patients were studied, more than 800 of whom received medications that may have interacted with their antidepressants. Analysis of these records of patients in these prospectively collected clinical trials failed to identify any adverse event linked to drug interactions.**[12] In the 8 years since the newer antidepressants became available in the United States, a large percentage of all prescribing physicians have used these medications, often coadministering them with medications on the list of potential drug interactions. Despite this extensive exposure, most physicians have seen few, if any, significant drug interactions involving these medications.

As already emphasized, pharmacology is the key to understanding potential drug interactions. **If the potential for a drug interaction exists because of the inhibition of a hepatic enzyme, the substrate will be eliminated more slowly, thereby producing a higher plasma level and a longer duration of action.** This may produce toxic effects if the coadministered substrate drug has a low therapeutic index, as do the TCAs. Adverse effects that do occur as a result of enzyme inhibi-

33

tion will occur within a few days or, at the very most, within a few weeks of starting the newly coadministered medication (or the antidepressant)—with a maximum effect occurring within 1 month for fluoxetine and within approximately 1 week for the other antidepressants once full dose levels are achieved. If the two medications have been administered at a steady dose for longer than five times the half-life of the medication with the longer half-life, new symptoms attributed to toxicity as a result of enzyme inhibition are unlikely to occur.

The toxic effects of these enzyme-mediated drug interactions are not new effects. They are the ordinary toxic effects of excessive dosing of the coadministered drug (the substrate for the inhibited P-450 enzyme) and are similar to the normal variations seen in genetically determined poor metabolizers.

These facts help put the issue of possible drug interactions involving the newer antidepressants squarely back into the hands of prescribing physicians. Physicians can be reassured that the routine techniques used in managing the dosing of the antidepressants for many years are appropriate to handle potential drug interactions. **The old advice of "start low and go slow" applies to coadministered medications, as does the advice that each patient must be dosed and possible side effects noted as the dose is raised.** If there is a drug interaction involving the P-450 system, it will produce a higher plasma level of the substrate than expected at a particular dose. **Coadministration of drugs is not necessarily dangerous or unwise; however, a lower-than-normal dose of the coadministered medication must be prescribed to produce the expected clinical result.**

Enzyme inhibition produces the same clinical result as does genetic polymorphism (i.e., a state of enzyme deficiency). Variability of individual response to most medications is common and can usually be handled with routine clinical guidelines, although added caution is indicated for medications with low therapeutic indexes (such as TCAs). **Coadministered substrates may require determinations of plasma levels, but for many medications (including the newer antidepressants and most other psychotropics), there is such a poor correlation between either therapeutic or adverse effects and plasma levels that laboratory tests are not usually needed.** Coadministered TCAs, however, may justify determinations of plasma levels because of their low therapeutic indexes.

Table 2.4
Newer Antidepressants and Potentially Important Drug Interactions

Antidepressant	Enzyme	System Inhibited	Potential Drug Interactions
Fluoxetine	2D6*		Secondary-amine antidepressants, haloperidol, type 1C antiarrhythmics
	2C		
	3A4	Phenytoin, diazepam	Carbamazepine, alprazolam, terfenadine
Sertraline	2D6*		Secondary amine TCAs, antipsychotics, type 1C antiarrhythmics
	2C	Tolbutamide and diazepam	
	3A4	Carbamazepine	
Paroxetine	2D6*		Secondary-amine TCAs, antipsychotics, type 1C antiarrhythmics, trazodone
Fluvoxamine	1A2*		Theophylline, clozapine, haloperidol, amitriptyline, clomipramine,
	2C	imipramine	
Diazepam	3A4*		Carbamazepine, alprazolam, terfenadine, astemizole ‡
Nefazodone	3A4		Alprazolam, triazolam, terfenadine‡, astemizole ‡

* Evidence of inhibition in vitro

Inhibition suggested by clinical observation or results of pharmacokinetic studies

‡ Currently contraindicated for concomitant use with nefazodone

Reprinted by permission of the publisher from Nemeroff CB, DeVane CL, Pollock BG. Newer antidepressants and the cytochrome P-450 system. Am J Psychiatry. 1996;153:311–320. Copyright 1996 by the American Psychiatric Association.

Effects of SSRIs on TCA Serum Levels:

To explore the interaction between SSRIs and TCAs, Figure [2.1] shows the effects of coadministration of fluoxetine and desipramine on 25 patients. It illustrates the serum level of desipramine after the addition of fluoxetine and whether or not new adverse events appeared. **According to Baldessarini,**[16] **"the concentrations of these drugs in plasma that have been suggested to correlate best with satisfactory antidepressant responses range from 100 to 250 ng/mL. Toxic effects of these drugs can be expected when their concentrations in plasma rise above 500 ng/mL, and levels above 1 mg/mL can be fatal."**

The plasma levels of patients with good clinical responses to the TCAs ranged from approximately 75 ng/mL to 300 ng/mL before fluoxetine was added. After the addition of 20 mg fluoxetine, 4 of the 25 patients did not show any change in TCA serum levels, presumably because they were genetically poor metabolizers through the 2D6 enzyme; therefore, inhibition of this enzyme was not a factor in their TCA serum levels. Two of these patients were at the low end of the TCA plasma level spectrum before receiving fluoxetine, which suggests that alternative metabolic pathways for TCAs were being used by their hepatic enzymes. After fluoxetine was administered, many patients had TCA serum levels above the 500 ng/mL level that Baldessarini indicated as the threshold for toxic reactions.[16] **After coadministration of desipramine and fluoxetine, many patients had serum levels that did not produce any adverse events, despite being remarkably high** (up to the 1,000 ng/mL level, which can be fatal). **On the other hand, some patients with slight elevations in TCA serum concentrations did have new adverse events after coadministration of fluoxetine with desipramine.**

In essence, Figure 2.1 shows the striking individual variation in clinical response in terms of serum levels for the therapeutic effects of the TCAs as well as of the poor correlation between serum levels and side effects.

Pregnancy and Medications for Depression

Both anxiety and affective disorders occur at higher rates among women than among men and at higher rates among people in their middle years than among adolescents or the elderly. This demography translates into a high prevalence of significant anxiety and depression for women in childbearing ages. Even though pregnancy itself is not an unusually high-risk time in a woman's life, clinically significant anxiety and depression are common during pregnancy, especially for women whose history of these disorders preceded their pregnancies. The FDA uses a four-scale classification of teratogenicity, ranging from Category A (the least risk) to Category D (the highest risk). Published reports cover 500 exposures to TCAs over the past 35 years and 2,100 exposures to fluoxetine over the past nine years. The FDA places all of the newer antidepressants in Category C.

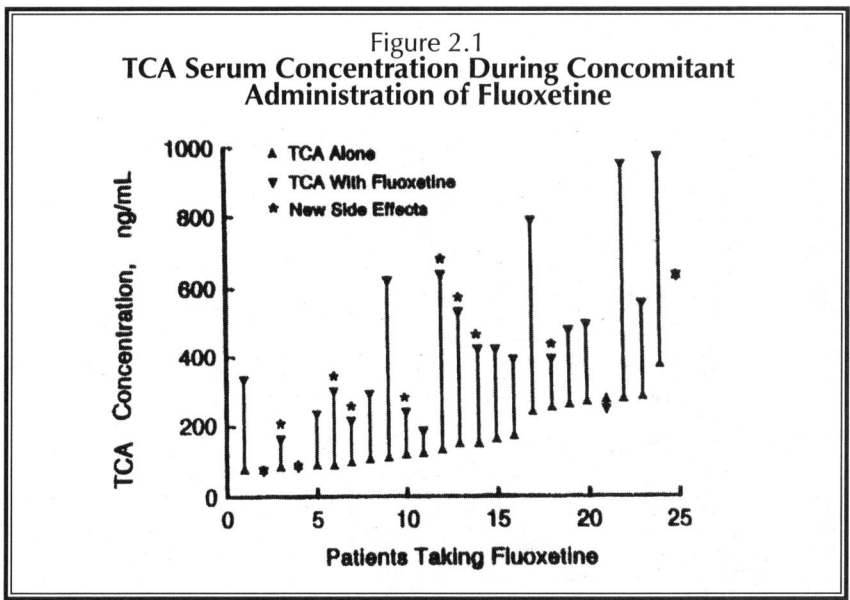

Figure 2.1
TCA Serum Concentration During Concomitant Administration of Fluoxetine

The medications used to treat both anxiety and depression are not known to be associated with added risk of fetal malformations, but caution dictates consideration of nonmedical approaches to these problems and the use of the safest medication at the lowest effective dose during pregnancy. On the other hand, women's health needs are poorly met by a "no medicine during pregnancy" stance when it comes to the treatment of anxiety and depression.[17]

I have found it helpful to refer pregnant patients and their spouses to a university genetic counseling center so that they can get an independent assessment of fetal risks to help them make their decisions. I also encourage consultation with their obstetricians and anyone else who can play a useful role. Then I remind patients that about 10% of fetuses have some abnormality at birth—with about 1% having a serious abnormality—unrelated to exposure to medications taken by their mothers. Parents need to weigh this risk and to consider how they will handle any problems that may arise in terms of blaming themselves or their physicians.

In striking a reasonable balance, it is important to consider the risk to the mother's health of untreated affective or anxiety disorders. Many women say that the only way they will go through a pregnancy is with medications because the pain they experience off medications is so great that they would choose an abortion as an alternative. These obviously are not easy decisions for physicians or patients; there is no simple formula. It is useful to keep in mind that psychoactive drugs are not known to cause a high risk to the fetus and that the illnesses from which the mothers suffer are painful, often crippling, as well as treatable with appropriate medications.

Clinical Failures with SSRIs

When a patient fails to respond to an SSRI in initial doses, the most appropriate responses are usually to extend the trial for at least 10 weeks and to increase the dose of the SSRI to the maximum recommended dose, if the drug can be tolerated by the patient. Most clinical failures with SSRIs and other antidepressants are the result of insufficient trials, often because of inadequate duration and sometimes because of inadequate doses. **If a patient cannot tolerate a maximum dose of a particular SSRI and does not respond well to lower doses, trying another SSRI is a reasonable next step.** If the patient tolerates a full dose of an SSRI for 10 weeks or longer, it is less likely (but not impossible) that switching to another SSRI will produce an improved response. In those situations, it may be desirable to switch to one of the newer antidepressants that is not an SSRI.

Augmentation Strategies:

In addition to the selection of alternative antidepressants in cases of poor clinical response to an SSRI, it is possible to follow specific aug-

Table 2.5
Selected TCA Drug Interactions

Drug	Interaction	Type of Data	Management
Phenothiazines, haloperidol	Increased TCA levels	1	Reduce dose of TCA
Anticholinergics	Anticholinergic toxicity	1	Monitor and reduce dose of TCA if needed
Valproate	Increased valproate levels	1	Use lower dose
Carbamazepine, barbiturates	Decreased TCA levels	1	Increase TCA dose if levels are low
Verapamil	Increased TCA levels	1	Check TCA levels and lower dose if needed
MAOI	Fatal reaction possible	1	See text
SSRIs	Increased TCA levels	1	Decrease TCA dose
Cimetidine	Increased TCA levels	1	Decrease TCA dose
Quinidine	Increased TCA levels	1	Monitor and reduce dose of TCA if needed
Epinephrine	Increased TCA levels	1	Use lower dose of TCA
Disulfiram	Increased TCA levels	2	Monitor TCA levels
Methylphenidate	Increased TCA levels	2	Monitor TCA levels
Methadone	Increased TCA levels	2	Monitor TCA levels

1 = in vivo studies/well established; 2 = multiple case reports and/or based on related compounds

Reprinted by permission of the publisher from Krishnan KRR, Steffens DC, Doraiswamy PM. Psychotropic drug interactions. Prim Psychiatry. 1996;1:21–45. Copyright 1996 by MBL Communications.

mentation strategies. Adding lithium, a stimulant such as dextroamphetamine sulfate (Dexedrine), or thyroid (in usual clinical doses) is a good first response for augmentation of inadequate antidepressant effects.[10] When using lithium for antidepressant augmentation, use typical clinical dosing even if the patient is not bipolar. When using thyroid, it may be wise to use T3, liothyronine (Cytomel), at doses of 25–50 mg/day for 7–14 days or longer to convert antidepressant nonresponders into responders.[18] If T3 augmentation is successful, the T3 should be continued for 2 or 3 months and then gradually tapered over several weeks. Augmenting agents, and responses to medication changes to reduce the sexual dysfunction sometimes induced by antidepressants, are likely to produce results within 3 weeks or less of the start of the trial; therefore, results of augmentation trials can be evaluated much more rapidly than the 6–10 weeks needed to determine maximum antidepressant and antianxiety effects of starting a new medication.

When these conservative augmentation strategies fail to produce adequate clinical responses, sophisticated clinicians may try concomitant use of an SSRI with a TCA. This combination can produce serious and even fatal side effects as a result of drug interactions if they are not anticipated and if clinical responses and dose levels are not handled skillfully.

The SSRIs are not the only medications that raise plasma levels of TCAs. Table 2.5 offers some of the commonly used medications that raise plasma levels of TCA as well as appropriate ways to handle each potential drug interaction. Table 2.6 presents a list of medications that interact with MAOIs.

SSRI-Induced Adverse Effects

Sexual Dysfunction:

The most common sexual dysfunctions seen with SSRIs are decreased sexual interest and inhibited orgasm, which occur in both men and women. Unlike the headaches and gastrointestinal side effects of the SSRIs, sexual dysfunction, when it occurs, is often an enduring adverse event.

Before withdrawing an effective SSRI because of sexual dysfunction, it is usually desirable to try some simple responses to the problem, including reducing the dose and implementing drug holidays for

Table 2.6
Selected MAOI Drug Interactions

Drug	Interaction	Type of Data	Management
Meperidine	Rapid, serious, or fatal reaction possible	1	Combination is contraindicated
Methadone	Minimal	1	Concurrent use needs careful monitoring
Phenylephrine	Hypertensive crisis	1	Contraindicated
TCAs	Fatal reaction possible	1	See text
SSRIs	Serotonin syndrome	1	Combination contraindicated (see text)
l-Tryptophan	Serotonin syndrome	1	Combination contraindicated
Tyramine	Hypertensive crises	1	See PDR for foods and drinks to avoid
Morphine	Decreased blood pressure	2	Concurrent use needs careful monitoring
Epinephrine, norepinephrine, or isoproterenol	Increased blood pressure	2	Concurrent use needs careful monitoring
Tranylcypromine	Hypertensive reaction with other MAOIs	2	Use caution if replacing tranylcypromine with other MAOIs
Fenfluramine	Confusion	2	Avoid combination
Reserpine	Hypomania	3	Avoid combination
Ginseng	Additive stimulant effect	3	Avoid combination
Dextromethorphan	Resembles serotonin syndrome	3	Avoid combination

1 = in vivo studies/well established; 2 = multiple case reports and/or based on related compounds; 3 = isolated case report

Reprinted by permission of the publisher from Krishnan KRR, Steffens DC, Doraiswamy PM. Psychotropic drug interactions. Prim Psychiatry. 1996;1:21–45. Copyright 1996 by MBL Communications.

1 or 2 days before intercourse. This side effect, like most others, may be promptly responsive to lowered plasma levels, even when the decreased level lasts only a few days. Some patients will experience an upsurge of anxiety or depression when the SSRI is stopped, even for a few days on such drug holidays, but many others will not. Medication holidays are not without risk. They may lead to discontinuation of the antidepressant, a serious adverse outcome.

An alternate way of handling SSRI-induced sexual dysfunction is to add bupropion (75 mg/day) to the SSRI regimen. Also, some patients experience reduction of sexual dysfunction while taking SSRIs when they add buspirone (BuSpar; 10 mg) either 1–2 hours before intercourse or 10–15 mg three or four times a day on a continuing basis along with the SSRI. **Bupropion, mirtazapine, and nefazodone are less likely to produce sexual dysfunction than are the SSRIs, so they are reasonable choices if sexual dysfunction leads to discontinuation of an SSRI.**

Nausea and Vomiting:

The SSRIs commonly produce nausea and sometimes vomiting, especially early in treatment. These side effects presumably are the result of the release of serotonin into the gut wall and typically subside within a few weeks of stable dosing. They also may be lessened by taking the SSRI with meals.

Activation and Sedation:

In some patients, all the newer antidepressants produce anxiety and insomnia (activation) and, somewhat paradoxically, they all can produce sedation in some patients. Occasionally, patients complain of both symptoms simultaneously. Regarding activation, it is useful to distinguish between agitation, which is a physical, behavioral symptom (such as restless pacing or another continuous activity) and anxiety, which is a feeling state associated with fear and worry. Anxiety is more common than agitation as a side effect of the antidepressants, but both agitation and anxiety can be either side effects of these drugs or, more often, symptoms of underlying depression or an anxiety disorder.

Patients with insomnia and anxiety should be asked whether the symptoms existed before the medication was started or whether they emerged (or worsened) after the medication was initiated. If the symptoms preceded the use of the medication (i.e., if they are the result of depression and a side effect of the medication), they are likely to be improved with continued treatment, even though it is common for these symptoms to become more severe in the first few days of treatment with an antidepressant. Because worry is a common manifestation of both depression and anxiety disorders, patients frequently worry about their use of antidepressants and other drugs. **Before medications are initiated, patients should be informed that they may experience side effects, especially early in treatment, and that these symptoms generally are not dangerous. In fact, side effects are signs that the drug is working and usually subside within a few weeks of using the medication. Thus, side effects can be a reason for hope for a good treatment outcome rather than signs of treatment failure.**

In general, fluoxetine and sertraline are more likely to produce activation than other agents, and paroxetine and nefazodone are more likely to produce sedation than other agents. On the other hand, it is important not to let these occasionally bothersome side effects weigh too heavily in the initial selection of an antidepressant, because most patients receiving fluoxetine and sertraline do not experience activation and many patients receiving paroxetine and nefazodone do not experience clinically significant sedation. Most patients who do experience these side effects find that the effects diminish over several weeks of continued therapy. If activation or sedation continues to be bothersome after 6–8 weeks of treatment at stable doses, it may be helpful to lower the dose of the antidepressant in an attempt to improve these side effects while the benefits of treatment are sustained.

In the first weeks of using an antidepressant, it is often useful to prescribe zolpidem tartrate (Ambien) if insomnia is a prominent symptom. In most cases, a reassuring and supportive physician who helps patients understand and cope with initial side effects and the relatively slow onset of therapeutic benefits of antidepressants can improve patient compliance with the antidepressant treatment long enough at a high enough dose to produce a good therapeutic result.[5]

Antidepressant Withdrawal

The benzodiazepines have been widely recognized for a powerful withdrawal syndrome that sometimes follows abrupt discontinuation.[7,19]

43

Although less dramatic than benzodiazepine withdrawal, symptoms following withdrawal of imipramine were first reported nearly 40 years ago.[20] Since then, withdrawal symptoms have been reported with other TCAs and the MAOIs. More recently, withdrawal has been reported following discontinuation of the SSRIs.[21]

Withdrawal symptoms following antidepressant withdrawal include many symptoms seen following benzodiazepine withdrawal, except that seizures have not been reported. Common symptoms of antidepressant withdrawal are flulike symptoms, such as fatigue, tremor, sweating, stomach distress, dizziness (lightheadedness rather than true vertigo), chills, and incoordination. Additional symptoms of antidepressant withdrawal include anxiety, arrhythmias, sleep disturbance, mania or hypomania, panic attacks, and delirium.[21]

The two most likely causes of antidepressant withdrawal symptoms are cholinergic rebound and serotonin mechanisms, either alone or in combination.[21] Cholinergic rebound is the most likely cause of TCA withdrawal because of the affinity of these medications for muscarinic acetylcholine receptors. Although the SSRIs show far less affinity for acetylcholine receptors, many of the withdrawal symptoms seen after discontinuation of the SSRIs are indistinguishable from those seen following discontinuation of the TCAs.[22,23]

The risk of antidepressant withdrawal is greater after more prolonged treatment and for younger patients.[21] Shorter elimination half-life also raises the risk.[24-26] **Antidepressant withdrawal symptoms are seldom severe and generally disappear over the course of a few days or weeks after stopping the antidepressant medication.** No medication has been shown to alleviate these withdrawal symptoms. As is the case for withdrawal symptoms related to opiates and benzodiazepines, antidepressant withdrawal symptoms are reduced by reinstitution of the original medication and by more gradual dose reduction over a period of a few weeks or longer.[27,28] Among the SSRIs, withdrawal symptoms are less likely to occur following the discontinuation of fluoxetine than sertraline, fluvoxamine, or paroxetine, presumably because of the much longer half-life of its active metabolite, norfluoxetine.

Conclusion

Many of the newer antidepressants (and all of the SSRIs) inhibit specific hepatic enzymes that metabolize other medications. When these enzymes are inhibited, the peak plasma levels and elimination half-lives of the coadministered medications are increased, sometimes by as much as three or more times the levels prior to addition of the antidepressant. For medications that have low therapeutic indexes and that potentially produce serious adverse events at high plasma levels, these drug interactions can pose clinically significant risks.

The most common problems of drug interactions with the newer antidepressants involve the 3A4 enzyme, which is inhibited by nefazodone and fluvoxamine, leading to increased plasma levels of alprazolam, triazolam, carbamazepine, and midazolam. Particularly worrisome is the interaction of the inhibition of 3A4 by terfenadine and astemizole, which can cause serious or even fatal adverse events. Less common, but better studied, are the interactions involving the 2D6 enzyme inhibited by fluoxetine, paroxetine, and sertraline. This enzyme is involved in the metabolism of the TCAs, which can produce increases in TCA plasma levels of 50%–400% with coadministration of other agents. Because of the low therapeutic indexes of the TCAs, this can be a significant, and even a fatal, problem.

Checklists of potentially interacting medications are now available. Because they are based on in vitro studies that fail to consider alternative metabolic pathways, these checklists overpredict drug interactions involving the newer antidepressants. When such interactions do occur, they are not new adverse reactions but familiar reactions to elevated plasma levels commonly seen in patients who genetically lack specific P-450 enzymes. When antidepressants are coadministered with other agents that may be metabolized by inhibited hepatic enzymes, the old adage of "start low and go slow" rings true.

Clinicians should look for the emergence of both therapeutic and adverse reactions to the gradual escalation of dose of the coadministered substrate medication. Once the prescribing physician is alert to the potential for drug interactions, doses can usually be managed clinically. Despite the controversy surrounding this issue, drug interactions involving the newer antidepressants are relatively uncommon in clinical practice and usually handled easily with routine clinical skills.

References

1. Thompson D, Oster G. Use of terfenadine and contraindicated drugs. JAMA. 1996;275:1339–1341.

2. Physicians' Desk Reference. 50th ed. Montvale, NJ: *Medical Economics*; 1996.

3. Nemeroff CB, DeVane CL, Pollock BG. Newer antidepressants and the cytochrome P-450 system. *Am J Psychiatry*. 1996;153:311–320.

4. Hardman JG, Limbird LE, eds. *Goodman and Gilman's The Pharmacological Basis of Therapeutics*. 9th ed. New York: McGraw-Hill; 1996.

5. Schatzberg AF, Siegel A, DuPont RL. The experts converse. SSRI treatment controversies: the elderly. *J Clin Psychiatry* INTERCOM. 1996;July:1–11.

6. Schatzberg AF, Cohen L, DuPont RL. The experts converse. SSRI treatment controversies: the anxious depressed patient. *J Clin Psychiatry* INTERCOM. 1996;October:1–11.

7. DuPont RL. Anxiety and addiction: a clinical perspective on comorbidity. *Bull Menninger Clin*. 1995;59(suppl A):A53–A72.

8. Wells BG, Mandos LA, Hayes PE. Depressive disorders. In: Dipiro JT, Talbert RL, Yee GC, et al., eds. *Pharmacotherapy: A Pathophysiologic Approach*. 3rd ed. Stamford, CT: Appleton and Lange; 1993:1395–1418.

9. Sternbach H. The serotonin syndrome. *Am J Psychiatry*. 1991;148: 705–713.

10. Nemeroff CB. Augmentation regimens for depression. *J Clin Psychiatry*. 1991;52(May suppl):21–27.

11. Preskorn SH, Alderman J, Chung M, et al. Pharmacokinetics of desipramine coadministered with sertraline or fluoxetine. *J Clin Psychopharmacol*. 1994;14:90–98.

12. Nemeroff CB. *P-450 enzyme systems, newer antidepressants and drug-drug interactions*. Presented to Continuing Medical Education, Inc., program on Clinical Controversies in Treating Depression; February 17, 1996; Bethesda, MD.

13. Hollander AAMJ, van Rooij J, Lentjes EGWM, et al. The effect of grapefruit juice on cyclosporine and prednisone metabolism in transplant patients. *Clin Pharmacol Ther*. 1995;57:318–324.

14. Harvey AT, Preskorn SH. Cytochrome P-450 enzymes: interpretation of their interactions with selective serotonin reuptake inhibitors, part I. *J Clin Psychopharmacol*. 1996;16:273–285.

15. Harvey AT, Preskorn SH. Cytochrome P-450 enzymes: interpretation of their interactions with selective serotonin reuptake inhibitors, part II. *J Clin Psychopharmacol*. 1996;16:345–355.

16. Baldessarini RJ. Drugs and the treatment of psychiatric disorders—depression and mania. In: Hardman JG, Limbird LE, eds. Goodman and Gilman's The Pharmacological Basis of Therapeutics. 9th ed. New York: McGraw-Hill; 1996;431–459.

17. Altshuler LL, Cohen L, Szuba MP, Burt VK, Girlin M, Mintz J. Pharmacologic management of psychiatric illness during pregnancy: dilemmas and guidelines. *Am J Psychiatry*. 1996;153:592–606.

18. Kaplan HI, Sadock BJ, Grebb JA. *Kaplan and Sadock's Synopsis of Psychiatry—Behavioral Sciences/Clinical Psychiatry, Seventh Edition*. Baltimore, MD: Williams & Wilkins; 1994.

19. Sellers EM, Ciraulo DA, DuPont RL, et al. Alprazolan and benzodiazepine dependence. *J Clin Psychiatry*. 1993;54(Suppl):64–74.

20. Mann AM, MacPherson A. Clinical experience with imipramine (G22355) in the treatment of depression. *Can Psychiatr Assoc J*. 1959;4:38–47.

21. Lejoyeux M, Ades J, Mourad I, Solomon J. Dilsaver S. *Antidepressant withdrawal syndrome: recognition, prevention, and management*. CNS Drugs. 1996;5:278–292.

22. Richelson E. Pharmacology of antidepressants—characteristics of the ideal drug. *Mayo Clin Proc*. 1994;69:1069–1081.

23. Barr LC, Goodman WK, Price LH. Physical symptoms associated with paroxetine discontinuation. *Am J Psychiatry*. 1994;151:289.

24. Berlin CS. Fluoxetine withdrawal symptoms. *J Clin Psychiatry*. 1996; 57:93–94.

25. Louie AK, Lannon RA, Ajari LK. Withdrawal reaction after sertraline discontinuation. *Am J Psychiatry*. 1994;151:450–451.

26. Frost L, Lal S. Shock-like sensations after discontinuation of selective serotonin reuptake inhibitors. *Am J Psychiatry*. 1995;152:810.

27. DuPont RL. A physician's guide to discontinuing benzodiazepine therapy. *West J Med*. 1990;152:600–603.

28. DuPont RL. A practical approach to benzodiazepine discontinuation. *J Psychiatr Res*. 1990;24:81–90.

3   Decision Making in the Use of Antidepressants: Treatment Considerations

Pedro L. Delgado, MD, and Alan J. Gelenberg, MD

Dr. Delgado is Associate Professor of Psychiatry and Associate Department Head for Research, and Dr. Gelenberg is Professor and Head, Department of Psychiatry, University of Arizona College of Medicine, Tucson, AZ.

Editor's Note

Antidepressants apparently are effective for treating disorders other than major depression, including dysthymia, generalized anxiety disorder, panic disorder, social phobia, obsessive-compulsive disorder, bulimia and anorexia nervosa, and posttraumatic stress disorder. Therefore, Drs. Delgado and Gelenberg suggest that these drugs in fact affect the core brain systems involved in modulating stress, probably by "restoring function." This viewpoint ties into the concept of psychological resilience, which posits that being depressed per se after significant stress is not a problem so much as how well the disturbance is managed and how successful recovery from a state of emotional disruption can become. Inadequate resilience can exist on a psychosocial level, a biological level, or both; accordingly, psychotherapy is directed to the psychosocial issues, and pharmacotherapy is used to restore the biological pathways necessary for recovery and maintenance of resilience in the face of future stressors.

As the authors point out, antidepressant medication should be started quickly when improvement is unlikely without it; possible harmful effects may arise otherwise (e.g., loss of job, marital disruption, suicide); there is a history of previous episodes; or there is a strong family history of mood disorder. Conversely, initiation of antidepressant pharmacotherapy is best postponed if symptoms are mild, the risk of harmful consequences is minimal, or depression appears secondary to recent severe life stressors, medical illness, or coadministered medication. Discontinuation of treatment (acute, continuation, maintenance) is described in detail, with many practical suggestions.

Introduction

The latter half of the 20th century has been marked by a dramatically increased understanding of mood disorders. In addition to increasing our understanding of the theoretical basis and pathophysiology of depression, 50 years of clinical research have refined our knowledge of brain function and the mechanism of action of antidepressant medications. Millions of persons who suffer from depression have already received the benefits of this research, with new treatment options under constant investigation.

The growth in knowledge and the availability of newer drugs have brought about an increase in the number of factors that should be considered when selecting appropriate antidepressant medications. This two-part chapter provides an overview of the decision-making process involved in the selection of appropriate medications for depression, including known benefits, potential side effects, and proper use. The first part explores the decision to use antidepressant medication and the treatment considerations for each phase of its use. The second part serves as a guide for choosing a medication, with an in-depth examination of the pharmacokinetics and side effects of the various classes of antidepressant agents.

It is important to note the limitations in our current concepts of antidepressant and depression. Antidepressant erroneously implies selectivity and specificity for depression. Antidepressants are effective in the acute treatment of milder mood disorders such as dysthymia[1,2] as well as other mental disorders such as generalized anxiety disorder,[3] panic disorder,[4-6] social phobia,[7] obsessive-compulsive disorder,[8,9] bulimia nervosa and anorexia nervosa,[10,11] and posttraumatic stress disorder.[12]

Antidepressant drugs affect the core brain systems that are involved in modulating stress.[13,14] The disorders for which antidepressant drugs are effective can be exacerbated by stress,[15] suggesting that such medication may simply restore function. The high rates of depressive relapse upon discontinuation of antidepressant drugs support this concept.[16-18]

The modern concept of major depression describes a syndrome with many likely etiologic factors. It is highly unlikely that only one type of abnormality, whether inherited or environmentally caused, is responsible for all forms of major depression, dysthymia, cyclothymia, and bipolar disorders. Specific types of cerebral infarcts,[19] hypothyroidism,[20] some of the porphyrias, acquired immunodeficiency syndrome,[21] and many types of drugs can cause symptoms indistinguishable from those found in depression of unknown etiology.

The limitations of both the concept of antidepressant and the heterogeneity of depression require that the action of antidepressants be compared, by analogy, with the nonspecific antiinflammatory effects of corticosteroids in the treatment of inflammatory conditions. **For the purpose of this chapter, antidepressant drugs are defined as those drugs for which efficacy has been shown in published clinical studies.** Depression is defined according to the DSM-IV[22] definition of major depression.

Choosing to Prescribe

Antidepressant Medication:

The decision to use antidepressant medication to treat a patient should follow a careful physical and psychological assessment and diagnosis. This usually can be accomplished in one visit, especially if medical, psychiatric, and substance abuse histories are available.[23,24] Once a diagnosis of major depression has been made, antidepressant medications are usually indicated. **Given the known efficacy and safety of these drugs, treatment of most patients should be initiated with the understanding that the choice of an agent may be significantly affected by presenting symptoms and concurrent psychiatric, medical, or substance abuse diagnoses.** Concomitant supportive, educational, or cognitive psychotherapy is usually indicated. Determining when to attempt a trial of psychotherapy before medication treatment is an issue that lies beyond the scope of this chapter, but in general, an indication for psychotherapy is based on clinical presentation, diagnosis, course of illness, past history, and severity.

Several situations call for immediate initiation of medication treat-ment. These situations, listed in Table 3.1, include conditions in which improvement is unlikely without medication treatment, where possible harmful consequences may arise if the depression is untreated (e.g., loss of job or risk of suicide), or where relapse and recurrence are highly likely outcomes. Other situations necessitating medication treatment include a strong family history of mood disor-ders or major depression with atypical features.

Medication treatment should be postponed if the diagnosis of major depression is unclear, if the symptoms are very mild, if the risk of harmful consequences of the depression is minimal, or if the patient is strongly averse to the use of pharmacotherapy. The most common of these situations occurs when a recent life stress raises the possibility that the presenting symptoms represent a moderate to severe form of an adjustment disorder or that the depression may be secondary to medical illness, concomitant medication, or substance abuse. The decision to initiate medication treatment in these patients should follow one or two further evaluations.

Table 3.1
Clinical Situations Usually Requiring Antidepressant Pharmacotherapy

Major Depression:
- with moderate to severe symptoms
- with potential for suicide or other harmful consequences
- with psychotic features (antipsychotic medication or electroconvulsive therapy usually required)
- with melancholia
- when maintenance treatment is planned or relapse likely
- with bipolar disorder (concomitant antimanic drug therapy usually required)
- with prior history of:
- poor inter-episode recovery
- prior medication response
- failure to respond to psychotherapy
- with obsessive-compulsive or panic disorder

Stages of Treatment

Mood disorders appear to be chronic, with high rates of relapse upon discontinuation of drug therapy; therefore, it is important that treatment be conceptualized as a long-term process.[16,25-31] Although medications restore function, they do not cure the disease.

Three stages of treatment have been proposed: an acute treatment phase, a continuation phase, and a maintenance phase (Figure 3.1).[27] The stages are defined in relation to the status of symptoms and involve the concepts of treatment response, relapse, remission, recurrence, and recovery.[18,27]

Response refers to a decrease in symptoms after initiation of drug treatment. Relapse involves the return of some symptoms of a disease during or upon cessation of treatment. Remission refers to a clinically meaningful diminution of the symptoms of a disease. Recurrence describes the return of symptoms after a remission. Recovery describes a more complete remission, implying the absence or near absence of symptoms.

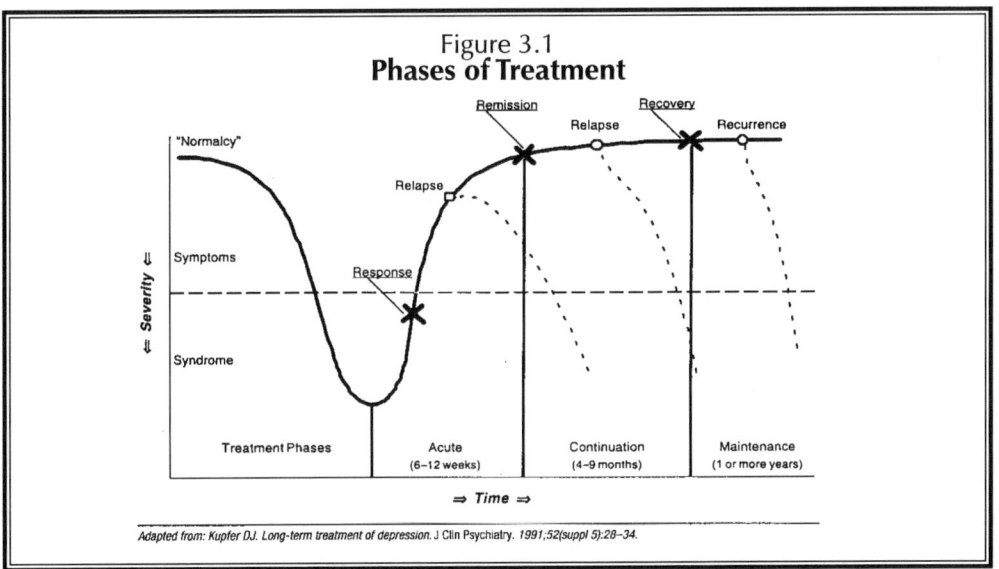

Figure 3.1
Phases of Treatment

Adapted from: Kupfer DJ. Long-term treatment of depression. J Clin Psychiatry. 1991;52(suppl 5):28–34.

Acute Treatment Phase:

The acute treatment phase begins with a clinical interview, diagnostic assessment, physical and neurological examinations, and appropriate clinical and laboratory studies.[23,24,32] **A decision to initiate treatment is based on the presence of diagnostic criteria for major depression or a manic episode. The goals of this phase include establishing a diagnosis, defining short-term and long-term multidisciplinary treatment plans, selecting the most appropriate medication, titrating** the dose to a therapeutic range, monitoring side effects, maintaining compliance, and determining the magnitude and quality of response. During this phase, which lasts 6–12 weeks, patients are usually seen for medication management every 1 or 2 weeks. If a satisfactory treatment response is achieved, the continuation phase follows. If a new treatment is initiated, a second acute treatment phase may ensue. An algo-

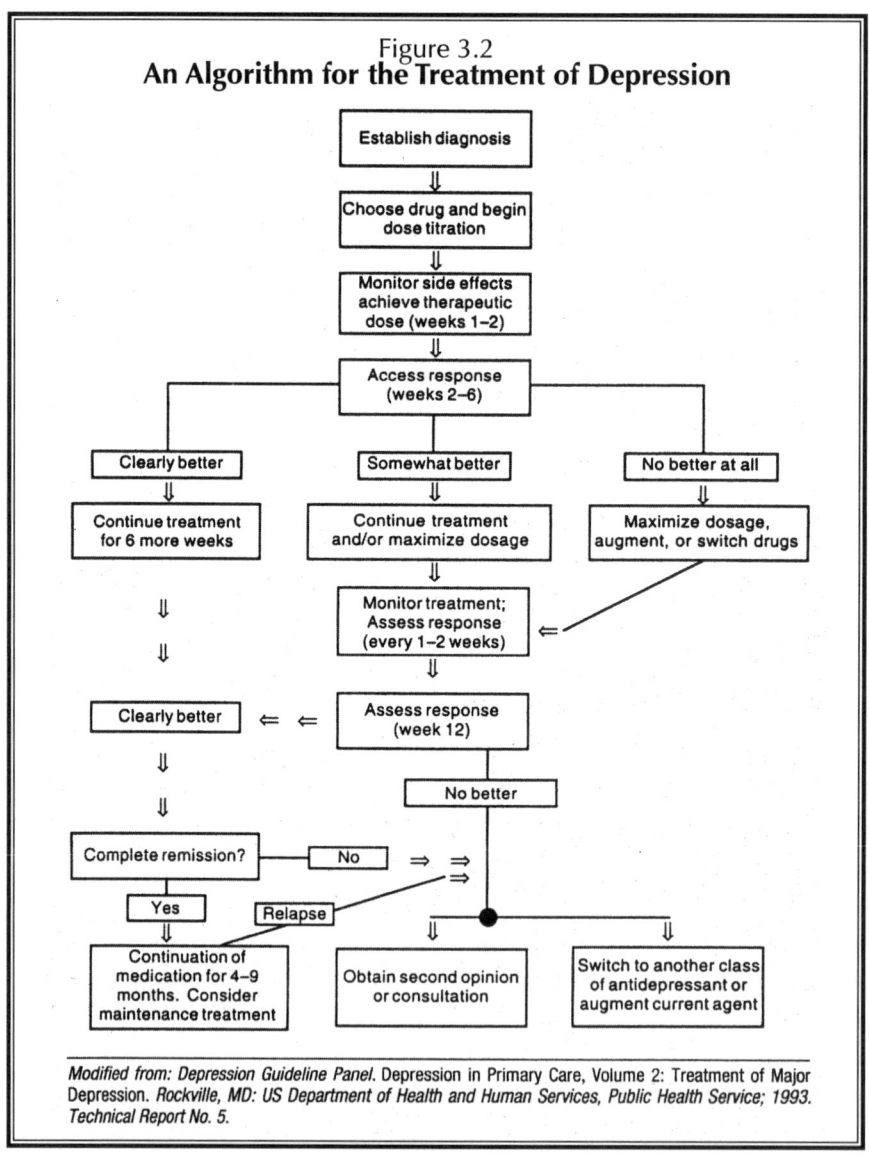

Figure 3.2
An Algorithm for the Treatment of Depression

Modified from: Depression Guideline Panel. Depression in Primary Care, Volume 2: Treatment of Major Depression. Rockville, MD: US Department of Health and Human Services, Public Health Service; 1993. Technical Report No. 5.

rithm for decision making has been suggested for antidepressant treatment phases,[23,32] a modified version of which is presented in Figure 3.2.

All current antidepressant medications require continuous dosing for an average of 10–21 days before major clinical improvement is evident. This time lag in action is unrelated to the time required to achieve therapeutic doses and may be the result of the time-dependent process of neuronal adaptation. **With most drugs, raising the dose beyond the usual therapeutic range does not speed up response but exacerbates side effects.** In some drugs, such as nortriptyline (Pamelor), with so-called therapeutic windows, higher-than-usual doses actually can be associated with a lower rate of response. These facts strongly support titration to the usual therapeutic dose range and necessitate patient monitoring of the response during the first 21 days of treatment.

The rate of dose titration is closely related to a medication's side-effect profile. The drugs with the greatest anticholinergic and antiadrenergic activity require the most careful titration. Because of the severity of side effects, the clinician may be unable to achieve therapeutic doses of medications, such as clomipramine (Anafranil), amitriptyline (Elavil), doxepin (Sinequan), amoxapine (Asendin), and trazodone (Desyrel). Conversely, for all selective serotonin-reuptake inhibitors (SSRIs) except fluvoxamine (Luvox), the therapeutic dose usually may be started at once. Because of nausea and asthenia, most investigators have titrated the dose of fluvoxamine over a 7–14-day period.

Because of the relatively soft side-effect profile associated with SSRIs, these medications are frequently prescribed at doses much higher than required. Such administration was common with fluoxetine (Prozac) **in the first few years after its introduction; gradually, it became apparent that 20 mg a day of fluoxetine was an adequate dosage for most patients. Doses of paroxetine** (Paxil) **and sertraline** (Zoloft) **often are raised too rapidly. Most investigators agree that dosages of 20 mg/day of paroxetine and 50–100 mg/day of sertraline are therapeutic. In older patients or in persons who are sensitive to side effects, starting doses of 5–10 mg of fluoxetine, 10 mg of paroxetine, or 25 mg of sertraline can be used.**

Assessment of treatment response should include an evaluation of current depressive symptoms as well as a determination of current level of function. Treatment response is clearly a continuous variable, with some patients having limited symptom relief. Other patients experience a complete restoration of normal function, and others develop a degree of improvement that is better than their prior best level of functioning.

Conceptual guidelines for defining treatment response have recently been published that draw an important distinction between partial remission and full remission.[18] **Partial remission involves a treatment response in which the patient no longer meets the full criteria for major depression or manic episode but continues to have more than minimal symptoms. Full remission is declared when a patient no longer meets criteria for major depression or manic episode and has no more than minimal symptoms.**[18] Factors that are important in assessing therapeutic response are listed in Table 3.2.

If the patient has shown no evidence of response after 3 or 4 weeks, then the dose should be titrated toward the maximum recommended dose that is tolerated. For tricyclic antidepressants and monoamine oxidase inhibitors, the dose can be increased in 3- or 4-day intervals, but for SSRIs the dose should be raised in 7–14-day intervals because most patients respond to the lower dose ranges. If the patient still has not achieved a partial response after a 4–6-week period, then a careful reevaluation of current treatment should be pursued. This involves reassessing the accuracy of the diagnosis, investigating dynamic psychosocial factors, discussing compliance issues with the patient, assessing the current dosage, and giving consideration to switching medications or augmenting the current regimen.

If a partial response has been achieved after a 4–6-week period, another waiting period of 12 weeks usually results in continued improvement and a full response. If the rate of improvement has reached a plateau after 12 weeks, consideration should be given to changing or augmenting medications. If improvement is continuing, the acute period should be extended until the response has reached a plateau.

The clinician should verify the plasma drug levels when assessing the reasons for a lack of response, when encountering a higher-than-expected degree of side effects or when suspecting toxicity. Evidence supports the presence of minimum therapeutic plasma levels for desipramine (Norpramin), imipramine (Tofranil), amitriptyline, and nortriptyline (Pamelor). Nortriptyline appears to have a therapeutic window and is less effective when plasma levels are above 150 ng/ml than when levels are between 50 and 150 ng/ml. **With desipramine, imipramine, and amitriptyline, plasma levels above 300 ng/ml are associated with a higher risk of potentially dangerous side effects, such as cardiac conduction abnormalities or seizures.**

Continuation Phase:

If a response is obtained, then the continuation phase begins, which consists of monitoring for completeness of response and for side effects. **Discontinuation of medication during or before this phase has been completed is asso-**

Table 3.2 **Assessing Therapeutic Response**
No longer meets criteria for major depressive or manic episodes
Presence or absence of specific symptoms
Level of functioning
Side effects

ciated with a high rate of relapse.[27,30] **Continuation treatment lasts 4–9 months and can be viewed as a consolidation phase.** A recent World Health Organization consensus meeting suggested that 6 months be the minimum period of time for continuation treatment.[17,33,34]

The primary tasks of the continuation phase are to monitor response, assess side effects, and establish compliance; the primary objective is to prevent relapse. If maintenance treatment is not planned, medication should be gradually tapered over a 4–6-week period at the end of this phase.

Several factors are associated with a higher risk of relapse and need to be considered before discontinuation of medication is started. **Patients with residual symptoms, significant psychosocial problems, or a history of prior relapse or recurrence are at increased risk for recurrence after continuation therapy.** Because of the high rates of recurrence of major depression, most patients should be strongly encouraged to consider maintenance treatment.

Maintenance Phase:

Maintenance treatment is thought to be prophylactic, geared toward the prevention of recurrence; however, maintenance treatment is essential for continuing the response because the illness persists regardless of its true nature. **Patients with two or more prior episodes of major depression, those with more severe episodes, and those with a risk of suicide should be strongly encouraged to consider maintenance treatment. Patients with multiple mild episodes spaced in longer intervals and patients with complete interinterval recovery obviously may choose not to use maintenance treatment.**

Studies of maintenance treatment have taken on considerable importance because of recent findings of high rates of relapse and recurrence in patients with relatively uncomplicated major depression after continuation treatment.[16-18] The most studied medication in the maintenance treatment of major depression is imipramine. The recent study[17] by the Pittsburgh group that investigated the long-term effectiveness of maintenance treatment with imipramine has become the gold standard for future maintenance studies. This study and the earlier studies by the same group[16]—as well as the study by Prien and colleagues[18]—have made imipramine the drug against which other drugs should be compared. **The rate of relapse or recurrence during imipramine treatment is 20%–30%, whereas the rate during placebo treatment approaches 80% over a 1–3-year treatment period. Dosages of imipramine below the usual therapeutic range** (150–300 mg a day, plasma level >150 ng/ml) **lead to a higher rate of relapse, suggesting that maintenance treatment should employ full antidepressant doses.**[17]

The majority of patients with a mood disorder will have more than one episode. Recurrence rates for depression are estimated to be at least 50% for patients with one episode of major depression and 80%–90% if the person has had two episodes.[27,35] **Of the patients who have been treated successfully for major depression, 70%–90% will experience a recurrence of illness when active medication is replaced by a placebo during a 3-year maintenance phase, as opposed to only 15%–20% of those taking a full dose of imipramine during the same period of time.**[18] In a prospective 10-year epidemiologic follow-up study of young depressed patients, 78% relapsed during the follow-up period.[35] These high rates of recurrence and relapse have highlighted the need for consideration of the efficacy of antidepressant treatments in the continuation and maintenance phases of treatment.

To manage medications, clinicians should see patients every 4–12 weeks during the first year of maintenance treatment and at intervals

of 6–12 months thereafter. The frequency of visits during this phase should be individualized on the basis of psychosocial factors, compliance, and presence of symptoms and side effects. **Rates of depressive relapse appear to be higher when antidepressant drugs are discontinued rapidly, compared with lower rates when drugs are tapered over 3–4 weeks.**[27,36] **Therefore, if medication is discontinued, it should be tapered over a 4-week period.**

Summary

Antidepressant drugs are highly effective in the acute and maintenance treatment of major depression. Although the disorders are usually chronic and the vulnerability to the illness remains, most patients who use antidepressants can live relatively normal lives with minimal treatment-related side effects.

References

1. Hellerstein DJ, Yanowitch P, Rosenthal J, et al. A randomized double-blind study of fluoxetine versus placebo in the treatment of dysthymia. *Am J Psychiatry*. 1993;150:1169–1175.

2. Koscis JH, Frances AJ, Voss CB, et al. Imipramine for treatment of chronic depression. *Arch Gen Psychiatry*. 1987;45:253–257.

3. Rickels K, Dosning R, Schweizer E, Hassman H. Antidepressants for the treatment of generalized anxiety disorder: a placebo-controlled comparison of imipramine, trazodone, and diazepam. *Arch Gen Psychiatry*. 1993;50:884–895.

4. Evans L, Kenardy J, Schneider P, Hoey H. Effect of a selective serotonin uptake inhibitor in agoraphobia with panic attacks: a double-blind comparison of zimelidine, imipramine, and placebo. *Acta Psychiatr Scand*. 1986;73:49–53.

5. Klein DF. Delineation of two drug-responsive anxiety syndromes. *Psychopharmacologia*. 1964; 5:397–408.

6. Klein DF, Fink M. Psychiatric reaction patterns of imipramine. *Am J Psychiatry*. 1962;119:432–438.

7. Versani M, Nardi AE, Mundim FD, et al. Pharmacotherapy of social phobia: a controlled study with moclobemide and phenelzine. *Br J Psychiatry*. 1992;161:353–360.

8. Goodman WK, Price LH, Rasmussen SA, et al. Efficacy of fluvoxamine in obsessive-compulsive disorder: a double-blind comparison with placebo. *Arch Gen Psychiatry*. 1989;46:36–44.

9. Pigott TA, Pato MT, Bernstein SE, et al. Controlled comparisons of clomipramine and fluoxetine in the treatment of obsessive-compulsive disorder. *Arch Gen Psychiatry*. 1990;47:926–932.

10. Goldbloom DS, Olmstead MP. Pharmacotherapy of bulimia nervosa with fluoxetine: assessment of clinically significant attitudinal change. *Am J Psychiatry*. 1993;150:770–774.

11. Walsh JI, Stewart JW, Roose SP, et al. Treatment of bulimia with phenelzine: a double-blind placebo-controlled study. *Arch Gen Psychiatry*. 1984;4:1105–1109.

12. Davidson JRT, Kudler HS, Saunders WB, et al. Predicting response to amitriptyline in post-traumatic stress disorder. *Am J Psychiatry*. 1993;150:1024–1029.

13. Chalmers DT, Lopez JF, Akil H, Watson SJ. Molecular aspects of the stress axis and sertonergic function in depression. *Clin Neurosci*. 1993;1(3):122–128.

14. Henn FA, Edwards E, Muneyyirci J. Animal models of depression. *Clin Neurosci*. 1993;1(3):152–156.

15. Chrousos GP, Gold PW. The concepts of stress and stress system disorders: overview of physical and behavioral homeostasis. *JAMA*. 1992;267:1244–1252.

16. Frank E, Kupfer DJ, Perel JM, et al. Three-year outcomes for maintenance therapies in recurrent depression. *Arch Gen Psychiatry*. 1990;47:1093–1099.

17. Kupfer DJ, Frank E, Perel JM, et al. Five-year outcome for maintenance therapies in recurrent depression. *Arch Gen Psychiatry*. 1992;49:769–773.

18. Prien RF, Kupfer DJ, Mansky PA, et al. Drug therapy in the prevention of recurrences in unipolar and bipolar affective disorders: report of the NIMH Collaborative Study Group comparing lithium carbonate, imipramine, and a lithium carbonate–imipramine combination. *Arch Gen Psychiatry*. 1984;41:1096–1104.

19. Robinson RG, Chait RM. Emotional correlates of structural brain injury with particular emphasis on post-stroke mood disorders. *Crit Rev Clin Neurobiol*. 1985;1(4):285–318.

20. Sachar EJ, Puig-Antich J, Ryan ND, et al. Three tests of cortisol secretion in adult endogenous depression. *Acta Psychiatr Scand*. 1985;71:1–8.

21. Perry SW. Organic mental disorders caused by HIV: update on early diagnosis and treatment. *Am J Psychiatry*. 1990;147:696–710.

22. American Psychiatric Association. *Diagnostic and Statistical Manual of Mental Disorders*. 4th ed. Washington, DC: American Psychiatric Association; 1994.

23. American Psychiatric Association Work Group on Major Depressive Disorder. American Psychiatric Association practice guidelines: practice guidelines for major depressive disorder in adults. *Am J Psychiatry*. 1993;150:1–26.

24. Depression Guideline Panel. *Depression in Primary Care, I: Detection and Diagnosis*. Rockville, MD: Public Health Service; 1993. US Department of Health and Human Services technical report 5.

25. Angst J, Baastrup P, Grof P, et al. The course of monopolar depression and bipolar psychoses. *Psychiatr Neurol Neurochir*. 1973;76:489–500.

26. Keller MB, Shapiro RW, Lavori PW, et al. Recovery in major depressive disorder: analysis with the life table and regression models. *Arch Gen Psychiatry*. 1982;39:905–910.

27. Kupfer DJ. Long-term treatment of depression. *J Clin Psychiatry*. 1991;52(suppl 5):28–34.

28. Kraepelin E. *Manic Depression Illness*. Edinburgh: E & S Livingstone; 1921.

29. Montgomery SA, Montgomery DB. Prophylactic treatment in recurrent unipolar depression. In: Montgomery SA, Roullon F, eds. *Long-Term Treatment of Depression*. New York: John Wiley & Sons; 1992:53–72.

30. Prien RF, Kupfer DJ. Continuation therapy for major depressive episodes: how long should it be maintained? *Am J Psychiatry.* 1986;143:18–23.

31. Frank E, Prien RF, Jarrett DB, et al. Conceptualization and rationale for consensus definitions of terms in major depressive disorder: response, remission, recovery, relapse, and recurrence. *Arch Gen Psychiatry.* 1991;48:851–855.

32. Depression Guideline Panel. Depression in Primary Care, II: *Treatment of Major Depression.* Rockville, MD: Public Health Service; 1993. US Department of Health and Human Services technical report 5.

33. Altamura AC, Percudani M. The use of antidepressants for long-term treatment of recurrent depression: rationale, current methodologies, and future directions. *J Clin Psychiatry.* 1993;54(suppl 8):29–37.

34. WHO Mental Health Collaborating Centers. Pharmacotherapy of depressive disorders: a consensus statement. J Affective Disord. 1989;17:197–198.

35. Angst J. National history and epidemiology of depression: results of community studies. In: Cobb J, Goeting N, eds. *Prediction and Treatment of Recurrent Depression.* Southampton, England: Duphar Medical Relations; 1990:1–9.

36. Robinson DS, Lerfald SC, Bennett B, et al. Continuation and maintenance treatment of major depression with the monoamine oxidase inhibitor phenelzine: a double-blind placebo-controlled discontinuation study. *Psychopharmacol Bull.* 1991;27:31–39.

4 Current Status of Monoamine Oxidase Inhibitors in Psychiatric Practice

Kishore M. Gadde, MD, and K. Ranga R. Krishnan, MD

Dr. Gadde is Assistant Clinical Professor of Psychiatry and Dr. Krishnan is Professor of Psychiatry, Duke University Medical Center, Durham, NC.

Editor's Note

The role of monoamine oxidase inhibitors (MAOIs) in the pharmacologic treatment of psychiatric disorders has varied considerably over their 40-year history. MAOIs were among the earliest of antidepressants, though links to liver toxicity diminished the initial enthusiasm that surrounded them. Less hepatotoxic MAOIs were later discovered and use increased, only to decline again when a life-threatening interaction with certain foods and medications was observed. Risks have subsequently been reduced with the development of guidelines warning patients to avoid these substances while on MAOIs.

In this chapter, the authors describe reasons for a resurgence of interest in these medications. Although new antidepressants continue to be released, there remains a need for agents to treat refractory conditons. Also, research studies have begun to identify disorders and disorder subtypes that may respond preferentially to MAOIs. Controlled trials support the efficacy of MAOIs for depression (particularly the atypical subtype), panic attacks, and social phobia. Less rigorous evidence suggests the agents may be useful for symptoms of obsessive-compulsive disorder, posttraumatic stress disorder, and borderline personality disorder.

MAOIs require a thoughtful consideration of risks and benefits in each patient. The potential for improved response must be weighed

63

against the risks of adverse reactions. These risks are greater for the suicidal, cognitively impaired, or impulsive patients, and in other cases where compliance and judgment are an issue. Another change in the equation may lie ahead: a new generation of MAOIs, not yet available in the United States, may offer comparable efficacy with a substantially improved safety profile.

Introduction

Although monoamine oxidase inhibitors (MAOIs) have been available for 40 years, their utilization as antidepressants has been limited historically by various complexities associated with administering these medications in routine clinical practice. With the emergence of additional clinical indications, such as social phobia, and the availability of selective and reversible MAOIs (although not yet in the United States), there has been a resurgence of clinical interest in these drugs.

As was the case with many psychiatric medications, the recognition of MAOIs as antidepressants occurred serendipitously. In the 1950s, it was noted that iproniazid (Marsilid), an antituberculosis drug structurally similar to isoniazid, had antidepressant properties.[1,2] Although use of iproniazid was discontinued subsequently because of liver toxicity, it paved the way for development of MAOIs because it was recognized in the laboratory that iproniazid potently inhibited monoamine oxidase (MAO) enzymes in the brain. Over the years, use of the available irreversible MAOIs, phenelzine (Nardil), tranylcypromine (Parnate), and isocarboxazid (Marplan), has fluctuated considerably, but these drugs have rarely achieved the status of first-line agents for treatment of depression because of their potential to cause toxic reactions with many medications and several common foods.

Pharmacologic Aspects of MAOIs

MAO is an enzyme found in many human tissues, such as the liver, intestines, and central nervous system, in humans as well as in several other species. In the human brain, the highest activity of MAO is found in the hypothalamus. Two MAO subtypes, MAO-A and MAO-B, have been recognized to be important to psychiatric research. Although both forms of the enzyme are present in the brain and various other tissues, MAO-B is more abundant in the brain and MAO-A is more active in the gut. Both forms of MAO exert specific physiologic actions in the brain. MAO-A selectively deaminates serotonin and norepinephrine, whereas the substrates targeted by MAO-B are dopamine, phenylethylamine, phenylethanolamine, tyramine, and benzylamine.

The most important physiologic role of MAO is to regulate neuronal cytoplasmic concentrations of monoamine neurotransmitters by deaminating the latter in presynaptic terminals and cell bodies. With MAOI-induced inhibition, significant increases occur in the vesicular and cytoplasmic concentrations of various monoamine neurotransmitters, including serotonin, norepinephrine, and dopamine, with the greatest increase occurring in serotonin.[3] After several weeks of treatment with an MAOI, one finds down-regulation of β- and α2-adrenergic receptors and postsynaptic 5-hydroxytryptamine (5HT1 and 5HT2) serotonin receptors.

Three MAOIs, phenelzine, tranylcypromine, and selegiline (Eldepryl), are currently available in the United States. The classic MAOIs, phenelzine and tranylcypromine, long used as antidepressants, are inhibitors of both MAO isoenzymes, whereas selegiline, approved for use only in Parkinson's disease, is a selective inhibitor of MAO-B. All MAOIs available in the United States are irreversible inhibitors, meaning it would take several days for MAO physiologic activity to resume after the drugs are discontinued. **The distribution of isocarboxazid, another nonselective MAOI used for a number of years, has recently been discontinued by the drug's manufacturer, leaving phenelzine and tranylcypromine as the only MAOI antidepressants available in the U.S. market.** Various new-generation MAOIs with selective actions have been tested in clinical and nonclinical settings in recent years. Moclobemide (Aurorix, Maclamine, Manerix), a reversible inhibitor of MAO-A (RIMA), currently available in a number of European and Latin American nations, and Canada, has gained popularity in those markets because of its favorable safety profile. Moclobemide is not available for routine clinical use in the United States. Structurally, phenelzine and isocarboxazid are hydrazine compounds, whereas the rest are nonhydrazine compounds.

Clinical Uses of MAOIs

Depression:

Clinicians and investigators in Great Britain have long believed that MAOIs are particularly beneficial for patients with atypical features of depression.[4] In subsequent years, efforts were made to clearly define atypical depression accurately. *The Diagnostic and Statistical Manual of Mental Disorders, Fourth Edition*, definition of atypical depression places emphasis on well-preserved mood reactivity and also requires at least two of the following features: increased appetite, hypersomnia, a heavy feeling in the limbs, and a rejection-sensitivity trait. In several prospective controlled studies, MAOIs have been shown to be more efficacious in the treatment of depressed patients with the previously noted atypical features.[5-8] Conducted by the Columbia University group, these studies have typically compared the MAOI phenelzine with the tricyclic antidepressant (TCA) imipramine (Janimine, Tofranil). In addition to persons with atypical depression, those with bipolar anergic depression also may respond better to MAOIs than to TCAs, but further research is needed. In one study, Himmelhoch and colleagues[9] found that tranylcypromine was more effective than imipramine for this type of depression.

Thase and associates[10] have recently reviewed controlled studies of available MAOIs. They noted that in severely depressed patients with melancholic features, MAOIs may be less effective than TCAs, although this difference has been seen primarily in inpatient studies. **The greatest efficacy for MAOIs seems to be in patients with depression marked by reverse vegetative symptoms, yet these drugs are judged to be as effective as other antidepressants in endogenously depressed patients in outpatients settings; TCAs may have an edge in severely depressed hospitalized patients. MAOIs, on the other hand, may be somewhat superior to TCAs in alleviating depressions that have a prominent phobic anxiety component.** Because data are emerging that demonstrate selective serotonin-reuptake inhibitors (SSRIs) also may be effective for atypical depressions and phobic anxiety, clinicians are not likely to use MAOIs as first-line agents for these syndromes. **However, clinicians should not forget that there is always the likelihood that a patient for whom a number of antidepressants have failed may finally respond to an MAOI. About half of depressed patients resistant to TCAs respond to MAOIs, and the likelihood of**

success is even greater when the patients demonstrate atypical features.[11]

MAOIs are effective in long-term maintenance treatment. In a study[12] of geriatric outpatients, phenelzine was superior to nortriptyline (Aventyl, Pamelor) or placebo at 1 year. In another study of younger patients with primarily atypical features,[13] phenelzine was again superior to placebo during the maintenance phase. **The dropout rate for the MAOI group was high; this is not surprising because weight gain is often an unacceptable side effect during long-term MAOI treatment.**

Panic Disorder:

MAOIs are effective in alleviating panic attacks[14] and may be more effective than other agents in treating phobic anxiety.[15] Unlike TCAs and SSRIs, MAOIs do not seem to cause hyperstimulation and restlessness in patients with panic disorder at the initiation of therapy. However, because patients with panic disorder generally respond quite well to a variety of medications with a low risk/benefit ratio, including TCAs, SSRIs, and benzodiazepines, the available classical MAOIs are unlikely to be used—even as second-choice agents—for these patients.

Social Phobia:

As was the case with atypical depression, controlled and comparative studies conducted by the Columbia group have attested to the preferential efficacy of phenelzine in reducing symptoms of social phobia.[16] In a double-blind comparison study of 85 patients with social phobia, 64% of patients who received phenelzine were much improved after 8 weeks, compared with 30% of patients who received atenolol (β-blocker) and 23% of patients who received placebo. The preferential response to an MAOI was striking in patients with the generalized form of social phobia; this is not surprising considering that interpersonal sensitivity to rejection is a common feature of both patients with atypical depression and social phobia. Our clinical experience suggests that atypical depression is more common in persons with generalized social phobia, and such an episode often is triggered by rejection or criticism. MAOIs appear to reduce interpersonal rejection sensitivity in these patients. On the other hand, MAOIs do not seem to score an additional advantage over β-blockers and benzodiazepines in treating individuals with discrete performance anxiety.

A Brazilian group led by Versiani[17] conducted a double-blind comparison study of phenelzine, placebo, and moclobemide, a reversible MAO-A inhibitor currently not available in the United States. In this study of 78 patients with social phobia, 92% of patients who received phenelzine and 80% of patients who received moclobemide showed a marked positive response. Although phenelzine was slightly more efficacious than moclobemide, the latter was better tolerated. This group also investigated the effectiveness of tranylcypromine in an open-label study,[18] with positive results. To date, there are no double-blind comparisons of tranylcypromine for social phobia.

Generalized Anxiety Disorder:

Except in extremely resistant cases of generalized anxiety disorder, there is no definite role for MAOIs in patients with this condition because medications with a more benign risk profile such as azaspirones (e.g., puspirone) and benzodiazepines (e.g., chlordiozepoxide, clonazepam, diazepam) are clearly effective. Nevertheless, MAOIs may be indicated for patients with treatment-resistant generalized anxiety disorder with superimposed panic attacks.

Obsessive-Compulsive Disorder:

Although an open study of a small number of patients with obsessive-compulsive disorder and comorbid panic attacks showed phenelzine to be effective,[19] there have been no controlled trials with either classic MAOIs or newer reversible MAOIs in patients with obsessive-compulsive disorder. A double-blind comparison study of clorgyline, a selective but irreversible MAO-A inhibitor not currently available, found the drug to be ineffective compared with clomipramine (Anafranil).[20] SSRIs (e.g., paroxetine [Paxil]) remain the first-line drugs for this disorder. However, a small number of patients may respond well to MAOIs, particularly patients with obsessions and compulsions of symmetry.

Posttraumatic Stress Disorder:

There have been two controlled studies of efficacy of MAOIs in posttraumatic stress disorder (PTSD), both using phenelzine. **In one study[21] of 46 male Vietnam veterans treated for a mean duration of**

approximately 6 weeks, phenelzine was more effective than imipramine and placebo in reducing the intrusive symptoms of PTSD, although there were no major group differences in alleviation of global symptomatology. In another crossover trial of short duration (4 weeks), no differences were found between phenelzine and placebo in a small group of Israeli patients with PTSD resulting from a variety of traumas.[22] Because substance abuse is a frequent comorbid condition with PTSD, clinicians should be particularly cautious in prescribing MAOIs for these patients.

Borderline Personality Disorder:

Cowdrey and Gardner,[23] of the National Institute of Mental Health, compared five different treatments sequentially in 16 women with severe borderline personality disorder without major depression. In this study, the MAOI tranylcypromine was superior to alprazolam (Xanax), a neuroleptic (trifluoperazine [Stelazine]), and placebo in reducing core symptoms of borderline personality disorder. Carbamazepine (Tegretol) also was effective in this group. Soloff and colleagues[24] in Pittsburgh compared haloperidol (Haldol) (average dosage 4 mg/day) and phenelzine (average dosage 60 mg/day) for 5 weeks in a placebo-controlled study conducted in an inpatient setting. **Phenelzine was effective in reducing anger and hostility measures but not atypical depressive symptoms and hysteroid dysphoria, whereas haloperidol was found to be generally ineffective on most measures.**

Bulimia:

Phenelzine[25] and isocarboxazid are effective in reducing a few symptoms of bulimia. However, patients with bulimia and borderline personality disorder often cannot be trusted to adhere to dietary and other instructions. **Thus, MAOI use with this population should be restricted to patients who are able to form a good therapeutic alliance with their clinician and in whom dysphoric features are more prominent than poor impulse control.**

Parkinson's Disease:

Selegiline, an irreversible but selective MAO-B inhibitor, is currently approved for use in combination with carbidopa/levodopa (Sinemet) to help slow the progression of Parkinson's disease. At higher doses, this medication has demonstrated antidepressant efficacy,[26] but it loses its selectivity and inhibits MAO-A as well. Hence, there has been little interest in pursuing further investigations with this drug for primary depression.

Depression and Anxiety in Elderly Patients:

MAOIs are effective in elderly patients whose depressive symptoms are resistant to standard first-line treatments.[27] These agents, particularly phenelzine, may be helpful for depressed patients who also present with a high level of anxiety. The starting dosage should be no more than 7.5 mg/day, with a gradual increase as needed and tolerated up to 45 mg/day. Some clinicians who specialize in geriatric psychopharmacology[28] prefer tranylcypromine, which is less sedating than phenelzine. **The starting dosage for tranylcypromine is up to 5 mg/day or less with approximately 15 mg/day producing an optimal effect in most responders. Compared with phenelzine, tranylcypromine appears to cause less severe postural hypotension, which is a serious risk in elderly patients. Considerable time should be spent educating geriatric patients about the drug's side effects, interactions, and dietary issues. In the elderly population, MAOI use should be restricted for patients with treatment-resistant depression in inpatient settings or specialized clinics because of the following risks: (a) elderly patients are likely to be forgetful and may not follow dietary and drug restrictions, (b) there is a higher potential for stroke when hypertensive reactions occur, and (c) postural hypotension can result in falls and fractures.**

Miscellaneous Uses:

MAOIs have been found to reduce premenstrual dysphoria in women[29]; however, because SSRIs also seem to be effective and are easier to use than MAOIs, MAOIs are unlikely to be used for this problem. MAOIs also have been reported to reduce various types of pain syndromes (e.g., atypical facial pain). In a recent report,[30] the reversible MAO-A inhibitor moclobemide helped smoking cessation in highly dependent smokers.

Guidelines for Using MAOIs

Dosing:

Because selegiline is approved for use only in Parkinson's disease, we shall focus our discussion on the use of phenelzine and tranylcypromine, two MAOIs with psychiatric indications available in the U.S. market.

Phenelzine is typically started at 15 mg twice a day and increased to 45 mg/day after about 3–4 days. Over the next month, the dosage may be increased as needed and tolerated up to 60–90 mg/day, which is the therapeutic dosage for most adults. Orthostasis often dictates how quickly the dose can be increased. **For tranylcypromine, the starting dosage is 10 mg three times a day. The dosage may be increased by 10 mg every week, up to 40–50 mg/day.** Some patients with resistant and anergic forms of depression may need dosages in the range of 60–80 mg/day. Plasma levels do not help to predict treatment response with tranylexpromine.[31]

Adverse Effects:

Orthostatic hypotension is the most bothersome side effect of MAOIs. This problem is generally worse than the orthostasis seen with TCAs. Increasing fluid intake sometimes helps this problem. Support stockings also may be useful, particularly in older patients. To alleviate the impact of this side effect, increasing fluid intake, using support stockings (especially with older patients), and administering fludrocortisone acetate (Florinef) are options that may prove helpful. During the first few weeks, small amounts of coffee or caffeinated soft drinks also may help to combat orthostatic hypotension, but large quantities should be avoided. Although patients report dry mouth and constipation, these problems are milder than similar side effects of TCAs.

Orgasmic dysfunction is seen more commonly with MAOIs than with TCAs. **Cyproheptadine (Periactin), 4 mg, one or two pills taken 1 hour before sexual activity, helps to alleviate this problem in some patients.**

Sedation is seldom seen with tranylcypromine, which, however, can cause insomnia because of its stimulant effects. Phenelzine is more likely to cause sedation during the day, but insomnia at night can be a problem, too. **Trazodone** (Desyrel), **50–100 mg at bedtime, is helpful and generally safe at this dose for many patients experiencing insomnia with MAOIs.**[32]

Tingling sensations or needle-prick flashing pains are sometimes reported by patients taking MAOIs. These effects may be related to pyridoxine deficiency because MAOIs can interfere with the metabolism of the vitamin. In some patients, supplementing 50–100 mg/day of pyridoxine can reduce the symptoms.

The first MAOI, iproniazid, was taken off the market because of a high incidence of hepatotoxicity. This can still be a rare problem with the hydrazine compound phenelzine, but it is not common enough to warrant routine liver function tests. **However, clinicians should keep this in mind if patients present with persistent nausea, malaise, low-grade fever, and similar symptoms. Hepatotoxicity is almost never seen during treatment with tranylcypromine.** This nonhydrazine MAOI does not cause any major changes in cardiac electrophysiology[33] in persons who do not suffer from cardiac disease, whereas shortening of the QTC interval has been noted during treatment with phenelzine.

Special Considerations With MAOIs

Hypertensive Crises Linked to Certain Drugs and Foods:

The most difficult aspect of MAOI therapy is the associated risk of hypertensive crises resulting from consuming certain medications with sympathomimetic properties, including several over-the-counter cold medications such as pseudoephedrine, and certain types of foods rich in tyramine. Table 4.1 lists medications that are contraindicated for patients taking irreversible MAOIs. This is a short list, and many other medications can be problematic. **Patients should be advised to check with their physician about every new medication they are prescribed.**

The risks of certain drugs and foods should be carefully explained to patients. In addition to a verbal explanation, written or printed information should be provided. Patients should be given simple instructions about the symptoms of a hypertensive reaction. **Such reactions generally occur within 2 hours of ingesting a prohibited food or medication and take the form of a pounding headache, sweating, palpitations, stiff neck, or photophobia. If patients experience these symptoms, they should be advised to seek medical attention immedi-**

ately. Nifedipine (Adalat, Procardia), **10 mg every hour once or twice, generally lowers blood pressure effectively.** Although medications such as meperidine (Demerol) do not cause hypertensive crises,

---

Table 4.1
Drug Contradicted for Patients Receiving Irreversible MAOIs

Over-the-Counter cold
and cough medications
- ephedrine
- pseudoephedrine
- phenylephedrine
- dextromethorphan
- phenylpropanolamine

Stimulants
- methylphenidate
- dexamphetamine

Diet Pills
- prescription
- over-the-counter

Street Drugs
- cocaine
- speed

Anesthetics containing pressors

Narcotics
- meperidine is most risky
- morphine is less dangerous
- codeine is generally safe

Centrally acting
antihypertensives
- reserpine
- guanethidine
- α–methyldopa

Serotenergic agents SSRIs
- clomipramine
- venlafaxine
- nefazodone
- fenfluramine
- dexfenfluramine
- sumatriptan (Imitrex)

Important: If a MAOI is stopped, drug restrictions should still be followed for 2 weeks.

---

they can be extremely dangerous when administered to patients taking an MAOI.

Patients should be advised to tell their other physicians that they are taking an MAOI. We have found it useful to have our patients carry or wear a Medic-Alert bracelet, which can be ordered through most pharmacies. For a small fee, this information can then be part of a pharmacy computer network. For an excellent review of MAOI drug interactions, readers are referred to a recent article by Livingston and Livingston.[34] **Of importance to psychiatrists, the concurrent use of all SSRI drugs with MAOIs is contraindicated.** Fatal reactions in the form of "serotonin syndrome" have occurred when the two classes of drugs were used together or within close proximity.

When prescribing an MAOI, clinicians have developed a tendency to present a long list of prohibited foods and other substances to their patients. Although the risk of hypertensive crises is real, gross overestimation of the risk with foods that may have caused one reaction in 40 years can provoke excessive fear and anxiety, adversely affecting compliance. **Only a few foods should be absolutely avoided.** Most reactions have occurred with aged cheese. Some foods listed in many textbooks are rarely used in the United States. With bananas, it is the peel that should not be eaten; the pulp is safe. In any case, it is not a custom for Americans to eat banana skins, which contain moderate to high amounts of vasoactive substances and monoamines. Similarly, with fava (broad) beans, the beans are safe, but the pods are not. Chocolate is not a problem unless it is consumed in huge quantities. Generally, foods containing less than 10 mg of tyramine (in normal portions) do not cause severe hypertensive reactions, except when consumed in large quantities. As a rule, fermented foods are likely to contain significant amounts of tyramine. With regard to alcohol, small quantities of white wine are not risky; however, Chianti is not recommended.

Gardner and associates[35] recently reviewed the historic MAOI diet and commented that users of MAOIs were being advised to restrict many "risky" foods without much scientific evidence. Based on a literature review as well as their own tyramine assay results, they recommend that the MAOI diet be simplified to improve patient compliance. The list in Table 4.2 incorporates these recommendations and our own clinical experience. **Patients should be reminded to continue the dietary restrictions for 2 weeks after discontinuation of an MAOI.**

Medically Ill Depressed Patients:

Because of their potential to cause weight gain and exaggerate hypoglycemic responses,[36] MAOIs are not favored in the treatment of depression in patients with diabetes. **Unlike TCAs, MAOIs do not cause significant electrocardiographic changes, and the risk for cardiac arrhythmias is minimal; however, because these drugs can cause significant orthostatic hypotension, it is wise to avoid using them in patients with cardiovascular disease. Phenelzine should be avoided in patients with liver disease because of its potential, albeit rare, to** cause hepatotoxicity. Because selegiline can help both parkinsonian symptoms and depression,[37] this drug should be considered in depressed patients with Parkinson's disease. However, it is important to remember that selegiline loses its MAO-B specificity at the

---

Table 4.2
Assesing Therapeutic Response

Foods to Avoid Completely
- Aged cheese (all cheeses except cottage, farmer, ricotta and cream)
- Pickled or aged meats (fermented and dry sausage, pepperoni, salami), poultry or fish (herring), or caviar
- Spoiled meat, poultry, or fish (such as that left in the refrigerator too long)
- Fava (broad bean pods
- Concentrated yeasts extracts (avoid Marmite or brewer's yeast tablets; yeast used in baking is safe)
- Sauerkraut
- Soy sauce and soy-bean condiments
- Tap beer, red wine, sherry, chianti, liquerus
- Liver (beef or chicken)
- Banana peel

Foods to Avoid in Large Quantities
- White wine, bottled or canned beer, vodka, gin
- Ripe avocados
- Anchovies
- Chocolate
- Meat tenderizers
- Beverages containing caffeine

Important: If an MAOI is stopeed, dietary restrictions should still be followed for 2 weeks.

---

high doses required for treating depression; hence, all the usual MAOI precautions and restrictions apply.

Anesthesia:

Most anesthesiologists insist that MAOI therapy be stopped at least 2 weeks before surgery. However, Stack and colleagues[38] reviewed the literature and argued that such requirements were unreasonable because MAOIs are often used to treat most difficult cases of depression, and most fatal reactions have occurred only with meperidine. **Regardless,** most clinicians agree that it is prudent to stop MAOI therapy for as long as possible 2 weeks before surgery. Meperidine seems to elicit an excitatory (type 1) reaction, which presents as agitation, hypertension or hypotension, hyperthermia, and convulsions leading to a coma. This is not related to tyramine but is thought to be because of meperidine's serotonin-reuptake blockade.

Most other narcotic analgesics, including morphine, have caused a type 2 response in the presence of MAO inhibition; this type of reaction manifests as respiratory depression and hypotension. Fentanyl (Sublimaze) is generally safe to use, and codeine also does not cause problems. The anesthetic gases are generally safe. Use of benzodiazepines also is not associated with complications. All local anesthetics are safe to use in patients taking MAOIs; hence, patients can undergo dental work provided sympathomimetic drugs are not used. Indirect-acting sympathomimetics such as ephedrine should be avoided. Direct-acting sympathomimetics such as adrenaline and noradrenaline generally do not elicit any serious reactions.

A more likely situation in psychiatric practice is a severely depressed and suicidal patient who is taking an MAOI, with only partial response, and requires electroconvulsive therapy (ECT). A 2-week waiting period, off the MAOI, is the conservative approach, but psychiatrists also should consider the risk of depression itself for patients who must be managed without an antidepressant. Remick and colleagues[39] argued that a 2-week washout period before employing ECT is an unnecessary caution. These investigators compared two patients taking an MAOI and two not receiving an MAOI at the time of administration of ECT. Although the sample size was quite small, the two patients receiving an MAOI underwent a total of 28 shock treatments, whereas the two patients not receiving an MAOI underwent [21] treatments. All four patients received intravenous methohexital (Brevital) anesthesia with succinylcholine; atropine was not given. No significant problems emerged in the two patients receiving MAOIs. It would be reassuring if these results could be replicated with larger groups of patients.

Therapeutic Alternatives

Combined MAOI and TCA Therapy:

It is fascinating and intriguing that there have been no serious reactions reported in the literature when an MAOI and a TCA are started together, usually at low doses.[40] Most fatal reactions have occurred when a TCA is added to an MAOI or started soon after discontinuing an MAOI. Imipramine is the agent incriminated most often in such cases. Amitriptyline appears to be safer than imipramine in this combination approach. It is unwise to use clomipramine in combination with an MAOI. Adverse reactions include agitation, fever, delirium, and convulsions, similar to a meperidine–MAOI reaction. There are few case reports of serious adverse reactions when an MAOI is added to a TCA. Interestingly, patients taking an MAOI–TCA combination seem to be at a lower risk for tyramine-mediated hypertensive crises. Although this combination therapy has not proved to be superior to either class of drug alone, there have been several reports in the literature of large groups of patients with refractory depression who finally responded to the combination after multiple trials failed.[41] Nevertheless, this type of treatment is associated with considerable risk and should be conducted only by experienced psychopharmacologists.

Switching from One MAOI to Another:

Switching from phenelzine to tranylcypromine is risky. Reactions characterized by severe hypertension and tachycardia have been reported when switches are made from one drug to another drug with less than a 2-week washout period. The risk may be lower when switching from tranylcypromine to phenelzine. Nevertheless, it is prudent to wait at least 1 week, preferably 2 weeks, when switching from one irreversible MAOI to another one.

Serious reactions in the form of serotonin syndrome have been noted in patients who were switched from an SSRI to an MAOI without a washout period. Similar unfortunate reactions have been reported when an SSRI was started immediately after discontinuation of an MAOI. We recommend the following guidelines:

1. Never use MAOIs and SSRIs together.

2. When switching from an MAOI to an SSRI, allow at least a 2-week washout period.

3. When switching from an SSRI to an MAOI, also allow a 2-week washout period. The ex-ception is fluoxetine (Prozac), which requires a 5-week washout period because of its unusually long elimination half-life.

4. When switching from venlafaxine (Effexor) to an MAOI, a washout period of 7–10 days should be sufficient.

All the above guidelines also apply to selegiline use.[42] The newer reversible inhibitors of MAO-A drugs seem to be generally safe in combination with SSRIs.[43,44] However, there has been at least one case report of a fatal serotonin syndrome following a combined overdose of moclobemide, clomipramine, and fluoxetine.[45]

Reversible Inhibitors of MAO-A:

Moclobemide and brofaromine, which belong to a new class of MAOIs known as reversible inhibitors of MAO-A (RIMAs), have become popular in Europe and elsewhere because of their safety profile, if not their greater efficacy. Both agents are nonhydrazine compounds. While moclobemide is available in many countries for routine clinical use, brofaromine is currently off the market. These drugs are devoid of significant tyramine interactions, thus making dietary restrictions minimal or unnecessary. **In comparative trials, the efficacy of moclobemide was similar to that of imipramine, clomipramine, amitriptyline, doxepin** (Adapin, Sinequan), **and fluoxetine. The efficacy of moclobemide also has been noted in patients with endogenous depression.[46] In the treatment of atypical depression, moclobemide has been reported to be slightly superior to fluoxetine.[47]**

Studies comparing RIMAs with nonselective irreversible MAOIs have generally reported equal efficacy for the newer drugs.[48–50] However, the Danish University Antidepressant Group,[51] which previously had shown that SSRIs are weaker than TCAs in the treatment of severe depression, have also found moclobemide to be less effective than clomipramine in a controlled multicenter study. **Although the combination of a standard MAOI and an SSRI is a liability for serious** reactions, the combination of fluoxetine and moclobemide has been used with no serious problems in a 6-week trial of patients who responded only partially to SSRI or TCA monotherapy.[44]

Moclobemide has been shown to be an effective maintenance therapy for depression[52] with few dropouts. However, these findings are from an open-label study, and positive results in maintenance studies with placebo would be more reassuring. In addition to depression, RIMAs also have demonstrated their usefulness in patients with various anxiety disorders, thus showing a broad spectrum of efficacy similar to that of older MAOIs. In a recent report, brofaromine and fluvoxamine (Luvox) for panic disorder were compared. Both drugs showed similar efficacy. The study was double blind but not placebo controlled.[53] Furthermore, brofaromine has been demonstrated to be effective in patients with social phobia.[54,55]

Summary

Although the classic MAOIs currently available in the United States are seldom used today as first-line agents for any specific psychiatric condition because of their complex dietary and drug interactions, these agents have demonstrated their efficacy beyond doubt in patients with all types of depression as well as in patients with a number of anxiety disorders. Atypical depression and generalized social phobia are two syndromes that seem to respond preferentially to MAOIs. RIMAs, a new class of MAOIs currently not available in the United States, appear to have better toxicity profiles than the older agents. If the newer drugs stand the test of time and show efficacy similar to that of classic MAOIs, there is a strong possibility that these drugs can gain wide acceptance, similar to that of SSRIs, among clinicians.

References

1. Ayd FJ Jr. A preliminary report on Marsilid. *Am J Psychiatry*. 1957;114:459.

2. Crane GE. Iproniazid (Marsilid) phosphate, a therapeutic agent for mental disorders and debilitating disease. *Psychiatr Res Rep*. 1957;8:142–152.

3. Murphy DL, Garrick NA, Aulakh CS, et al. New contributions from basic science to understanding the effects of monoamine oxidase inhibiting antidepressants. *J Clin Psychiatry*. 1984;45:37–43.

4. Sargant W. Drugs in the treatment of depression. *BMJ*. 1961;1:225–227.

5. Liebowitz MR, Quitkin FM, Stewart JW, et al. Antidepressant specificity in atypical depression. *Arch Gen Psychiatry.* 1988;45: 129–137.

6. Quitkin FM, McGrath PJ, Stewart JW, et al. Atypical depression, panic attacks, and response to imipramine and phenelzine: a replication. *Arch Gen Psychiatry.* 1990;47:935–941.

7. Quitkin FM, Harrison W, Stewart JW, et al. Response to phenelzine and imipramine in placebo nonresponders with atypical depression. *Arch Gen Psychiatry.* 1991;48:319–323.

8. McGrath PJ, Stewart JW, Nunes EV, et al. A double-blind crossover trial of imipramine and phenelzine for outpatients with treatment-refractory depression. *Am J Psychiatry.* 1993;150:118–123.

9. Himmelhoch JM, Thase ME, Mallinger AG, et al. Tranylcypromine versus imipramine in anergic bipolar depression. *Am J Psychiatry.* 1991;148:910–916.

10. Thase ME, Trivedi MH, Rush AJ. MAOIs in the contemporary treatment of depression. *Neuropsychopharmacology.* 1995;12:185–219.

11. Thase ME, Rush AJ. Treatment-resistant depression. In: Bloom FE, Kupfer DJ, eds. *Psychopharmacology: The Fourth Generation of Progress.* New York: Raven Press; 1995:1081–1097.

12. Georgotas A, McCue RE, Cooper TB. A placebo-controlled comparison of nortriptyline and phenelzine in maintenance therapy of elderly depressed patients. *Arch Gen Psychiatry.* 1989;46:783–786.

13. Robinson DS, Lerfald SC, Bennett B, et al. Continuation and maintenance treatment of major depression with the monoamine oxidase inhibitor phenelzine: a double-blind placebo-controlled discontinuation study. *Psychopharmacol Bull.* 1991;27:31–39.

14. Tyrer PJ, Candy J, Kelly D. A study of the clinical effects of phenelzine and placebo in the treatment of phobic anxiety. *Psychopharmacologia.* 1973;32:237–254.

15. Sheehan DV, Ballenger J, Jacobson G. Treatment of endogenous anxiety with phobic, hysterical, and hypochondriacal symptoms. *Arch Gen Psychiatry.* 1980;34:51–59.

18. Liebowitz MR, Schneier F, Campeas R, et al. Phenelzine vs. atenolol in social phobia: a placebo-controlled comparison. *Arch Gen Psychiatry.* 1992;49:290–300.

19. Versiani M, Nardi AE, Mundim FD, et al. A controlled study with moclobemide and phenelzine. *Br J Psychiatry.* 1992;23:353–360.

20. Versiani M, Mundim FD, Nardi AE, et al. Tranylcypromine in social phobia. *J Clin Psychopharmacol.* 1988;8:279–283.

21. Jenike MA, Surman DS, Casem NH, et al. Monoamine oxidase inhibitors in obsessive-compulsive disorder. *J Clin Psychiatry.* 1983;44:131–134.

22. Insel TR, Murphy DL, Cohen RM, et al. Obsessive-compulsive disorder: a double-blind comparison of clomipramine and clorgyline. *Arch Gen Psychiatry.* 1983;40:605–612.

23. Frank JB, Koster TR, Giller EL, et al. A randomized clinical trial of phenelzine and imipramine for posttraumatic stress disorder. *Am J Psychiatry.* 1988;145:281–285.

24. Shestazsky M, Greenberg D, Lerer B. A controlled trial of phenelzine in posttraumatic stress disorder. *Psychiatr Res.* 1988;24:149–155.

25. Cowdrey RW, Gardner DL. Pharmacotherapy of borderline personality disorder. *Arch Gen Psychiatry.* 1988;45:111–119.

26. Soloff PH, Cornelius J, George A, et al. Efficacy of phenelzine and haloperidol in borderline personality disorder. *Arch Gen Psychiatry.* 1993;50:377–385.

27. Walsh BT, Stewart JW, Roose SP, et al. A double-blind trial of phenelzine in bulimia. *J Psychiatr Res.* 1985;19:485–489.

28. Sunderland T, Cohen RM, Molchan S, et al. High-dose selegiline in treatment-resistant older depressive patients. *Arch Gen Psychiatry.* 1994;51:607–615.

29. Georgotas A, Stokes PE, Krakowski M, et al. Hypothalamic-pituitary-adrenalocortical function in geriatric depression: diagnostic and treatment implications. *Biol Psychiatry.* 1984;19:685–693.

30. Jenike MA. The use of monoamine oxidase inhibitors in the treatment of elderly, depressed patients. *J Am Geriatr Soc.* 1984;32:571–575.

31. Glide R, Harrison W, Endicott J, et al. Treatment of premenstrual dysphoric symptoms in depressed women. *J Am Med Wom Assoc.* 1991;46:182–185.

32. Berlin I, Said S, Spreau-Varoquaux O, et al. A reversible monoamine oxidase A inhibitor (moclobemide) facilitates smoking cessation in heavy, dependent smokers. *Clin Pharmacol Ther.* 1995;58: 444–452.

33. Mallinger AG, Himmelhoch JM, Thase ME, et al. Plasma tranylcypromine: relationship to pharmacokinetic variables and clinical antidepressant actions. *J Clin Psychopharmacol.* 1990;10:176–183.

34. Nierenberg AA, Keck PE. Management of Monoamine oxidase inhibitor-associated insomnia with trazodone. *J Clin Psychopharmacol.* 1989;9:42–45.

35. O'Brien S, McKeon P, O'Regan M. A comparative study of the electrocardiographic effects of tranylcypromine and amitriptyline when prescribed singly and in combination. *Int Clin Psychopharmacol.* 1991;6:11–17.

36. Livingston MG, Livingston H. Monoamine oxidase inhibitors: an update on drug interactions. *Drug Saf.* 1996;14:219–227.

37. Gardner DM, Shulman KI, Walker SE, et al. The making of a friendly MAOI diet. *J Clin Psychiatry.* 1996;57:99–104.

38. Bressler R, Johnson D. New pharmacological approaches to therapy of NIDDM. *Diabetes Care.* 1992;15:792–805.

39. Klassen T, Verhey FR, Sneijders GH, et al. Treatment of depression in Parkinson's disease: a meta-analysis. *J Neuropsychiatry.* 1995;7:281–286.

40. Stack CG, Rogers P, Linter SPK. Monoamine oxidase inhibitors and anaesthesia: a review. *Br J Anaesth.* 1988;60:222–227.

41. Remick, RA, Jewesson P, Ford RWJ. Monoamine inhibitors in general anesthesia: a reevaluation. *Convulsive Ther.* 1987;3:196–203.

42. White K, Simpson G. The combined use of MAOIs and tricyclics. *J Clin Psychiatry.* 1984;45:67–69.

43. Sethna ER. A study of refractory cases of depressive illness and their response to combined antidepressant treatment. *Br J Psychiatry.* 1974;124:265–272.

44. Gelenberg AJ. Selegiline plus antidepressants. *Biol Ther Psychiatry Newslett.* 1995;18:20.

45. Joffe RT, Bakish D. Combined SSRI-moclobemide treatment of psychiatric illness. *J Clin Psychiatry*. 1994;55:24–25.

46. Ebert D, Albert R, May A, et al. Combined SSRI-RIMA treatment in refractory depression: safety data and efficacy. *Psychopharmacology*. 1995;119:342–344.

47. Power BM, Pinder M, Hackett LP, et al. Fatal serotonin syndrome following a combined overdose of moclobemide, clomipramine, and fluoxetine. *Anaesth Intensive Care*. 1995;23:499–502.

48. Woggon B. The role of moclobemide in endogenous depression: a survey of recent data. *Int Clin Psychopharmacol*. 1993;7:137–139.

49. Lonnqvist J, Sihvo S, Syvalahti E, et al. Moclobemide and fluoxetine in atypical depression: a double-blind trial. *J Affect Disord*. 1994;32:169–177.

50. Gabelic I, Kuhn B. Moclobemide (Ro 11-1163) versus tranylcypromine in the treatment of endogenous depression. *Acta Psychiatr Scand Suppl*. 1990;360:63.

51. Larsen JK, Gjerris A, Holm P, et al. Moclobemide in depression: a randomized multicentre trial against isocarboxazid and clomipramine emphasizing atypical depression. *Acta Psychiatr Scand*. 1991;84:564–570.

52. Nolen WA, Haffmans PMJ, Bouvy PF, et al. Monoamine oxidase inhibitors in resistant major depression: a double-blind comparison of brofaromine and tranylcypromine in patients resistant to tricyclic antidepressants. *J Affect Disord*. 1993;28:189–197.

53. Danish University Antidepressant Group. Moclobemide: a reversible MAO-A inhibitor showing weaker antidepressant effect than clomipramine in a controlled multicenter study. *J Affect Disord*. 1993;28:183–189.

54. Moll E, Stabl M, Wegscheider R, et al. Long-term treatment with moclobemide: an open-label non-comparative multiple-distributed study in patients with a major depressive episode as defined by DSM-III. *Psychopharmacology*. 1992;106S:120–122.

55. van Vliet IM, den Boer JA, Westenberg HGM, et al. A double-blind comparative study of brofaromine and fluvoxamine in outpatients with panic disorder. *J Clin Psychopharmacol*. 1996;16:299–306.

56. Fahlen T, Nilsson HL, Borg K, et al. Social phobia: the clinical efficacy and tolerability of the monoamine oxidase-A and serotonin uptake inhibitor brofaromine: a double-blind placebo-controlled study. *Acta Psychiatr Scand*. 1995;92:351–358.

57. van Vliet IM, den Boer JA, Westenberg HGM. Psychopharmacologic treatment of social phobia: clinical and biochemical effects of brofaromine, a selective MAO-A inhibitor. *Eur Neuropsychopharmacol*. 1992;2:21–29.

5   Benzodiazepines: Behavioral and Pharmacologic Basis of Addiction, Tolerance, and Dependence

Norman S. Miller, MD

Dr. Miller is Associate Professor of Psychiatry and Neurology and Chief, Division of Addiction Programs, Department of Psychiatry, The University of Illinois at Chicago.

Editor's Note

For the past two decades, benzodiazepines have been at the forefront of controversy concerning their risk-benefit ratio. Among the clinical problems are addiction, (i.e., nonmedical use, physiological tolerance, dependence arising within medical use) and withdrawal. In addition, benzodiazepines can lead to memory impairment, sedation, psychomotor effects, and emotional blunting. This chapter by Dr. Miller combines the basic pharmacology at the receptor level of benzodiazepine addiction with practical clinical guidelines for the management of patients with benzodiazepine-related problems. Also presented is a rationale for the differences in risk-benefit ratios between the various benzodiazepines and some newer benzodiazepine-like compounds.

Behavioral Basis of Addiction

Epidemology and Diagnosis:
Benzodiazepine Use and Addiction in Medical Populations

The scope of the problem of addiction to benzodiazepines in medical populations has yet to be determined. Studies that find low rates of benzodiazepine dependence in general do not assess for adverse consequences from benzodiazepine use.[1] **Rather, symptomatology such as** anxiety and depression, which are related to and induced by benzodiazepine use, dependence, and addiction, are frequently ascribed to other medical and psychiatric illnesses (e.g., generalized anxiety or panic disorder).[2-4] Because benzodiazepines are used in a medical context, there is a resistance by physicians and patients to identify patients who might be using benzodiazepines addictively and experiencing phan-nacologic tolerance and dependence. The stigma of addictive use in a therapeutic context is often prohibitive to performing an evaluation for addictive use of benzodiazepines.In a medical setting, preoccupation with acquisition and compulsive use of benzodiazepines may not be ascribed to addictive use but to pharmacologic compliance with a regular dosing regimen. **In this setting, addiction entails preoccupation with, compulsive use of, and relapse to use of a substance despite adverse consequences. Withdrawal symptoms may be interpreted as anxiety resulting from anxiety disorders.**

As benzodiazepine doses increase, assessments of addiction or pharmacologic dependence are often made, even though dose increases can indicate pharmacologic tolerance and not necessarily addiction. One study that found diagnoses (as described in the *Diagnostic and Statistical Manual of Mental Disorders, third edition revised*) of benzodiazepine dependence in all patients studied (n = 131) concluded that "persistent use of alprazolam (Xanax) and/or lorazepam (Ativan) for therapeutic purposes did not represent abuse or addiction, as the terms are usually understood, because the subjects did not appear to escalate their doses."[5] However, the patients had resistance to discontinuing benzodiazepines because of an inability to cut back or stop using these drugs, which is an indication of either addiction or pharmacologic dependence.

Benzodiazepine Use and Addiction in Special Populations

Nonmedical use of benzodiazepines often occurs in populations of alcoholics and drug addicts, who appear to be particularly vulnerable to the development of addiction to and dependence on benzodiazepines. Survey data indicate that alcoholics and drug addicts constitute 25% of general medical populations and 50% of general psychiatric populations.[6-8] The contemporary alcoholic is frequently a user or addict of multiple drugs; as many as 80% of the alcoholics under the age of 30 are addicted to at least one other drug, which may include benzodiazepines.[3,6,8] **Studies indicate that 30%-50% of opiate addicts are addicted to high-dose benzodiazepines as well.[8] Cocaine addicts also addictively use benzodiazepines.[9]** The addictive use is an extension of their addictive use and an attempt to ameliorate the anxiety from stimulant use. Physicians are the largest source of benzodiazepines for all populations, whether medical or nonmedical use occurs.[6,10-13]

One reason it is difficult to apply the criteria for diagnostic diagnoses for benzodiazepine addiction, tolerance, and dependence is that the nosology for substance-related disorders fails to clearly differentiate addiction from pharmacologic dependence; it includes both under the term dependence syndrome. Use of a single diagnostic category makes it difficult to interpret reports regarding "benzodiazepine dependence and addiction."[9,14] **The distinction between addiction and pharmacologic dependence is critical for understanding and assessing liability for addiction as a consequence of benzodiazepine use in clinical practice.**[9,14-16] Studies have not examined the relationship between addictive use and the subsequent development of adverse consequences associated with continued benzodiazepine use (e.g., loss of control), which are included in criteria 3, 4, 5, 6, and 7 for substance dependence in the fourth edition of the *Diagnostic and Statistical Manual of Mental Disorders* (DSM-IV).[16]

Physiologic Tolerance and Dependance:

The criteria in DSM-IV for physiologic tolerance and dependence in substance dependence are a need to markedly increase doses to achieve desired effect (i.e., the development of tolerance to the sedative effect) and a need to take the medication to avoid withdrawal symptoms (e.g., anxiety from physiologic dependence).[16] Pharmacologic tolerance and dependence can develop independently of addictive use. **Many chronic users of benzodiazepines manifest pharmacologic tolerance and dependence without the preoccupation with, compulsive use of, and relapse to benzodiazepines. On the other hand, pharmacologic tolerance and dependence can develop as a result of addiction because of regular and chronic benzodiazepine use.**

Withdrawal:

Symptoms of substance-induced anxiety similar to those found in anxiety disorders can be expected during acute withdrawal in chronic users of benzodiazepines.[17-19] **Acute withdrawal symptoms because of pharmacologic dependence must be ruled out before suggesting an anxiety disorder is the cause of anxiety symptoms.** The DSM-IV criteria for anxiety disorders require the exclusion of substance-induced anxiety syndromes; "the anxiety disorder is not due to the direct physiological effects of a substance (e.g., a drug of abuse, a medication)."

Controlled studies have provided information regarding the onset, prevalence and clinical characteristics of pharmacologic dependence.[7,18-22] For clinical practice, pharmacologic tolerance and withdrawal follow known pharmacokinetic parameters. The withdrawal syndrome from long-term benzodiazepine use can be identified by a predictable and inevitable course. **Pharmacologic dependence to any preparation of benzodiazepines develops within weeks of regular use. However, the onset is quicker for short-acting than long-acting preparations, particularly those that have pharmacologically active metabolites. Severity is greater in short-acting than in long-acting preparations of benzodiazepines and with higher doses and longer duration of** use (see Table 5.1).[7,18-25]

Table 5.1
Sedative/Hypnotics

Benzodiazepines	Nonbenzodiazepines	Glycerol
Short-acting Agents	Zolpidem	Meprobamate
Triazolam	Buspirone	Piperidinedione
Oxazepam	Barbiturates	Glutethimide
Temazepam	Amobarbital	Quinazoline
Lorazepam	Butabarbital	Methaqualone
Alprazolam	Butalbital	Chloral Derivatives
Long-acting Agents	Pentobarbital	Chloral Hydrate
Chlordiazepoxide	Secobarbital	Ethchlorvynol
Diazepam	Phenobarbital	Placidyl
Halazepam		Glutethimide
Clorazepate		Doriden
Prazepam		Methypryton
Clonazepam		Nodular
Flurazepam		Paral

The most common symptom of acute withdrawal is anxiety, followed by fear, depression, headache, tremor, sensory disturbances, diaphoresis, insomnia, tension, fatigue, gastrointestinal disturbances, seizures, and delirium.[7,15,18–20,26] The signs and symptoms of withdrawal can be categorized (see Table 5.2), and separated into acute and protracted states. **The acute withdrawal for short-acting preparations peaks in 2-3 days and has a duration of 5-7 days; for long-acting preparations, the peak period is 4-5 days, and the duration is 9-11 days.**[15,27,28]

Table 5.2
Signs and Symptoms of Benzodiazepine Withdrawal

Symptoms of Hyperexcitability	Gastrointestinal Symptoms
Agitation	Abdominal pain
Anxiety	Constipation
Hyperactivity	Diarrhea
Insomnia	Nausea
Neuropsychiatric Symptoms	Vomiting
Ataxia	Cardiovascular Symptoms
Depersonalization	Chest pain
Depression	Flushing
Fasciculations	Palpitations
Formication	Genitourinary Symptoms
Headache	Incontinence
Hyperventilation	Loss of libido
Malaise	Urinary urgency, frequency
Myalgia	
Paranoid Delusions	
Paresthesias	
Pruritus	
Tinnitus Tremor	
Visual Hallucinations	

The onset of symptoms of acute withdrawal from short-acting benzodiazepines begins within hours. Alprazolam produces anxiety symptoms within 2 hours of the last dose, and triazolam (Halcion) produces insomnia within 3 hours of the bedtime dose. With short-acting preparations, the onset of seizure activity is 2-3 days from the last dose, and delirium with hallucinations and delusions may occur 3-4 days after cessation of use. The onset of withdrawal from long-acting benzodiazepines, such as diazepam (Valium), begins 1-2 days after the last dose, seizures can occur within 5-7 days, and delirium may follow within 8-9 days.[15,27,28]

Protracted Withdrawal:

A protracted withdrawal syndrome can occur following long-term benzodiazepine use and is reported more frequently with short-acting than with long-acting preparations.[29] It begins after acute withdrawal and can be viewed as a continuation of acute withdrawal with the addition of other signs and symptoms, particularly neuropsychiatric symptoms. The protracted withdrawal can last for months or even years and can be particularly distressing to the patient. **The signs and symptoms of benzodiazepine withdrawal are similar to those of anxiety disorders and therefore exclusionary criteria are necessary to differentiate between the two.** The protracted withdrawal syndrome may be responsible for poor compliance with the discontinuation of the benzodiazepine, as well as for the misdiagnosis of new or persistent symptoms as an anxiety disorder. **Protracted withdrawal should be treated with antidepressants, psychotherapy, and eventually addiction treatment if indicated.**[17,30] Additional benzodiazepines are not indicated because they prolong protracted withdrawal.

Behavioral Addiction:

The potential to develop an addiction to sedatives, hypnotics, and anxiolytics can be assessed by examining the reinforcing effects of these drugs, based on the finding that reinforcing effects are positively correlated with drug self-ingestion in addictive use in humans.[31]

Animal Studies of Benzodiazepine Self-Administration

Studies have shown that benzodiazepines function as reinforcers in animals.[32-34] Reinforcing effects have been demonstrated in several different species including rats, baboons, rhesus monkeys, and humans. Thus, as with other drugs of addiction, there is a broad biological basis for the reinforcing effects of benzodiazepines that is not limited to the human species.[35]

Human Studies of Benzodiazepine Self Administration

Benzodiazepines have been shown to be reinforcers in self-administration studies in humans who have histories of sedative, alcohol, or multiple-drug addiction.[25,31-34,36-40] **In those individuals addicted to other sedatives or hypnotics, several benzodiazepines, including diazepam (Valium), lorazepam (Activan), oxazepam (Serax), and triazolam (Halcion), were self-administered to a greater extent than placebo and other medications.**[41] In methadone-maintenance patients, diazepam can serve as a reinforcer and is often used addictively. Although alprazolam self-administration has not been examined directly in methadone-maintenance patients, it and other benzodiazepines also are used addictively by this population.[35]

Benzodiazepines are reinforcing for a variety of psychiatric and other populations.[42] In anxious subjects who seek treatment, a significant proportion find diazepam to be a positive reinforcer.[43]

Reinforcing responses to benzodiazepines have been shown by normal volunteers who drink lightly (fewer than five drinks per week) and moderately (an average of 11 drinks per week),[44] abstinent alcoholics and sons of alcoholics,[42] as well as occasional users of sedatives without physical dependence and abnormal users.[45] Barbiturates, meprobamate, and methaqualone appear to have more euphoric or reinforcing properties than benzodiazepines.[42]

The potential for abuse and addiction appears to be different for different benzodiazepines. Diazepam, lorazepam, triazolam, and alprazolam (Xanax) have relatively high liability for abuse and addiction, whereas oxazepam, chlorazepate (Tranxene), and chlordiazepoxide (Librium) have slow onset and lower addiction potentials. **The quicker the onset of drug effects, the greater the addiction liability of the drug.**[42]

Pharmacologic Basis of Actions

Physical Addiction and Withdrawal:

Addictive behavior can be separated from physical withdrawal in animal model studies. The mesolimbic system consists of projections of dopamine neurons in the ventral tegmental area (VTA) to the nucleus accumbens. Self-administration studies in animals show that stimulation of neurons in the ventral tegmental area will result in reinforced drug use that mimics addictive drug use in humans. **The locus ceruleus (LC) is the site of physical withdrawal and consists of neurons containing norepinephrine that project widely to diffuse brain sites. The LC is responsible for stress-related behavior and fires in response to sedatives** (e.g., alcohol, opiates, benzodiazepines). The ventral tegmental area and LC are both affected by drugs of addiction, including benzodiazepines, although they contribute differently to the addiction and physical withdrawal.

Although the LC and mesolimbic dopamine system can influence each other, they appear to regulate distinct aspects of drug addiction. The LC mediates physical opiate dependence but plays a minor role in opiate reinforcement, whereas the mesolimbic dopamine system mediates the reinforcing properties of many drugs of addiction but plays little role in physical dependence. This is illustrated by a recent study in which an opiate-receptor antagonist was administered locally into discrete brain regions of opiate-dependent animals.[46] Antagonist administration into the LC resulted in a dramatic physical withdrawal syndrome but had little effect on measures of drug reinforcement. Conversely, antagonist administration into the nucleus accumbens resulted in a dramatic change in drug reinforcement but little physical withdrawal.

New Classification for Pharmacologic Tolerance and Dependence:

The actions of benzodiazepines, barbiturates, and ethanol have been linked in a different manner to the γ-aminobutyric acid (GABA) receptor complex, which forms a chloride channel gated by GABA, the major inhibitory neurotransmitter in the vertebrate brain.[47] There are three classes of GABA receptors, $GABA_A$, $GABA_B$, and $GABA_C$. $GABA_A$ and $GABA_B$ classes include the majority of inhibitor receptors expressed in the central nervous system, where sedatives and anxiolytics act.[48]

$GABA_B$ and $GABA_C$ are resistant to the action of benzodiazepines; thus, this discussion will be confined to $GABA_A$ receptors.

Pharmacologic tolerance and dependence cannot always be predicted by the half-life of a benzodiazepine. A newer classification based on modification of $GABA_A$ receptor subtypes that are coded according to different receptor actions, drug binding affinity, and intrinsic action may be more revealing in understanding the development of tolerance and dependence to benzodiazepines. **Full, selective, and partial agonists can be classified according to binding affinity and intrinsic activity at GABA$_A$ receptors: Full agonists bind to most GABA$_A$ receptor subtypes and have high intrinsic activity, selective agonists act only at some receptor subtypes with high intrinsic activity, and partial agonists act at all receptors but with lower intrinsic activity.** Full agonists (e.g., diazepam, alprazolam) **show the highest liability to produce tolerance, dependence, and addiction.** Selective agonists (e.g., zolpidem [Ambien]) **and partial agonists** (e.g., imidazenil, bretazenil), **not on the market, have a lower liability for tolerance, dependence, and addiction.** Both zolpidem and triazolam are equally short-acting, but zolpidem, a selective agonist, shows less dependence liability than triazolam, a full agonist. A single benzodiazepine may be both a full and selective agonist and have a short and long half-life depending on the pharmacologic activity of its metabolites (see Table 5.3). (Diazepam is a full agonist with short duration of action, but its metabolites are selective agonists with long duration of action.)

Classes of Benzodiazepines According to Recognition Sites on GABA Receptors

FULL AGONISTS: FLUNITRAZEPAM (FULL ALLOSTERIC MODULATORS-FAM)

Full agonists (FAM) (benzodiazepines and nonbenzodiazepines) have high affinity for the specific recognition sites associated with most GABAA receptors (i.e., can maximize the opening frequency of chloride channels elicited by GABA) (see Table 5.3). Flunitrazepam (Rohypnal) is an example of a potent FAM that has a high-addiction potential. Its rapid onset and potent sedative effects are potentiated by ethanol." Incidences of rape have been reported in which Rohypnal was used to compromise the victim.

PARTIAL AGONISTS: IMIDAZENIL (PARTIAL ALLOSTERIC MODULATORS-PAM)

Partial agonists (PAM) act to bind at all benzodiazepine recognition sites with high affinity but low intrinsic activity.[50] The term partial allosteric modulator refers to GABA-dependent ligands that (a) have a high affinity for benzodiazepine recognition sites located on GABA$_A$ receptors; (b) have low intrinsic activity and fail to maximize GABA action in every GABA$_A$ receptor subtype on which they have been

Table 5.3
Pharmacological Profile Classifications Of Drugs Acting On Benzodiazepine Recognition Sites

Drug	Occurrence of maximal amplification of GABA action	Cognition impairment	Antagonisms of cognition impairment	Ataxia, sedation, ethanol potentiation	Anxiolytic, anticonvulsant, sleep inducer	Tolerance liability	Classification
never	NO	YES	NO	YES	NO	PAM	
Flumazenil	inactive	NO	YES	NO	NO	NO	A
Zolpidem	in some subtypes	?	NO	YES	WEAK	YES	SAM
Alpidem	in some subtypes	?	NO	YES	WEAK	?	SAM
Abecarnil	in some subtypes	?	NO	WEAK	WEAK	?	SAM
Diazepam	in many subtypes	YES	NO	YES	YES	YES	FAM
Alprazolam	in many subtypes	YES	NO	YES	YES	YES	FAM
Triazolam	in many subtypes	YES	NO	YES	YES	YES	FAM

A = Antagonist; PAM = partial allosteric modulator; SAM = selective allosteric modulator; FAM = full allosteric modulator tested; (c) not only fail to cause the cognitive action, sedation, and ataxia elicited by full allosteric modulators but, because of their high affinity for the receptor, they can antagonize these actions; (d) fail to potentiate ethanol and barbiturates; (e) maintain anxiolytic and anticonvulsant activity; and (f) fail to produce addiction, tolerance, and dependence. RO198022 and divaplon may be similar to imidazenil, but bretazenil is not because it is metabolized into metabolites with high intrinsic activity on $GABA_A$ receptors.

Partial agonists are clinically useful because of their less severe side-effect profile (i.e., less sedation, ethanol potentiation, and ataxia) and because they have less potential for abuse and addiction.[51–54] Imidazenil has a long duration of action and is given in small doses. It can inhibit the cognitive and ataxic action of benzodiazepines in monkeys. Imidazenil's high affinity and limited intrinsic activity, associated with lack of production of pharmacologically active metabolites, makes it a clinically attractive anxiolytic agent.

ANTAGONISTS: FLUMAZENIL (BLOCKS ALLOSTERIC MODULATION-BAM)

Antagonists are high-affinity ligands for benzodiazepine recognition sites that are completely devoid of intrinsic activity and do not modulate the action of GABA. Because of their high affinity for benzodiazepine recognition sites, they can prevent GABA modulation elicited by positive or negative allosteric modulators, and prevent the amplification of the GABA-gated opening of chloride channels like imidazenil.

Flumazenil is one of several[1,4]benzodiazepine derivatives (like imidazenil) with high affinity for benzodiazepine recognition sites. Because of its lack of activity, it acts as a competitive antagonist. It is the only benzodiazepine receptor antagonist currently available for clinical use. It blocks many of the actions of benzodiazepines but does not antagonize the CNS effects of other sedatives, hypnotics, ethanol, opioids, or general anesthetics. **Flumazenil is approved for use in reversing the CNS-depressant effects of benzodiazepine overdose and can decrease the actions of these drugs in anesthetic and diagnostic procedures.** Although the drug reverses the sedative effects of benzodiazepines, antagonism of benzodiazepine-induced respiratory depression is less predictable.[55] **Transient improvement in mental status has been reported with flumazenil when used in patients with hepatic encephalopathy.**[56] When given intravenously, flumazenil acts rapidly but has a short half-life (0.7-1.3 hours) because of rapid metabolite inactivation. Because all benzodiazepines have a longer duration of action than flumazenil, sedation commonly recurs, requiring repeated administration of the antagonist. Adverse effects of flumazenil include agitation, confusion, dizziness, and nausea. Flumazenil may cause a severe precipitated abstinence syndrome in patients who have developed physical benzodiazepine dependence. In patients who have ingested benzodiazepines with tricyclic antidepressants, seizures and cardiac arrhythmias may occur following flumazenil administration.

INVERSE AGONISTS: BETA-CARBOLINE (NEGATIVE ALLOSTERIC MODULATORS-NAM)
The inverse agonists (such as beta-carboline-3-carboxylic acid ethyl ester [B-CCE]) have the opposite action of the benzodiazepines, decreasing GABA-mediated chloride responses. Inverse agonists oppose GABA-induced inhibitory effects, thereby increasing arousal and activation and promoting seizures by increasing neuronal excitability.[57,58]

SELECTIVE AGONISTS: ZOLPIDEM (SELECTIVE ALLOSTERIC MODULATORS-SAM)
Although a number of compounds have been classified as partial allosteric modulators, they actually belong to another class of benzodiazepine recognition site ligands called selective allosteric modulators. Selective agonists act on some or many subtypes of the $GABA_A$ receptors. This class includes diazepam metabolites, abecamyl, Y23684, CL218872, and zolpidem, which are ligands with clear-cut evidence of their selective allosteric modulator profile on native or recombinant $GABA_A$ receptors. Diazepam and alprazolam are described elsewhere.

$GABA_A$ Receptors:
The discovery in 1975 that benzodiazepines have a high affinity for binding to the neuronal membranes was interpreted by investigators to indicate that the drugs were acting on a receptor for an unknown neurotransmitter.[57] Later, the original theory, that benzodiazepines exert their actions by acting on $GABA_A$ receptors and facilitating GABA action on these receptors, was confirmed by purifying a GABA receptor subunit that included GABA and benzodiazepine binding sites that were saturable and stereospecific on $GABA_A$ receptors.[58] This finding occurred at about the same time that the public and physicians were becoming alarmed about benzodiazepine abuse and dependence.[58,59] The

cloning of 13 GABA receptor subunits belonging to four families (a,b,g, and d) and the expression of various recombinant subtypes of $GABA_A$ receptors have demonstrated that GABA and benzodiazepines have different intrinsic activities at various GABA receptor subtypes.

The anxiolytic and sedative and hypnotic effects of benzodiazepines are specifically related to the benzodiazepine-induced amplification of GABA action at GABA receptors leading to GABA-mediated inhibition of postsynaptic neurons.[57,60] The high-affinity recognition sites through which benzodiazepines exert their action are located on the extracellular domain of the $GABA_A$ receptor. The GABA receptor is an ionotropic receptor that includes five different transmembrane subunits that define a chloride channel[61-63.] Each subunit has four transmembrane domains, one of which defines the selectivity of the ionic pore. $GABA_A$ receptors presumably are assembled from five subunits of various molecular forms derived from four subunit families (a,b,g and d); each of these families is encoded by multiple genes. Because 16 genes are currently known to encode the subunits that are pentamerically assembled in $GABA_A$ receptors, an astonishing structural diversity of these receptors may be expressed in the CNS. It has been proposed that more than 800 structurally different $GABA_A$ receptors are theoretically compatible with the mRNAs expressed in various CNS structures that encode the subunits for this receptor.[63] The relative quantities of these mRNAs differ in various brain structures.[64,65] They can change in the same structure during ontogenesis [66-68] and also under several experimental conditions (e.g., during denervation action of glutamate and during the expression of tolerance to benzodiazepines and ethanol).[54,69-71] GABA potency and the extent of GABA inhibition amplification elicited by anxiolytic modulators of GABA action at $GABA_A$ receptors are influenced by the structure of the subunits assembled to form the $GABA_A$ receptor.

Benzodiazepine Receptor Sites

Stereospecifically binding to B-$GABA_A$ receptor subunits promotes the binding of two molecules of GABA, which leads to the direct opening of the chloride-selective ion channels defined by the receptor. Electrochemical gradients cause the influx of chloride ions into neurons, which hyperpolarizes the cell membranes and increases the neuron resistance to excitatory depolarization.[47,48] The extent of neuronal firing inhibition elicited by activated GABAergic receptors depends on their location in the target neuron. In the pyramidal cells, GABA$_A$ receptors are expressed in somata, close to the axon hillock and at the base of dendrites. Benzodiazepines act only by potentiating the effects of GABA at these GABA$_A$ receptors by increasing the frequency with which chloride channels are opened. **None of the actions of benzodiazepines on the CNS is independent of GABA.**[47] Also, GABA can increase the binding affinity of benzodiazepines to the recognition site on GABA$_A$ receptors. This is known as the "GABA shift."[72]

Endogenous ligands for the benzodiazepine-binding site located at the GABA$_A$ receptor have been identified and named endozepines. Their intrinsic activity is like that of the FAMs and NAMs for benzodiazepines that can amplify or reduce GABA action at the GABA$_A$ receptor.[73]

Barbiturates are positive modulators of GABA$_A$ responses that bind to a site on the GABA complex that is distinct from the binding site of benzodiazepines. Benzodiazepines bind on the receptor extracellular domain while barbiturates bind to the receptor channel domains. Barbiturates increase the duration of the opening time of the chloride channel.[72] While benzodiazepines act on GABA$_A$ receptors only in the presence of GABA, barbiturates (and also endogenous neurosteroids) in high concentrations can directly open chloride channels and increase chloride ion flux. This action may explain the anesthetic activity of barbiturates and neurosteroids and the absence of this activity in benzodiazepines. Alcohol also may increase the flow of chloride ions through GABA-gated chloride channels, causing sedation. Alcohol's sedating actions are mediated via an attenuation of GABA receptor phosphorylation and the consequent inhibition of ligand-induced GABA receptor desensitization.[48]

Tolerance and Dependence to Benzodiazepines at GABA Receptors:

If benzodiazepines are administered for an extended period of time, tolerance occurs, detracting from their therapeutic usefulness, virtually preventing their introduction in the treatment of epilepsy, and reducing their effectiveness in the treatment of psychiatric and medical disorders. Pharmacologic tolerance is characterized by a down regulation of GABAergic transmission, leading to a reduction in benzodiazepine-induced amplification of GABA-elicited chloride currents.[74] The tolerence is because of a change in the structure of $GABA_A$ receptors characterized by a shift in the expression of mRNA encoding to a- and γ-subunits of $GABA_A$ receptors and associated with a decrease in $\alpha 1$- and an increase in $\alpha 5$-protein expression in specific brain areas of tolerant rats.[52,69-71] Using a 14-day treatment schedule with increasing doses of diazepam to induce tolerance in rats, the amount of mRNA in $\alpha 1$-, $\beta 2S$-, and $\delta 2L$-subunits decreases while that of $\alpha 5$ increases in the fronto-parietal motor cortex and in the hippocampus[52] (see Table 5.4). These changes appear to lead to rearrangements of the $GABA_A$ receptor subunit assembly to form $GABA_A$ receptor subtypes with a decreased sensitivity to the positive modulation of GABA specificity of benzodiazepine modulation. Rats treated chronically with imidazenil in doses equivalent to diazepam, a PAM (which amplifies, to a smaller extent, the GABA-elicited hypopolarization in various types of GABA receptors), elicited neither tolerance nor changes in the mRNA encoding $\alpha 1$-, $\gamma 2$-, and $\alpha 5$-subunits or their transmembrane product expression.[52]

Independent investigations suggest that a regulated dynamic state

Table 5.4
Phenobarbital Withdrawal Conversion For Benzodiazepines

Phenobarbital Benzodiazepine	Dose (mg)	Withdrawal Conversion (mg)
Alprazolam (Xanax)	0.5–1.0	30
Chlordiazepoxide (Librium	25	30
Clonazepam (Klonopin)	2	30
Chlorazepate (Tranxene)	15	30
Diazepam (Valium)	10	30
Flurazepam (Dalmane)	30	30
Lorazepam (Ativan)	2	30
Temazepam (Restoril)	15	30
Triazolam (Halcion)	0.25–0.50	30
Quazepam (Doral)	15	30
Estazolam (ProSom)	2	30

may control the assembly and expression of GABA$_A$ receptor subunits.[75,76] This regulated flexibility appears to attenuate the consequences of an enduring amplification of GABA-gated chloride currents elicited by protracted treatment with FAMs. Both GABA and several allosteric modulators of GABA action have different intrinsic activities on the GABA$_A$ receptor subtypes. The extent of GABA-signalling amplification by benzodiazepines depends on the presence of certain a- and γ-subunits. The development of pharmacologic tolerance may reflect changes in subunit assembly to compensate for a persistent increase in synaptic GABA concentration or for the enduring maximal amplification of GABA currents elicited by chronic benzodiazepine treatment.[52,69-71,75,77-81]

Efficacy and Liability

Recent Findings:

Important studies have examined the efficacy of long-term benzodiazepine use. In different controlled studies, patients were randomly assigned to benzodiazepine, placebo, or imipramine medications to study (a) effects of abrupt discontinuation,[21] (b) effects of gradual taper,[82] (c) comparison of alprazolam and imipramine[83], and (d) short- and long-term outcome after drug taper[22]

Conclusions regarding the effects of abrupt discontinuation included that baseline clinical measures (taken before benzodiazepine discontinuation) **revealed significant anxiety and depressive psychopathology despite long-term anxiolytic treatment. At 5 weeks, only 46% of long half-life (LHL) and 38% of short half-life (SHL) users were able to resist benzodiazepines.** Patients who were successfully abstinent from benzodiazepines had achieved lower anxiety and depression levels at the conclusion of 5 weeks than they had demonstrated at baseline while receiving benzodiazepines.

Conclusions regarding the effects of gradual taper included that a gradual taper was well-tolerated and was defined by the absence of withdrawal seizures, psychosis, other serious withdrawal symptoms, and inpatient management. However, 90% of both LHL and SHL benzodiazepine-treated patients experienced significant withdrawal symptoms.[82] Sixty-eight percent of LHL and 56% of SHL users could not tolerate the taper to completion and resumed daily dosage of benzodiazepines. At 5 weeks, 56% of LHL and 53% of SHL users were free of benzodiazepines. Benzodiazepine-free patients were lower in their level of anxiety and depressive symptoms at 5 weeks taper than at baseline while receiving benzodiazepine therapy.[82]

Both alprazolam (Xanax) and imipramine (Tofranil) demonstrated efficacy during the acute treatment of panic disorder on most measures of panic and nonpanic anxiety, as well as measures of phobic avoidance and panic-related social and occupational disability. Alprazolam appeared to have greater patient compliance than imipramine.[83]

The treatment outcome viewed in the short-term clearly favored alprazolam (because of apparent increased compliance that can be attributed either to efficacy or to pharmacologic dependence and/or addictive use), but treatment outcome viewed in the long-term was influenced little by the specific original treatment regimen employed in the double-blind study. **Over the long-term, patients originally treated with imipramine or placebo did as well at follow-up as patients treated with alprazolam. Importantly, the imipramine therapy did not cause the problems of addiction, pharmacologic dependence, and difficulty with discontinuation that can result from long-term alprazolam therapy.**[22]

Adverse Effects

The adverse effects of benzodiazepine use are consequences of use, addiction, tolerance, and dependence. Acute and chronic effects may be subtle. Clinicians and patients may have difficulty recognizing them and attribute the adverse consequences of benzodiazepine use to other clinical conditions.

Memory Impairment:

Benzodiazepines (except imidazenil, a partial agonist) **can induce anterograde amnesia following acute use because they impair the ability to learn new information. Also, long-term memory impairment can follow chronic use when benzodiazepines disrupt the process by which information is transferred from short-term memory to long-term memory storage** (the consolidation phase).[84,85] In general, the incidence of anterograde (for ensuing events) amnesia rises with increased dose, faster absorption, intravenous administration, and higher potency (partial and selective agonists are less active). Tolerance to the antegrade amnesia occurs but is not complete. In chronic users, transient amnestic effects can occur related to postdose, peak benzodiazepine levels.

Benzodiazepines also can produce a blackout, which is an impaired ability to recall events within a specified time-span that results in short-term memory loss (anterograde amnesia) **while cognitive and motor functions remain intact.**[84,85] Anterograde amnesia is the inability to form a new memory that normally begins with the acquisition of recall of immediate mental experiences (i.e., a blackout in unrecorded life events). Full agonist benzodiazepines-especially alprazolam and triazolam-are chiefly implicated. The true incidence is unknown. It is hypothesized that most patients who suffer from this disorder would conclude that nothing worth remembering has happened if they were unable to recall events, rather than concluding that they experienced a drug-induced cognitive dysfunction.[85]

Sedation:

Drowsiness and sedation are common side effects in most users. However, the majority of studies show that tolerance to these effects develops within days to weeks of regular daily dosing, although it often is not complete. Also, the impairment and tolerance may not be consistent from person to person and may depend on dose and time of drug administration.[84] **In general, sedation is a dose-related extension of the sedative and hypnotic effects of benzodiazepines. When benzodiazepines are taken at night as hypnotics, sedation may persist the next day in the form of "hangover" effects, particularly with longer lasting preparations.**

Psychomotor Effects:

The psychomotor effects of benzodiazepines, including ataxia, dysarthria, lack of coordination, diplopia, vertigo, dizziness, muscle weakness, and confusion, are common and appear related to dose and individual susceptibility.[84] Acute doses cause impairment in tasks that require vigilant readiness to detect and respond to changing stimuli.[85] Benzodiazepine-induced psychomotor impairment negatively affects driving skills, especially in the first days of use or when the dosage is increased. Chronic use of benzodiazepines may increase the risk of being involved in a serious traffic accident.[85]

The elderly who use alcohol, take high doses of benzodiazepines, and use other drugs (such as anticholinergics) seem to have increased sensitivity to the cognitive and psychomotor effects of benzodiazepines.[84,85] In the elderly, benzodiazepines with a long half-life may cause more impairment of psychomotor function than do the agents with a short half-life. Such impairment poses a significantly increased risk of falls and hip fractures.[86]

Depression and Emotional Blunting:

Chronic benzodiazepine users, like alcoholics and barbiturate-dependent patients, are often depressed, and the depression may first appear during prolonged benzodiazepine use.[30] It is possible that benzodiazepines cause or aggravate depression through their sedative effects, and perhaps by reducing central monoamine activity.[87] **Anxiety and depression often coexist, and benzodiazepines are often prescribed for co-occurring anxiety and depression. Chronic use of benzodiazepines may induce suicidal tendencies in such patients.**[88,89] It has been suggested that this effect is because of benzodiazepine-induced depression and disinhibition of aggressive tendencies (paradoxical stimulation), which are then turned toward the self.[89] **For this reason, it is recommended that benzodiazepines should not be used to treat depression or anxiety associated with depression, particularly if associated with alcohol or other drug use.**

Emotional anesthesia, **the inability to feel pleasure or pain, is a common complaint of long-term benzodiazepine users. Such emotional blunting has similarities to the anhedonia seen in anergic depression and is probably related to the inhibitory effect of benzodiazepines on activity in emotional centers in the limbic system.** Former long-term benzodiazepine users often regret their lack of emotional response to important events during the period that they were taking the drugs.

Drug Interactions:

Benzodiazepines have additive effects with other CNS depressants, including other hypnotics, sedative antidepressants, neuroleptics, anticonvulsants, and sedative antihistamines. **The combined disinhibitory effects of alcohol and benzodiazepines also may be additive and contribute to aggressive behavior.** Patients prescribed benzodiazepines should be warned of these and other interactions. **Importantly, while use of benzodiazepines alone rarely results in a lethal overdose, their use in combination with alcohol and/or other sedative drugs can result in fatal overdoses from additive and synergistic actions.**

Adverse Effects in Pregnancy:

Benzodiazepines cross the placenta and, if taken regularly by the mother in late pregnancy, even in therapeutic doses, can cause neonatal complications. The fetus and neonate metabolize benzodiazepines slowly, and appreciable concentrations may persist in the infant up to 2 weeks after birth, resulting in the floppy infant syndrome (i.e., hyptonia, CNS depression, and failure to suckle). Infants regularly exposed to benzodiazepines in utero also may develop delayed withdrawal symptoms with hyperreflexia, irritability, crying, and feeding difficulties. **Benzodiazepines also are secreted in breast milk.**

Benzodiazepines in therapeutic doses appear to carry very little, if any, teratogenic risk. However, some reports suggest that chronic maternal use in therapeutic doses may impair intrauterine growth and increase the incidence of perinatal complications.[90] High-dose benzodiazepine users who also take other drugs and alcohol are at increased risk of teratogenesis and other complications.[91]

Alcoholism and Drug Addiction:

Studies have linked the use of benzodiazepines to suicide attempts when used concurrently with alcohol or other drugs. Moreover, adverse effects on mood during use and withdrawal have led some investigators to postulate a role for benzodiazepines alone in fostering suicidal thinking and action.[92] Substantial social and occupational impairment in alcoholics and drug addicts has been associated with benzodiazepine addiction as well.[93] Long-term use of benzodiazepines is almost always contraindicated in patients who have a history of prior or active addictive disorder.[84]

Socioeconomic Costs of Long-Term Use

The socioeconomic costs of long-term benzodiazepine use are potentially high. **The potential problems include increased risk of accidents at work, at home, or in traffic; increased risk of overdose if** combined with other drugs; increased risk of attempted suicide, especially in depressed patients; increased risk of aggressive behavior and assault; increased risk of shoplifting and other antisocial acts; contributions to domestic disharmony because of emotional and cognitive impairment; contributions to job loss, unemployment, and loss of work through illness; cost of hospital investigations, consultations, and admissions; dependence and abuse potential (therapeutic and recreational); cost of drug prescriptions; and costs of litigation. Each of the risks may be more or less problematic for a particular person. Together they add up to a considerable burden for many individuals and for their respective states. The costs could be minimized by careful prescribing.

Clinical Approach to Benzodiazepine Dependence

Tranquilizers, Sedatives, Hypnotics:
Intoxication (Pharmacologic Toxicity)

Tranquilizers (benzodiazepines), sedatives, and hypnotics (barbiturates, ethchlorvynol, glutethimide, and meprobamate) are depressants that suppress brain function. Manifestations of intoxication from sedatives and tranquilizers include sedation, slowed mentation and coordination, confusion, loss of consciousness, and coma. Depressants can cause hypotension, bradycardia, and slowed respiratory rate; as heart conduction slows, cardiac arrhythmias can occur. Prolonged slowing of the respiratory rate can lead to respiratory acidosis, respiratory arrest, and death.

Withdrawal (Pharmacologic Dependence)

The peak period of withdrawal for short-acting preparations of benzodiazepines (e.g., alprazolam) is 2–4 days, and the full duration of withdrawal is 4–7 days. The peak period of withdrawal for long-acting preparations (e.g., diazepam) is 4–7 days, with a full duration of 7–14 days. Signs of withdrawal are agitation; increased psychomotor activity; muscular weakness; tremulousness; hyperpyrexia; sweating; delirium; convulsions; tachycardia; elevated blood pressure; coarse tremor of tongue, eyelids, and hands; and status epilepticus. Symptoms of withdrawal are anxiety; euphoria; depression; incoherent thoughts; hostility; grandiosity; disorientation; tactile, auditory, and visual hallucinations; and suicidal ideation and thinking.

Signs, symptoms, and treatment of withdrawal from sedatives and hypnotics are similar to those for benzodiazepines.

Withdrawal from benzodiazepines is not usually marked by significant elevations in blood pressure and pulse as is withdrawal from alcohol. Supplemental PRN doses are usually not needed to address changes in vital signs. **The anxiety of withdrawal is usually controlled with a prescribed taper with a long-acting preparation, unless it appears objectively that the doses are too low.** The addict by definition is not able to control drug use and cannot reliably negotiate the schedule for tapering. Caution is urged, as drug-seeking behavior must be differentiated from anxiety of withdrawal and anxiety from other disorders. Only the anxiety of withdrawal, or other severe conditions, need to be treated with increased doses of benzodiazepines. Methods other than use of benzodiazepines for treating the anxiety from another disorder are indicated whenever possible. The prescriber must objectively assess the need for benzodiazepines and control the dispensing of the benzodiazepines or other medications used for withdrawal.

Treatment (Benzodiazepine Substitution)

Treatment of withdrawal is aimed at gradually tapering off the depressant drugs or substituting another depressant drug that shares pharmacologic cross-tolerance and dependence to suppress withdrawal symptoms. **Benzodiazepines have cross-tolerance and dependence with each other, other sedative and hypnotic drugs, and alcohol.** Therefore, benzodiazepines can be substituted for other benzodiazepines and barbiturates and vice versa. The conversion for equivalent doses can be calculated if doses are known before tapering (see Table 5.5). **A long-acting benzodiazepine is more effective than short-acting preparations in suppressing withdrawal symptoms and in producing a gradual and smooth transition to the abstinent state. In general, greater patient compliance and less morbidity can be expected from the use of the long-acting benzodiazepines** (see Table 5.6).

The duration of the tapering schedule is determined by the half-life of the benzodiazepine or barbiturate that is being withdrawn. **For short-acting benzodiazepines such as alprazolam, 7 to 10 days of a gradual taper with a long-acting benzodiazepine or barbiturate is often sufficient: 7 days for low-dose and short duration of use and**

Table 5.5
Opiate Detoxification

Heroin/morphine withdrawal (clonidine substitution)

Standing Dosing:
Clonidine
0.1 mg to 0.2 mg po QID for 3–4 days and taper over 4–7 days, or:

As Needed Dosing:
Clonidine
0.1 or 0.2 mg po every 4–6 hours PRN for signs and symptoms of
    withdrawal for 5–7 bdays.
(Peak doses are between 1 to 3 days.)
Check blood pressure before each dose, do not give if hypotensive
    (for that individual, e.g., 90/60).

Methadone Withdrawal (clonidine substitution)

Standing Dosing:
Clonidine
0.1 mg to 0.2 mg po qid x 14 days
0.1 mg to 0.2 mg po tid x 3 days
0.1 mg to 0.2 mg po bid x 3 days

As Needed Dosing:
Clonidine
0.1 mg to 0.2 mg po every 4–6 hours po PRN for signs and symptoms
of withdrawal (18–20) days.
Check blood pressure before each dose, do not give if hypotensive
(for that individual, e.g., 90/60).

Heroin/morphine Withdrawal (methadone substitution)

Methadone test dose of 10 mg po in liquid or crushed tablet. Additional
10 mg to 20 mg doses are given for signs and symptoms of withdrawal
every 4–6 hours after initial dose for 24 hours. Range for daily dose is
15–30 mg in 24 hours. Repeat total first day dose in single or two divided
doses (stabilization dose) for 2–3 days, then reduce by 5 mg to 10 mg per
day until completely withdrawn.

Methadone Withdrawal (methadone substitution)

Methadone test dose of 10 mg po in liquid or crushed tablet. Additional
10 mg to 20 mg doses are given for signs and symptoms of withdrawal
every 4–6 hours for 24 hours. Average dose is 20–30 mg in 24 hours.
Repeat total first day dose in single or two divided doses q.d. (stabilization
dose), then reduce by 1–5 mg per day until completely withdrawn.

10 days for high-dose and long duration of use. In the case of alpra-zolam, because of higher rates of withdrawal seizures, the use of phe-nobarbital substitution is recommended for the taper. For the long-acting benzodiazepines, 10-14 days of a gradual taper with a long-acting benzodiazepine or barbiturate is often sufficient, 10 days for low-dose and short duration, and 14 days for high dose and long duration of use. The doses can be given in q.i.d. or t.i.d. intervals. The long-acting preparations accumulate during the taper to result in a self-leveling effect of the blood level of the benzodiazepine or barbitu-rates over time (see Table 5.6).

Table 5.6
Benzodiazepine (barbiturate) Withdrawal

Benzodiazepine (barbiturate) Detoxification:

Short-acting:	7 to 10-day taper:
	Day 1, Diazepam 10 to 20 mg po QID with a gradual decremental reduction in dose to 5–10 mg po q.d. on last day; avoid PRN.
	Adjustments in dose according to clinical state may be indicated.
	Or
	7 to 10-day taper:
	Calculate barbiturate or benzodiazepine equivalence and give 50% of the original dose, and taper (if actual dose is known before detoxification).
	Avoid PRN.
Long-acting:	10 to 14-day taper:
	Day 1, Diazepam 10 to 20 mg po QID with a gradual taper to 5–10 mg po q.d. on last day. Avoid PRN. Adjustments in dose according to clinical state may be indicated.
	Or
	10 to 14-day taper:
	Calculate barbiturate or benzodiazepine equivalence and give 50% of the original dose and taper (if actual dose is known before detoxification).
	Avoid PRN.

Summary of Treatment for Addiction to Benzodiazepines and Other Drugs (Including Alcohol)

The treatment of benzodiazepine addiction begins with the detoxification from benzodiazepines and is aimed at the drug-seeking behavior as well as preoccupation with acquiring, compulsive use of, and relapse to benzodiazepines. Many of those who are addicted to benzodiazepines also are addicted to other drugs, including alcohol. Standard abstinence-based addiction treatment is effective for benzodiazepine addiction as well as other drug and alcohol addictions .

Evaluation studies of abstinence-based treatment show abstinence rates of 60% at **1 year, which increase to 80%–90% with continued treatment and participation in 12-step programs.** The abstinence-based methods include group and individual psychosocial therapies, cognitive behavioral techniques, and emphasis on abstinence from addicting drugs including alcohol. Continued long-term involvement in a recovery program (e.g., Alcoholics Anonymous or Narcotics Anonymous) is strongly encouraged.

The treatment of benzodiazepine addiction in the absence of other drug addictions is less clearly documented. The prevention of relapse to benzodiazepine use despite recurrence of adverse consequences requires continued monitoring, education, careful assessment and treatment of other psychiatric disorders, and distinguishing drug-seeking from complaints of psychiatric symptoms.

Summary

The diagnosis of benzodiazepine tolerance, dependence, and addiction is often problematic for the physician. The importance of differentiating tolerance and dependence from addiction to benzodiazepines is critical for their treatment. The biological basis of benzodiazepine effects forms the rationale for development of agents that do not induce tolerance and dependence. Future research is indicated for improving our identification and treatment of benzodiazepine tolerance, dependence, and addiction.

References

1 . DuPont RL, ed. Abuse of benzodiazepines: The problems and the solutions: A report of a committee of the Institute for Behavior and Health Inc. *Am J Drug Alcohol Abuse.* 1988;14(suppl 1).

2. Juergens SM. Sedative-hypnotics. In: Miller NS, ed. *Principles of Addiction Medicine.* Washington, D.C.: American Society of Addiction Medicine; 1994:1–10.

3. Miller NS, Gold MS. Introduction-Benzodiazepines: a major problem. *J Subst Abuse Treat.* 1991;8:3–7.

4. Shader RI, Greenblatt DJ. Use of benzodiazepines in anxiety disorders. *N Engl J Med.* 1993;328(19):1398-1405.

5. Romach M, Busto U, Somer G, Kaplan HL, Sellers E. Clinical aspects of chronic use of alprazolam and lorazepam. *Am J Psychiatry.* 1995;152(8):1161–1167.

6. Chan AWK. Effects of combined alcohol and benzodiazepines: a review. *Drug Alcohol Dependence.* 1984;13:315–341.

7. Juergens SM. Benzodiazepines and addiction. *Psychiatr Clin North Am.* 1993;16(l):75–85.

8. Miller NS, Mirin SM. Multiple drug use in alcoholics: practical and theoretical implications. *Psychiatric Annals.* 1989; 19:248–255.

9. Miller NS, Mahler JC. Addiction to and dependence on benzodiazepines. *J Subst Abuse Treat.* 1991;8:61–67.

10. Grantham P. Benzodiazepine abuse. Br J Hosp Med. 1987;37:999–1001.

11. Perera KMH, Tulley M, Jenner FA. The use of benzodiazepines among drug addicts. *Br J Addict.* 1987;82:511–515.

12. Schuster CL, Humphries RH. Benzodiazepine dependence in alcoholics. *Conn Med.* 1981;45:11–13.

13. Sellers EM, Marshman JA, Kaplan HL, et al. Acute and chronic drug abuse emergencies in metropolitan Toronto. *Int J Addict.* 1981; 16(2):283–303.

14. Juergens S. Alprazolam and diazepam: addiction potential. *J Subst Abuse Treat.* 1991; 8:43–5 1.

15. Busto U, Sellers EM. Phannacologic aspects of benzodiazepine tolerance and dependence. *J Subst Abuse Treat.* 1991; 8:29–33.

16. American Psychiatric Association. Substance-related disorders. In: *Diagnostic and Statistical Manual of Mental Disorders.* 4th ed. Washington, DC: Author; 1994.

17. Ashton H. Benzodiazepine withdrawal: an unfinished story. *Br Med J* [Clin Res]. 1984;25:385–398.

18. Busto U, Sellers EM. Pharinacokinetic determinants of drug abuse and dependence. A conceptual perspective. *Clin Pharmacokinet.* 1986;11:144–153.

19. Rosenberg HC, Chiu TH. Time course for development of benzodiazepine tolerance and physical dependence. *Neurosci Biobehav Rev.* 1985;9:123–131.

20. Lader M. Dependence on benzodiazepines. *J Clin Psychiatry.* 1983;44:121–127.

21. Rickels K, Schweizer E, Case G, Greenblatt DJ. Long-term therapeutic use of benzodi-azepines. Effects of abrupt discontinuation. *Arch Gen Psychiatry*. 1990;4:899–907.

22. Rickels K, Schweizer E, Weiss S, Zavodnick S. Maintenance drug treatment for panic disor-der. 11. Short- and long-term outcome after drug taper. *Arch Gen Psychiatry*. 1993;50:61–68.

23. Busto U, Sellers EM, Naranjo CA, Cappell H, Sanchez-Craig M, Sykora K. Withdrawal reac-tion after long-term therapeutic use of benzodiazepines. *N Engl J Med.* 1986;315(14):854–859.

24. Busto U, Simpkins J, Sellers EM. Objective determination of benzodiazepine use and abuse in alcoholics. *Br J Addict*. 1983;78:429–435.

25. Griffiths RR, Sannerud CA. Abuse and dependence on benzodiazepines and other anxi-olytic/sedative drugs. In: Meltzer HY, ed. *Psychopharmacology, The Third Generation of Progress*. New York: Raven Press; 1987:1535–1541.

26. Health and Human Services Department, Alcohol, Drug Abuse, and Mental Health Administration. National Institute on Drug Abuse. Sedatives and antianxiety agents. In *Drug Abuse and Drug Research: The Second Triennial Report to Congress from the Secretary, Department of Health and Human Services.* DHHS Publication ADM 87–1486. 1987.

27. Alexander B, Perry PJ. Detoxification from benzodiazepine: schedules and strategies. *J Subst Abuse Treat*. 1991;8:9–17.

28. DeVane CL, Ware MR, Lydiard RB. Pharmacokinetics, pharmacodynamics, and treatment issues of benzodiazepines: alprazolam, adinazolam, and clonazepam. *Psychopharmacol Bull.* 1991;27(4):463–473.

29. Ashton H. Protracted withdrawal syndromes from benzodiazepines. *J Subst Abuse Treat.* 1991;8:19–28.

30. Ashton H. Benzodiazepine withdrawal: outcome in 50 patients. *Br J Addict.* 1987;82:665–671.

31. Roache JD. Addiction potential of benzodiazepines and non-benzodiazepine anxiolytics. *Adv Alcohol Subst Abuse.* 1990;9:103–128.

32. Woods JH, Katz JL, Winger G. Abuse liability of benzodiazepines. *Pharmacol Rev.* 1987;39:251–419.

33. Woods JH, Katz JL, Winger G. Benzodiazepines: use, abuse, and consequences: a review. *Pharnacol Rev.* 1992;44:151–347.

34. Ator NA, Griffiths RR. Self-adminisration of barbiturates and benzodiazepines: a review. *Pharinacol Biochem Behav.* 1987;27:391–398.

35. Roache JD, Meisch RA. Findings from self-administration research on the addiction poten-tial of benzodiazepines. *Psychiatric Annals.* 1995;25:153–157.

36. Ciraulo DA, Barnhill JG, Greenblatt DJ, et al. Abuse liability and clinical pharmacokinetics of alprazolam in alcoholic men. *J Clin Psychiatry.* 1988;49:333–337.

37. Ciraulo DA, Sands BF, Shader RI. Critical review of liability for benzodiazepine abuse among alcoholics. *Am J Psychiatry.* 1988; 145:1501–1506.

38. de Wit H, Griffiths RR. Testing the abuse liability of anxiolytic and hypnotic drugs in humans. *Drug Alcohol Depend.* 1991;28:83–1 1 1.

39. Roache JD, Griffiths RR. Abuse liability of anxiolytics and sedative/hypnotics: methods assessing the likelihood of abuse. In: Mello NK, Fischman MW, eds. *Testing for Abuse Liability of Drugs in Humans.* Washington, DC: U.S. Government Printing Office, National Institute on Drug Abuse Research Monograph #92. 1989:123–146.

40. Roache JD, Meisch RA, Henningfield JE, Jaffe JH, Klein S, Sampson A. Reinforcing effects of triazolam in sedative abusers: correlation of drug liking and self-administration measures. *Pharmacol Biochem Behav.* 1995;50(2):171–179.

41. Zawertailo LA, Busto U, Kaplan HL, Sellers EM. Comparative abuse liability of sertraline, alprazolam, and dextroamphetamine in humans. *J Clin Psychopharmacol.* 1995;15(2):117–124.

42. Ciraulo DA, Sarid-Segal 0. Benzodiazepines: abuse liability. In: Roy-Byme PP, Cowley DS, eds. *Benzodiazepines in Clinical Practice: Risks and Benefits.* Washington, DC: American Psychiatric Press; 1991:157–174.

43. de Wit H, McCracken SM, Uhlenhuth EH, Johanson CE. Diazepam preference in subjects seeking treatment for anxiety. *NIDA Res Monogr.* 1987;76:248–254.

44. de Wit H, Pierri J, Johanson CE. Reinforcing and subjective effects of diazepain in nondrug-abusing volunteers. *Pharmacol Biochem Behav.* 1989;33:205–213.

45. Cole JO, Chiarello RJ. The benzodiazepines as drugs of abuse. *J Psychiatr Res.* 1990;24(suppl 2):135–144.

46. Koob GF, Maldonado R, Stinus L. Neural substrates of opiate withdrawal. *Trends Neurosci.* 1992:15;186–191.

47. Roy-Byme PP, Nutt DJ. Benzodiazepines' biological mechanisms. In: Roy-Byme PP, Cowley DS, eds. *Benzodiazepines in Clinical Practice: Risks and Benefits.* Washington, DC: American Psychiatric Press; 1991:5–18.

48. Zorumski CF, Isenberg KE. Insights into the structure and function of GABA-benzodiazepine receptor: ion channels and psychiatry. *Am J Psychiatry.* 1991;148:162–173.

49. Smith DE, Wesson DR. Benzodiazepine dependency syndromes. *J Psychoactive Drugs.* 1983;15(1–2):85–95.

50. Ducic I, Puia G, Vicini S, Costa E. Triazolam is more efficacious than diazepam in a broad spectrum of recombinant GABAA receptors. *Eur J Pharmacol.* 1993;244:29–35.

51. Busto U, Kaplan HL, Zawertailo L, Sellers EM. Pharmacologic effects and abuse liability of bretazenil, diazepam, and alprazolam in humans. *Clin Pharmacol Ther.* 1994;55(4):451–463.

52. Giusti P, Ducic 1, Puia G, et al. Imidazenil: a new partial postive allosteric modulator of γ-aminobutyric acid (GABA) action at GABAA receptors. *J Pharmacol Exp Ther.* 1993;266(2):1018–1028.

53. Guidotti A, Costa E. *Partial allosteric modulators of GABAA receptors in drug abuse medication.* Unpublished proposed project, 1996.

54. Impagnatiello F, Pesold C, Longone P, et al. Modifications of γ-aminobutyric acidA receptor subunit expression in rat neocortex during tolerance to diazepam. *Mol Pharmacol.* 1996;49:832–841.

55. Votey SR, Bosse GM, Bayer MJ, Hoffman JR. Flumazenil: a new benzodiazepine antagonist. *Ann Emerg Med.* 1991;20(2):181–188.

56. Bansky G, Meier PJ, Riederer E, Walser H, Ziegler WH, Schmid M. Effects of the benzodiazepine receptor antagonist flumazenil in hepatic encephalopathy in humans. *Gastroenterology.* 1989;97(3):744–750.

57. Haefely W, Kulcsdr A, M6hler H, Pieri L, Polc P, Schaffner, R. Possible involvement of GABA in the central actions of benzodiazepines. In: Costa E, Greengard P, eds. *Mechanisms of Action of Benzodiazepines.* Series: Advances in Biochemical Psychophartnacology. Vol. 14. New York: Raven Press; 1975:131–151.

58. Squires RF, Braestrup C. Benzodiazepine receptors in rat brain. *Nature.* 1977;266:732–734.

59. Paul S, Marancos P, Skolnick P. The benzodiazepine-GABA chloride ionophore receptor complex: common site of minor tranquilizer action. *Biol Psychiatry.* 1981;16:213–228.

60. Costa E, Guidotti A, Mao CC. Evidence for involvement of GABA in the action of benzodiazepines: studies in rat cerebellum. In: Costa E, Greengard P, eds. *Mechanisms of Action of Benzodiazepines.* Series: Advances in Biochemical Psychopharmacology. Vol. 14. New York: Raven Press; 1975:113–130.

61. Barnard EA. The molecular biology of $GABA_A$ receptors and their structural determinants. In: Biggio G, Sanna E, Costa E, eds. $GABA_A$ *Receptors and Anxiety: From Neurobiology to Treatment.* Series: Advances in Biochemical Psychopharmacology. Vol. 14. New York, Raven Press; 1995:1–16.

62. Macdonald RL, Olsen RW. $GABA_A$ receptor channels. *Ann Rev Neurosci.* 1994; 17:569–602.

63. Wisden W, Seeburg PH. GABAA receptor channels: from subunits to functional entities. *Curr Opin Neurobiol.* 1992;2:263–269.

64. Wisden W, Laurie DJ, Monyer H, Seeburg PH. The distribution of 13 $GABA_A$ subunit mRNAs in the rat brain. 1. Telencephanon, diencephalon, mesencephalon. *J Neurosci.* 1992; 12:1040–1046.

65. Haffis BT, Charlton ME, Costa E, Grayson DR. Quantitative changes in a1 and a5 γ-aminobutyric acid type A receptor subunit mRNAs and proteins after a single treatment of cerebellar granule neurons with N-methyl-D-aspartate. *Mol Pharmacol.* 1994;45(4):637–648.

66. Bovolin P, Santi M-R, Memo M, Costa E, Grayson DR. Distinct developmental patterns of expression of rat a1, α5, γ2S, and γ2L γ-aminobutyric acid A receptor subunit mRNAs in vivo and in vitro. *J Neurochem.* 1992;59:62–72.

67. Fritschy J-M, Paysan J, Enna A, M6hler H. Switch in the expression of rat $GABA_A$-receptor subtypes during postnatal development: an immunohistochemical study. *J Neurosci.* 1994; 14(9):5302–5324.

68. Zheng T, Santi M-R, Bovolin P, Marlier LNJ-L, Grayson DR. Developmental expression of the a 6 $GABA_A$ receptor subunit mRNA occurs only after cerebellar granule cell migration. *Dev Brain Res.* 1993;75:91–103.

69. Kang 1, Miller LG. Decreased GABAA receptor subunit mRNA concentrations following chronic lorazepam administration. *Br J Phannacol.* 1991; 103:1285–1287.

70. Primus RJ, Gallager DW. $GABA_A$ receptor subunit mRNA levels are differentially influenced by chronic FG 7142 and diazepam exposure. *Eur J Pharmacol Mol Pharmacol Sect.* 1992;226:21–28.

71. Zhao T-J, Chiu TH, Rosenberg HC. Reduced expression of γ-aminobutyric acid type A/benzodiazepine receptor γ2 and α5 subunit mRNAs in brain regions of flurazepam-treated rats. *Mol Pharmacol.* 1994;45(4):657–663.

72. Vicini S, Mienville J-M, Costa E. Actions of benzodiazepine and b-carboline derivatives on g-aminobutyric acid-activated Cl- channels recorded from membrane patches of neonatal rat cortical neurons in culture. *J Pharmacol Exp Ther.* 1987;243(3):1195–1201.

73. Rothstein JD, Garland W, Puia G, Guidotti A, Weber R, Costa E. Purification and characterization of naturally occurrinig benzodiazepine receptor ligands. *J Neurochem.* 1992;58:2102–2115.

74. Zheng TM, Zhu WJ, Puia G, et al. Changes in y-antinobutyrate type A receptor subunit mRNAs, translation product expression, and receptor function during neuronal maturation in vitro. *Proc Natl Acad Sci USA.* 1994;91:10952–10956.

75. Ducic I, Caruncho HJ, Zhu WJ, Vicini S, Costa E. g-aminobutyric acid gating of Cl-channels in recombinant GABAA receptors. *J Pharmacol Exp Ther.* 1995;272:438–445.

76. Farb DH, Borden LA, Chan CY, Czajkowski CM, Gibbs TT, Schiller GD. Modulation of neuronal function through benzodiazepine receptors: biochemical and electrophysiological studies of neurons in primary monolayer cell culture. *Ann N Y Acad Sci.* 1984;435:1–3 1.

77. Costa E, Thompson DM, Auta J, Guidotti A. Imidazenil: a potent benzodiazepine partial positive modulator of GABAergic transmission virtually devoid of tolerance liability. *CNS Drug Rev.* 1995; 1(2):168–189.

78. Ducic I, Puia G, Vicini S, Costa E. Triazolam is more efficacious than diazepam in a broad spectrum of recombinant $GABA_A$ receptors. *Eur J Pharmacol.* 1993;244:29–34.

79. Korpi ER, Kleingoor C, Kettenmann H, Seeburg PH. Benzodiazepine-induced motor impairment linked to point mutation in cerebellar $GABA_A$ receptor. *Nature.* 1993;361:356–359.

80. Puia G, Ducic I, Vicini S, Costa E. Molecular mechanisms of the partial allosteric modulatory effects of bretazenil at g-aminobutyric acid type A receptor. *Proc Natl Acad Sci USA.* 1992;89:3620–3626.

81 .Puia G, Vicini S, Seeburg PH, Costa E. Influence of recombinanty–aminobutyric acid–A receptor subunit composition on the action of allosteric modulators of γ–aminobutyric acid-gated Cl- currents. *Mol Phannacol.* 1991;39:691–696.

82. Schweizer E, Rickels K, Case G, Greenblatt DJ. Long-term therapeutic use of benzodiazepines:II. Effects of gradual taper. *Arch Gen Psychiatry.* 1990;47:908–915.

83. Schweizer, E., Rickels, K., Weiss, S., Zavodnick, S. Maintenance drug treatment of panic disorder. 1. Results of a prospective, placebo-controlled comparison of alprazolam and imipramine. *Arch Gen Psychiatry.* 1993;50:51–60.

84. American Psychiatric Association. *Task Force Report on Benzodiazepines.* Washington, DC: Author; 1990.

85. Homer DW. Benzodiazepines: cognitive and psychomotor effects. In: Roy-Byrne PP, Cowley DS, eds. *Benzodiazepines in Clinical Practice: Risks and Benefits.* Washington, DC: American Psychiatric Press; 1991:113–130.

86. Ray WA, Griffin MR, Downey W. Benzodiazepines of long and short elimination half-life and the risk of hip fracture. *JAMA.* 1989;262:3303–3307.

87. Nutt DJ. Benzodiazepine dependence: new insights from basic research. In: Hindmarch I, Beaumont G, Brandon S, Leonard BE, eds. *Benzodiazepines: Current Concepts. Chichester:* John Wiley & Sons; 1990:19–42.

88. Priest RG, Montgomery SA. Benzodiazepines and dependence: a college statement. *Bull Royal College Psychiatrists.* 1988;12:107–108.

89. Committee on Safety of Medicines. Benzodiazepines, dependence and withdrawal symptoms. *Curr Prob.* 1988;21:1–2.

90. Laegreid L, Oleg'ard R, Conradi N, Hagberg G, Wahlstr6m J, Abrahamsson L. Association between congenital malformations and matemal consumption of benzodiazepines. A case-control study. *Dev Med Child Neurol.* 1990;32:432–441.

91. Bergman U, Rosa FW, Baum C, Wiholm BE, Faich GA. Effects of exposure to benzodi-azepine during fetal life. *Lancet.* 1992;340:694–696.

92. Miller NS, Gold MS. The psychiatrist's role in integrating pharmacologic and nonpharmaco-logic treatments for addictive disorders. *Psychiatr Ann.* 1992;22:436–440.

93. Juergens SM, Morse RM. Alprazolam dependence in seven patients. *Am J Psychiatry.* 1988; 1455:625–627.

6   Rational Copharmacy for Treatment Resistant Bipolar Disorder

Philip G. Janicak, MD, and Elizabeth A. Winans,
PharmD, BCPP

*Dr. Janicak is Professor of Psychiatry and Medical Director , and
Dr. Winans is Clinical Assistant Professor of Pharmacy Practice,
Psychiatric Institute, University of Illinois at Chicago.*

Editor's Note

Although lithium may prove effective in mild cases of bipolar disorder, there are several instances of this pernicious disorder that require a more robust and creative treatment approach. In light of the fact that only approximately 50% of patients respond to lithium and given the advances in the pharmacotherapy of schizoaffective disorders, it is important to consider the relative strengths of newer interventions while using lithium as a starting point for comparison and evaluation. In the course of treating patients with bipolar disorder, depressed phase, mixed states, episodes associated with psychotic features, manias in the elderly, secondary mania, and episodes associated with substance and/or alcohol abuse constitute characteristics of the disorder that thwart the conventional pharmacotherapy.

In this chapter, Drs. Janicak and Winans focus on lithium, valproate, and carbamazepine and offer guidelines on their use in this uniquely challenging patient population. Adverse side effects are noted, and it becomes clear that divalproex sodium is a superior monotherapy. The authors also quite conscientiously note the correlation between thyroid deficiencies and bipolar disorder. Baseline thyroid function tests, including thyroid stimulating hormone, are an essential part of the laboratory workup for a bipolar patient. Thyroid stimulating hormone, levthyroxine, is often a powerful adjunct to psychotropic interventions. The rapid onset of antimanic response, often seen in patients administered this drug, make it especially attractively, as this can eliminate the need for copharmacy in certain situations. However, when copharmacy is necessary, in severe cases of manic or depressive episodes, judicious use of benzodiazepines to militate against psychotic symptoms is often preferred because of their less intrusive side-effects. The authors also recommend the use of the newer antipsychotics, particularly olanzapine, quetiapine, and risperidone, in severe cases.

Introduction

Bipolar disorder can be one of the most challenging conditions to manage, with single drug therapy generally insufficient to control more severe episodes.[1] **Indeed, since half of all bipolar patients may not experience an adequate response to lithium, there is a need to develop more effective strategies, including alternative agents and optimal drug combinations.** Our review will focus on the relative merits of the primary mood stabilizers (i.e., lithium [Esklaith], valproate [Depakene and Depakote], and carbamazepine [Tegretol]), emphasizing their concurrent use with other psychotropics in the management of acute episodes of bipolar mania or depression.

Lithium

For over a quarter of a century lithium has been the standard drug therapy for bipolar disorder, primarily because of the quantity and the quality of evidence supporting its role as an effective maintenance/prophylactic treatment. Lithium alone is most effective for classic, milder forms of acute mania. It is not as effective for (a) the depressed phase, (b) mixed states,[2-4] (c) episodes associated with psychotic features, (d) manias in the elderly, (e) secondary mania,[5] and (f) episodes associated with substance and/or alcohol abuse.[6] In the context of acute treatment, however, lithium is not as effective for more severe episodes, has a narrow therapeutic index, and causes numerous troublesome complications. Indeed, 75% of patients on this agent will experience adverse effects, usually involving the renal, gastrointestinal, thyroid, and/or neurological systems.[7]

Acute Treatment of the Manic Phase:

Until very recently, the published literature on lithium treatment for acute mania totaled only 46 patients evaluated in prospective random-assignment, double-blind placebo controlled trials. In these studies **lithium was superior to placebo for the acute treatment of a manic episode.**[8–10] More recently, Bowden and colleagues conducted a multi-center study of divalproex which also included a lithium and a placebo treatment arm (i.e., 74 on placebo and 36 on lithium).[11] Marked improvement, defined as at least a 50% reduction in the manic syndrome subscale score, derived from the Schedule for Affective Disorders and Schizophrenia (SADS), occurred in 49% of the lithium group versus only 25% of the placebo group ($p<0.025$). This study significantly increased the number of lithium-treated acutely manic patients evaluated under placebo-controlled conditions, reaffirming its benefit in a substantial proportion.

Acute Treatment of the Depressive Phase:

Although there are few well-controlled studies, the existing data support the role of lithium as an effective antidepressant in *some* patients with bipolar disorder.[12] The role of antidepressants in altering the course of this illness, however, remains an issue of some dispute and has yet to be resolved conclusively.[13]

Although there is evidence that adding lithium to ongoing antidepressant therapy can improve response, there is little evidence on the outcome with combined treatment started simultaneously. Recently, Ebert and his collaborators randomly assigned two groups of 20 bipolar patients with melancholic depression to lithium plus amitriptyline (Elavil) or placebo plus amitriptyline.[14] The two-drug combination produced a better result that was statistically significant—with 17 versus 12 patients improving, respectively. Although confirmation is still needed, **this study seems to suggest that bipolar depressed patients may fare better with a combination mood stabilizer/antidepressant used at the outset of treatment.**

Suicide

Bipolar disorder is associated with a high mortality rate.[15] In particular, suicide rates during the depressed phase are significantly increased compared to the general population. For example, in a subsequent analysis of the National Institute of Mental Health (NIMH) Collaborative Study on Depression data, the rate of suicide in lithium-treated patients was 5.2 (7 suicides in 827 patients studied; 5,600 patient-years), whereas the expected rate was 1.3.[16] In a classic review of mortality associated with bipolar disorder before the discovery of effective treatments, Guze and Robins found that suicide accounted for at least 12% of all deaths.[17] There is greater risk for suicide as patients recover from an episode (particularly depression), perhaps because they then have to face some of the same problems that may have precipitated or been aggravated by the episode. For example, Weeke found that 40% of suicides occurred within 6 months of the first admission.[18]

Coppen et al., however, reported that long-term treatment with lithium reduces the risk of suicide substantially, in addition to the overall excess mortality seen in these patients.[19] Lenz studied 700 patients treated with lithium (430 for at least 5 years) and found that **the mortality rate did not differ from the general population but rose significantly after lithium was discontinued** (to a level approximately two times greater than expected).[20] In a collaborative study of lithium treatment centers involving 471 patients, there were 2 suicides in the first year, a rate substantially higher than in the general population.[21] In the later years of the study, however, there were only 2 suicides total, which constituted a rate no higher than that expected in the general population. Recently, Nilsson investigated 362 patients with a primary mood or schizoaffective disorder with or without lithium prophylaxis.[22] **Similar to the NIMH results, he found the suicide rate on lithium was substantially higher than the suicide rate of the general population, but the suicide rate off lithium produced a standardized mortality rate 29 times that of the general population and much higher than for those patients undergoing pharmacotherapy.**

Clinical Management:

The standard lithium workup includes a thorough medical and laboratory evaluation with an **emphasis on assessing renal, cardiac, and thyroid function.** Thus, thyroid status must be monitored and other drugs that interfere with thyroid function should be avoided. Renal function should also be followed and sodium or potassium depleting agents used cautiously.

Every effort should be made to achieve the highest tolerated lithium levels before considering an alternate agent or combination strategy. Levels in the range of 0.8–1.2 µEq/L to obtain optimal results and to minimize the need for adjunctive medications, unless adverse effects preclude such concentrations. Patients unable to tolerate the recommended therapeutic range may occasionally benefit from concentrations as low as 0.3–0.6 µEq/L, while others may tolerate and only respond to higher levels in the range of 1.2–1.5 µEq/L.

Adverse Effects:

For a variety of reasons, lithium may not be tolerated by patients even when it is effective in controlling their mood disorders.

Central Nervous System

A recent report suggests that cognitive sequelae may frequently go unrecognized.[23] The authors found that 9 out of 10 measures of cognition, creativity, and fine motor performance improved significantly when patients were taken off lithium, shedding further light on its potential for deleterious central nervous system (CNS) effects. In addition, when certain drugs are used concurrently, the incidence of lithium neurotoxicity may increase. Such agents include (a) conventional neuroleptics, (b) carbamazepine, (c) methyldopa, and (d) verapamil (Calan). Lithium-induced tremors may also be potentiated by selective serotonin re-uptake inhibitors (SSRIs).[24] Finally, toxic levels of lithium can cause confusion, seizures, and coma.

Renal System

The most common renal complication is nephrogenic diabetes insipidus (or polyuria-polydipsia) which occurs in about 5%–20% of patients on long-term lithium treatment. This can also occur with lithium intoxication and often persists for several weeks following drug discontinuation. There is also lingering controversy concerning the long-term effect on kidney function. Although two recent reviews[25,26] concluded that lithium does not lead to declines in glomerular filtration rates or to renal failure, Gitlin found that 3 out of 82 (3.7%) bipolar patients treated with lithium and monitored for at least 2 years developed serum creatinine levels greater than 2.0 mg/100 ml, with one patient progressing to chronic renal failure.[27] Even if this complication is related to lithium treatment, the overall incidence has been remarkably low over 40 years of clinical experience.

Cardiac System

Given reports of cardiac rhythm disturbances associated with lithium administration, an electrocardiogram should be obtained when clinically indicated, especially in the elderly and those at risk for heart disease. To clarify the question of bradycardia, a systematic 24-hour home monitoring study of sinus node dysfunction was done in 50 patients treated with lithium for at least 12 months.[28] **Forty-five patients completed the study, with 78% manifesting bradycardia** (i.e., less than 50 beats per minute); **generally, depression in sinus node functioning was mild.** In addition, the authors surveyed all patients in a given area placed on pacemakers because of sinus node disease and found that only three were on long-term lithium. **Although infrequent, sick sinus syndrome can lead to death and must be taken seriously.**

Pregnancy

Exposure in utero has been associated with Epstein's anomaly, a defect of the tricuspid valve. Lithium use, administered in the most appropriate dosing strategy during the perinatal period, must take into consideration several factors, including (a) **stage of pregnancy or postpartum status;** (b) **prior severity of episodes;** and (c) **relative risk of drug exposure to the fetus or the nursing neonate.** The best data indicate that **a decision to continue lithium during pregnancy is complicated and requires a review of the relative risks and benefits to both mother and fetus.**[29] Indeed, the ravages of bipolar disorder may be more deleterious than the risks of continuing lithium.

Drug Interactions:

Lithium is also involved in many significant drug interactions. **Agents that frequently *decrease* serum lithium levels, *possibly diminishing its efficacy,* include caffeine, verapamil, theophylline, aminophylline, osmotic diuretics, and carbonic anhydrase inhibitors. Drugs that may *increase* serum lithium levels, *possibly predisposing to toxicity,* include nonsteroidal anti-inflammatory agents, thiazide** diuretics and the nonthiazide diuretic indapamide, certain antibiotics (e.g., oral tetracycline), methyldopa, enalapril (as well as other ACE inhibitors), and fluoxetine.

Conclusion:

Although lithium has clearly revolutionized the treatment of bipolar disorder, it has many drawbacks. The most important of these include:

- A significant proportion of patients are not adequately helped or cannot tolerate its adverse effects.

- It is relatively ineffective for more severe acute manic or depressed episodes

- It has a narrow therapeutic index.

- It has the potential for long-term adverse effects, especially involving the thyroid and renal systems.

Thus, there is often a need to increase its efficacy by the judicious use of copharmacy or by developing alternative monotherapies.

Valproate

In the past few years, compelling clinical data have emerged supporting the mood-stabilizing properties of valproate.[31] The two most important studies include a Pope et al. report in which 36 previously lithium-resistant (i.e., nonresponsive and/or nontolerant) patients were treated for 3 weeks with the divalproex formulation of valproate (Depakote) or placebo in a random-assignment, double-blind design.[31] Divalproex was significantly more effective than placebo, with 12 of 17 patients responding to this agent, versus only 6 of 13 to placebo. Of note, an early high plasma level of divalproex (i.e., days 2–6) was found to predict response, while rapid cycling, predominant euphoria or dysphoria, family history of mood disorder, increased manic severity, and electroencephalographic abnormalities did not.[31] The second report by Bowden et al.[11] provides the strongest evidence for the efficacy of valproate in acute mania. This was a three-week multicenter study of 179 patients that compared divalproex to placebo, with the addition of a lithium arm that served as an active control.[11] A meta-analysis of these two placebo-controlled trials demonstrates a highly superior efficacy for active drug treatment versus placebo (see Table 6.1). **Other reports also suggest that valproate may be helpful in sub-groups of bipolar patients often resistant to lithium.** For example, Calabrese et al. in a prospective, longitudinal, naturalistic open design examined 101 **valproate-treated** *rapid cycling* **bipolar patients and found that predictors of good antimanic response included decreasing or stable episode frequencies and nonpsychotic episodes.**[33,34] Papatheodorou and Kutcher, in a preliminary open trial of 6 bipolar *adolescents* treated with divalproex, found that 5 had marked improvement and 1 had some improvement.[35,36] Other recent open-trial reports indicate that this agent may be effective and **well tolerated in elderly patients, those with concurrent substance and/or alcohol abuse, and those with organic mood disorders.**[37,38]

Table 6.1
Divalproex Versus Placebo in Acute Mania

Studies	N	Divalproex	Placebo	Difference
Pope et al. (1991)	36	71%	29%	42%
Bowden et al. (1994)	139	64%	32%	32%
Total	175	65%	32%	33%

Chi square=18.3; df=1; p=0.00002
Adapted from Janicak et al. (1995)

Acute Treatment of the Depressive Phase:

Open-label studies have found a response rate to valproate similar to the placebo rate in controlled studies of standard antidepressants.[39]

Clinical Management:

Routine laboratory tests at baseline should include **CBC and liver function tests. To treat acute mania, the divalproex formulation is usually started at 750–1000 mg on a b.i.d. or t.i.d. schedule with doses titrated up every few days to achieve blood levels in the range of 50–125 mcg/ml** (some patients may require slightly higher levels), **or until side effects prohibit further increases.**[40] For most patients, an adequate trial typically requires total doses ranging from 1000–2500 mg/day.

Keck et al. reported that divalproex also may be safely administered using a loading dose strategy.[41] In this study, patients tolerated 20 mg/day in divided doses for 5 days, with rapid onset of antimanic response. Such rapid response might also avoid or at least minimize the need for adjunctive copharmacy.

Adverse Effects:

The more common adverse effects associated with valproate include (a) gastrointestinal distress, (b) weight gain, (c) benign tremors, (d) CNS effects (e.g., sedation), (e) bruising, and (f) temporary alopecia.

Gastrointestinal symptoms (e.g., nausea, emesis) were more common with the valproic acid (valproate) formulation, but **divalproex** (an enteric-coated combination of valproate and valproic acid) **has significantly diminished this problem.** In addition, although it is **extremely rare, acute pancreatitis can occur.** Since **weight gain** can be significant with all mood stabilizers, including divalproex, it is important to stress the need for an aggressive weight management program at the beginning of treatment.

Hepatic System

Fatal hepatotoxicity **with divalproex is a rare, idiosyncratic, non-dose-related phenomenon occurring in approximately 1 of 40,000 cases.** The risk is almost entirely in epileptic patients under the age of two who have additional medical problems and/or mental retardation and are receiving multiple anticonvulsants. **Review of the pediatric neurologic literature reveals that elevated temperature, anorexia, and vomiting are the most frequent signs of impending hepatic toxicity, although lethargy and increased seizures also occur. Most of the cases develop in the first 90 days of treatment. Given the complications, we suggest that baseline liver enzymes be obtained and then monitored at least once during the first several weeks of treatment and every 6–12 months thereafter.** Baseline elevations in the absence of hepatic dysfunction should be monitored more frequently. If liver function tests continue to demonstrate an increase in enzymes, or there is present or past evidence for hepatic disease, this agent should be avoided or discontinued. Most importantly, patients should be carefully instructed to immediately report symptoms such as easy bruising, malaise, and jaundice.

Other Adverse Effects

Tremors secondary to valproate may respond to a dose reduction, when it is feasible, or to the addition of a β–blocker such as propranolol or atenolol. Although **hematological dyscrasias** such as transient thrombocytopenia have been reported, Tohen and colleagues recently found no life-threatening cases of more severe blood dyscrasias in 2,228 patients receiving divalproex or carbamazapine.[42]

Hair loss **may be minimized by the addition of vitamins containing selenium** (50 mg/day) **and zinc sulfate** (50 mg/day).

Pregnant women and women of childbearing age should be counseled that **valproate has teratogenic potential,** including a 1%–2% incidence of neural tube defects in embryos exposed to this agent in the first trimester. Thus, adequate precautions to prevent conception should be reviewed, and daily folate should be prescribed and valproate discontinued if pregnancy occurs.[43]

Significant drug interactions are less common with this agent. Since it is highly protein bound, however, it can displace other agents such as carbamazepine, as well as alter its metabolism, increasing serum levels of the active epoxide metabolite.[10,11,44] This latter effect may alter the ratio of parent compound to active metabolite and, possibly leading to increased toxicity.

Carbamazepine

Although this drug has been widely used to treat bipolar disorder, **in contrast to lithium and valproate, there have been no double-blind, placebo-controlled, parallel design studies evaluating its efficacy for bipolar disorder.**[1] Whereas several studies support a role for carbamazepine, they have methodological shortcomings, including the use of concomitant psychotropics, heterogeneous diagnostic categories, very small sample sizes, and brief treatment durations. As a result, the data are not sufficient to warrant FDA-approved labeling of this agent for the treatment of bipolar disorder.

Acute Treatment of the Depressive Phase:

Some studies have found carbamazepine superior to placebo for an acute bipolar depressive episode.[45-48] Two of these compared carbamazepine to placebo and a third compared carbamazepine plus placebo to carbamazepine plus lithium. In this last study, of 13 bipolar depressed patients who did not benefit from carbamazepine alone, six improved on the combination.

Clinical Management:

Carbamazepine is usually started at 400–600 mg/day in divided doses, with increases every few days unless side effects preclude further increments or desired clinical response is achieved. Until tolerance to side effects develops, titration may need to be slowed or even reversed.

Like lithium and *unlike* valproate, this agent has a relatively narrow therapeutic index. Although therapeutic blood levels for carbamazepine as an anticonvulsant are between 4 and 12 mcg/ml, the ideal range for carbamazepine as a mood stabilizer is unknown. Because of this uncertainty, it is more important to titrate dose based on clinical response and adverse effects. Standard clinical practice is to achieve a range of 8–12 mg/ml; some patients may require levels up to 15 mcg/ml, if side effects are tolerated.[44] Plasma levels should be monitored more frequently during the first few months because carbamazepine can accelerate its own metabolism (i.e., autometabolism), often leading to a clinically significant decrease in levels during the early phases of treatment.

Adverse Effects:

Common side effects associated with carbamazepine include gastrointestinal distress, sedation, and dizziness. Ataxic gait, hyponatremia (especially in the elderly), and more serious skin reactions (e.g., Stevens-Johnson syndrome) are relatively uncommon but can occur. Contraindications to the use of carbamazepine include a history of bone marrow depression, narrow angle glaucoma, and the use of a monoamine oxidase inhibitor within the previous two weeks. Because carbamazepine can slow the atrioventricular conduction system, it should be used cautiously when combined with tricyclic antidepressants or in those with significant cardiovascular disorders.

In this context, it also may lead to more serious cardiac complications when taken in an overdose.

In the hematological/hepatic systems, carbamazepine often produces a benign leukopenia, and there is a slight (i.e., 1 in 40,000) risk of aplastic anemia. **As the optimal time frame for repeating hematological measures is controversial, it is reasonable to obtain a complete blood count (CBC) at baseline, biweekly for 2 months, and every 6–12 months thereafter.** More importantly, patients should be counseled to contact a physician immediately in the event of fever, sore throat, petechiae, malaise, or other signs and symptoms of hematological dysfunction. **Because carbamazepine may also produce hepatotoxicity, liver function should be monitored at baseline and then on an annual basis.**

Overdose:

Though uncommon, fatal carbamazepine toxicity does occur. Overdoses are characterized by neurologic symptoms such as diplopia, dysarthria, ataxia, vertigo, nystagmus, or coma. Infrequently, cyclic coma with biphasic fluctuations of consciousness, seizures, respiratory depression, cardiac conduction defects, and the need for artificial ventilation may occur.[49,50] **Plasma levels are only moderately correlated to severity, but levels over 15 mcg/ml in children or 20 mcg/ml in adults should be considered potentially toxic.** Charcoal hemoperfusion, plasmapheresis, and gastric lavage with activated charcoal have been used, but the benefit of the plasmapheresis procedure has been questioned.[51]

Drug Interactions:

A major issue to consider when using carbamazepine in combination with other agents is its many significant drug interactions. Most involve the induction of microsomal CYP450 enzymes (e.g., 2D6, 1A2, 3A4, 2C9/10), which cause an accelerated elimination of drugs normally metabolized by this system.[52] **Plasma levels of various coprescribed drugs** (e.g., certain anti-psychotics, antidepressants, oral contraceptives, and anti-coagulants), **may be decreased to a clinically significant degree.** This may require appropriate dose adjustments to compensate for their lowered plasma levels.

Carbamazepine levels, in turn, may be *decreased by* barbiturates, phenytoin (Dilantin), and primidone (Mysoline). Carbamazepine levels may be *increased by* valproate; selective serotonin reuptake inhibitors (SSRIs), especially fluoxetine and fluvoxamine (Luvox); erythromycin; propoxyphene; cimetidine (Tagamet); isoniazid; and calcium channel blockers. As noted earlier, the combination of carbamazepine and lithium may enhance the risk of neurotoxicity, although the mechanism underlying this phenomenon is uncertain. **Finally, we do not recommend using carbamazepine in conjunction with clozapine** (Clozaril); theoretically this combination could further suppress bone marrow activity.

Electroconvulsive Therapy (ECT)

ECT is most often utilized to treat severe depressive episodes (both unipolar and bipolar), but the existing data indicate that it is also effective for acute mania. Furthermore, unlike the available pharmacotherapy, **ECT appears to be equally effective for both manic and depressive phases of bipolar disorder.** Although its exact mechanism of action is unknown, ECT has several effects in common with anticonvulsant mood stabilizers, including (a) raising the seizure threshold, (b) decreasing seizure duration and neurometabolic response, and (c) decreasing amygdaloid kindling.

In a recent review of the literature, Mukherjee et al. found that **ECT was associated with marked clinical improvement or remission in 80% of those treated for acute manic episodes.**[53] Data also suggest that **ECT is effective for those who have responded poorly to pharmacotherapy,** whereas **possible predictors of *nonresponse* to ECT include anger, irritability, and suspiciousness.**[54] In addition, several uncontrolled studies suggest that ECT is equal or superior to both anti-psychotics and lithium in the treatment of acute mania.[55,56] For example, Small and colleagues randomly assigned manic patients to ECT or lithium for eight weeks.[57] Both groups benefited, but the ECT-treated group demonstrated a significantly greater improvement by the end of the study. These data are difficult to interpret, however, since ECT-treated patients also received lithium, and many initially assigned to the lithium group were also receiving ECT in the later phases of the study.

Clinical Management:

Although bilateral and unilateral nondominant stimulus electrode placements have been used in depressive episodes, **there is debate over the optimal method of administering ECT for acute mania.** Mukherjee and colleagues found unilateral nondominant ECT to be effective, whereas Milstein et al. observed that bilateral electrode placement was required for optimal benefit.[58,59] **When possible, all medications** (especially lithium and heterocyclic antidepressants) **should be discontinued during a course of treatment to minimize the risk of cardiac or neurological toxicity. One exception may be the combined use of an antipsychotic and ECT.** For example, preliminary data indicate that the concurrent use of clozapine (and, by generalization, perhaps other novel antipsychotics such as olanzapine [Zyprexa] and risperidone [Risperdal]) and ECT may be used safely and benefit previously treatment-refractory patients.[60]

The existing evidence indicates that ECT is a safe and effective alternative treatment for acute manic or depressive episodes and may benefit those who are unresponsive to or intolerant of drug therapy, pose an immediate danger to themselves, or are pregnant. We believe that the adverse effects associated with this therapeutic modality (e.g., CNS or cardiovascular effects) are far outweighed by the potential benefit in those patients who require ECT. Although the nature of the disorder and the administration procedures make prospective blinded studies difficult, we believe that this modality has stood the test of time and may be effective when medications fail.

Other Anticonvulsants

Other novel anticonvulsants also have been considered for their potential mood-stabilizing properties.

Lamotrigine **has recently become available and is approved as an** *adjunctive* **agent for partial seizures in patients over 16 years of age.** It also may play a role as a monotherapy for partial seizures or an adjunct for other types of seizures and may also benefit younger children (<16 years of age). **Early reports indicate that this agent also may be effective for the depressed phase of bipolar disorder, though its role for the manic phase is less certain.**[61-63] Its adverse effect profile is considered acceptable, but **life-threatening rashes** (e.g., exfoliative skin reactions) **are reported to occur in 0.1%–2% of patients** (primarily pediatric groups). Further, **because coadministered valproate may increase the risk for such events, this combination usually should be avoided. Starting with low doses** (e.g., 25 mg/day) **and gradually titrating up** (e.g., with biweekly dose increases) **should help reduce the potential for rashes and neurological side effects** (e.g., dizziness, diplopia, ataxia, headaches, and blurred vision). **Maximum dose is usually 500 mg/day in adults and 2–8 mg/kg/day for children,** as dictated by response and adverse effects.

Gabapentin (Neurontin) **is used primarily as an** *adjunct* **treatment for refractory partial seizure disorders.**[64] Preliminary data indicate that **this agent may have antimanic and mood stabilizing effects.**[65-67] Gabapentin has **several potential advantages** over other mood stabilizers, including:

- A more benign side-effect profile.
- No need for routine blood or plasma level monitoring.
- Neurological side effects that are dose related and usually transient.
- Renal metabolism, leading to significantly fewer pharmacokinetic interactions.
- Minimal impact on the CYP450 microenzyme system.

Typical starting doses in adults are 300–900 mg/day. The therapeutic dose range has been reported to be between 600 and 5,000 mg/day.[68]

Adjunctive Antipsychotics Therapies

Antipsychotics were the treatment of choice for bipolar mania prior to the introduction of lithium. **Clinical experience has shown that in some cases, these agents may be the only effective therapy as well as the only practical** (i.e., depot preparation) **treatment in noncompliant patients. Although our meta-analysis of five well-designed studies comparing** *neuroleptics alone* **to** *lithium alone* **for acute mania clearly demonstrates the superior efficacy of lithium, over 50% of those on an antipsychotic alone also responded.**[69-73] More recently, Rifkin and associates compared three doses of haloperidol for up to 6

Table 6.2
Key Information About Mood Stabilizers Used in the Copharmacy of Bipolar Disorder

LITHIUM

Effectiveness:	• Milder forms of mania • Reduction in suicides with maintenance • More effective than antipsychotics
Neurotoxicity:	• May be increased with traditional antipsychotics (e.g. haloperidol), carbamazepine, methyldopa, verapamil • Tremors are potentiated by simultaneous use of SSRIs
Reduced serum level:	• Caffeine, verapamil, theophylline, aminophylline, osmotic diuretics, carbonic anhydrase inhibitors
Increased serum level:	• Non-steroidal anti-inflammatory agents, thiazide diuretics, indapamide, antibiotics (e.g. tetracycline), methyldopa, ACE inhibitors, fluoxetine

VALPROATE

Effectiveness:	• Acute mania • Rapid cycling • Lithium resistance/intolerance
Drug-drug interactions:	• Very few (e.g., carbamazepine, phenytoin)

CARBAMAZEPINE

Effectiveness:	• Acute Bipolar Mania**
Contraindications:	• History of bone marrow depression (Do not combine with clozapine) • Narrow angle glaucoma • Do not combine with MAOIs • Use caution with drugs affecting cardiovascular system such as tricyclics • Reduces plasma levels of antipsychotics, antidepressants, oral contraceptives, anticoagulants, theophylline (accelerates metabo lism of drugs metabolized by cytochrome P-450 enzymes)
Reduced serum level:	• Caused by barbiturates, phenytoin, primidone
Increases serum level:	• Caused by valproate, fluoxetine, fluvoxamine, erythromycin, propoxyphene, cimetidine, isoniazed, calcium channel blockers

LAMOTRIGINE

Effectiveness:	• Mania** • Bipolar depression**
Complications:	• Rashes which may be life threatening when combined with valproate

GABAPENTIN

Effectiveness:	• Mania** • Mood stabilization**

THYROID AUGMENTATION

Effectiveness:	• Rapid cycling**

**not established by double-blind, controlled studies

weeks as the only treatment in 47 acutely manic patients.[74] They found that 72% of subjects responded, excluding dropouts (most occurring in the first two weeks and being evenly distributed across all dose groups).

Ideally, patients should be treated with a *primary mood stabilizer* alone during an acute manic episode. These patients are often difficult to manage, however, and there may be a time lag before the primary mood stabilizer is fully effective, frequently making mono-drug therapy unfeasible. In such cases, an antipsychotic is often administered concurrently, and then tapered and discontinued once the primary agent has taken full effect, usually within a few weeks. Important clinical questions related to the *adjunctive use* of anti-psychotics include the comparative efficacy of various agents and the optimal dose of these medications. For example, we compared bioequivalent doses of the high-potency agent thio-thixene (Navane) and the low-potency agent chlorpromazine (Thorazine) used as adjuncts to lithium and found that moderate doses of either antipsychotic were sufficient to control acute manic symptoms.[75] Cookson et al. came to a similar conclusion, finding no difference between chlorpromazine and pimozide (Orap) for the treatment of acute mania.[76] The Rifkin et al. study noted earlier found 10, 30, or 80 mg/day of haloperidol to be equieffective (i.e., survival analysis showed no difference among the three dosing regimens). This is particularly noteworthy and parallels recent findings that lower doses of haloperidol to treat schizophrenic and schizoaffective patients may be as effective as moderate to high doses. [77]

Unfortunately, antipsychotics when used alone or as adjuncts are still given in higher-than-necessary acute doses and then often maintained at these inappropriately high levels.[78] Efforts to avoid such regimens involve a more careful determination of the minimal effective dose and adjunctive anxiolytics to further decrease exposure to antipsychotics, at times bypassing them altogether. Related to this question is the issue of *increased neurotoxicity* resulting from the combination of lithium and a conventional neuroleptic, particularly haloperidol.[79] Whether these cases represent neuroleptic malignant syndrome, lithium-induced neurologic dysfunction, or a true interaction between lithium and haloperidol (or other antipsychotics) is still not entirely clear. As noted earlier, lower doses of antipsychotics in combination with various mood stabilizers may be more effective and safer. When lithium is combined with conventional neuroleptics, especially potent agents such as haloperidol, patients should be monitored carefully for early signs of neuroleptic malignant syndrome and/or neurotoxicity.[80]

The role of *novel antipsychotics*, either as primary or adjunctive treatments, has yet to be fully explored. For example, there have been reports that clozapine, olanzapine, and risperidone may possess thymoleptic as well as antipsychotic properties.[81-83] If these observations are confirmed by controlled trials, agents such as clozapine, risperidone, olanzapine, and quetiapine may play an important and perhaps unique role for refractory mood disorders.

In summary, antipsychotics continue to play a crucial role in the management of both acute and chronic symptoms of bipolar disorder. Since adverse drug reactions are frequent, and at times potentially severe, these agents should be used only when necessary. **Strategies to maximize their benefit while minimizing adverse events include:**

- Prescribing *lower doses* of antipsychotics used as adjuncts for acute and maintenance management.

- Using *depot* preparations when pharmacokinetic or compliance issues exist.

- Prescribing *novel agents* (such as clozapine, olanzapine, risperidone) that may benefit certain treatment refractory patients.

- Using *anxiolytics* as an alternative or adjunct to minimize exposure to antipsychotics.

Benzodiazepines

Benzodiazepines play an important role in the treatment of bipolar disorder, with recent evidence suggesting that their use for sleep restoration may induce a rapid antimanic response.[84] As mentioned earlier, since benzodiazepines may attenuate nonspecific symptoms associated with an acute manic episode (particularly insomnia, agitation, hyperactivity, and anxiety), they may be used in lieu of more aggressive antipsychotic dosing to supplement the effects of a primary mood stabilizer. Thus, because of their more benign adverse effect profile, benzodiazepiness should be considered as an alternative to antipsychotics. However, **they should be used cautiously in patients who also suffer from comorbid alcohol and/or other substance abuse problems, which as many as 50% of bipolar patients do over the course of their illness.**

Chouinard's group reported on 16 agitated psychotic patients with manic symptoms who were randomly assigned to receive either clonazepam (Klonopin) (1–2 mg) or haloperidol (HPDL) (5–10 mg) at 0, 0.5, and 1.0 hours. After 2 hours both agents were found to have decreased manic symptomatology; however, **haloperidol produced beneficial effects more rapidly than clonazepam.**[85]

In the best study to date comparing the efficacy of different benzodiazepiness, Bradwejn et al. used clonazepam or lorazepam (Ativan) in a two-week double-blind study.[86] **Both medications were given in doses up to 24 mg/day** (mean doses were about 12 mg/day), and **lorazepam was found to be more effective than clonazepam.** In a second phase of the study, lithium was added for an additional two-week period. **Eight of 13 patients treated with lorazepam plus lithium remitted as compared to only 4 of 11 patients receiving the lithium-clonazepam combination.** Concerns about behavioral disinhibition were not borne out by this study or by most other reports in the literature. **One concern is the possible depressogenic effects of clonazepam, which should be monitored closely when this agent is utilized.**[87]

Thyroid Hormone

Endocrine disturbances have been associated with mood disorders but are usually correctable if recognized. However, **long-term lithium therapy can predispose patients to develop goiter and/or hypothyroidism.** At first, some patients may develop subtle mood changes as opposed to overt physiological signs and symptoms. Recognizing and correcting this endocrine perturbation is usually necessary for optimal management of symptoms. In this context, baseline thyroid function tests, including thyroid stimulating hormone, are an essential part of the laboratory workup for a bipolar patient.

Treatment-resistant and rapid cycling bipolar patients may have an increased frequency of thyroid dysfunction. In this context, **Kusalic found that 6 of 10 rapid cyclers had hypothyroidism based on their**

thyrotropin-releasing hormone tests.[88] Furthermore, the average number of mood episodes per year decreased by over 75% (i.e., 9.7 versus 2.2) after levthyroxine (Synthroid) was added to their treatment regimen. In addition, several case reports involving this population found that high doses of the thyroid hormone levothyroxine sodium (T₄) were clinically beneficial. For example, Bauer and Whybrow conducted a blind, placebo crossover trial of high-dose T4 augmentation of standard medication regimens in 11 treatment-resistant rapid cyclers.[89] In this trial T4 was used to produce *supranormal levels of circulating hormones*. Response was not related to the baseline thyroid status: Ten patients had substantial reductions in the severity of their depression and/or mania, as well as improvement in their quality of life.

Copharmacy Strategies

For classic manic presentations, it is best to start treatment with lithium or valproate, attaining adequate blood levels as quickly as possible. A *loading dose strategy* (e.g., 15–20 mg/day beginning on the first day of treatment) with the divalproex formulation may accelerate response and avoid the use of other agents. If the patient is agitated, adjunctive benzodiazepines are preferable to antipsychotics. During a depressive episode, lithium alone is usually not sufficient and patients will often require concurrent antidepressant therapy. This may further complicate their management, however, since there is the possibility of propelling patients into a manic episode, a rapid cycling course, or a more treatment-resistant phase of their illness.[90,91] In a manic episode, if insufficient response occurs and patients are also receiving antidepressants, they should be discontinued. Thyroid supplementation may be appropriate, especially if thyroid stimulating hormone is elevated or there is a blunted TSH response to stimulation and manic or depressive symptoms are not responding to other standard pharmacotherapies.

If response is still insufficient, or if the patient has moderate to severe manic or depressive symptoms (e.g., psychosis), an antipsychotic may be added to the primary mood stabilizer and/or benzodiazepine using *a low-dose titration schedule* to minimize side effects. Due to their relatively benign adverse-effect profiles, olanzapine,

risperidone, or quetiapine would be our first choice, despite limited clinical experience with them. We recommend lower doses that should only be increased if they prove inadequate over a several-day trial.

With other-than-classic presentations (e.g., *rapid cycling, mixed states, comorbid substance abuse, organic mood syndromes, or lithium-unresponsive/intolerant patients*), **valproate is our first choice.** This is based on its tolerability, the quality of studies, and the FDA-approved labeling of this agent for the treatment of bipolar disorder. **If necessary, it can be used in combination with lithium, benzodiazepines, and/or conventional or novel antipsychotics, chosen on the basis of target psychopathologic features.** Patients who do not respond to valproate may respond to carbamazepine, as recently reported by Nurnberg and colleagues.[92] If needed, valproate and carbamazepine may be combined, with or without lithium, but careful attention should be given to the potential for clinically relevant drug interactions. **Some patients may benefit from the combination of valproate and carbamazepine, with or without lithium. For patients who remain nonresponsive, clozapine may be initiated and, if necessary, combined with valproate and/or lithium, but *not* with carbamazepine.**

If a patient is in immediate danger, has previously responded to ECT, or has medical contraindications to pharmacotherapy, this somatic treatment may be the preferred choice for either the manic or the depressive phase. Finally, **the combination of a novel antipsychotic, such as clozapine or risperidone, with ECT may produce additional benefit in patients insufficiently responsive to either therapy alone.**

Conclusion

Because lithium has been the mainstay of treatment for bipolar disorders and NIMH funding has been lacking, there have been few systematic efforts to develop new treatments. Although indications are being developed for established compounds (e.g., valproate), others have little hard data to support their use (e.g., carbamazepine, verapamil). All existing primary drug therapies are often insufficient when given as a monotherapy. Thus, adjunctive copharmacy is generally the rule in managing bipolar patients. Given this reality, a careful risk/benefit evaluation should be the primary guide in choosing a specific approach.

References

1. Janicak PG, Davis JM, Ayd FA, Preskorn S. Advances in the Pharmacotherapy of Bipolar Disorder. *Principles and Practice of Psychopharmacotherapy Update.* 1995;1(3):1–20.

2. Krasuski JS, Janicak PG. Mixed states: issues of terminology and conceptualization. *Psychiatric Annals.* 1994:24:269–277.

3. Krasuski JS, Janicak PG. Mixed states: current and alternate diagnostic models. *Psychiatric Annals.* 1994;24:371–379.

4. Swann AC. Mixed or dysphoric manic states: psychopathology and treatment. *J Clin Psychiatry.* 1995;56(suppl 3):6–10.

5. Evans DL, Byerly MJ, Greer RA. Secondary mania: diagnosis and treatment. *J Clin Psychiatry.* 1995;56(suppl 3):31–37.

6. Brady KT, Sonne SC. The relationship between substance abuse and bipolar disorder. *J Clin Psychiatry.* 1995;56(suppl 3):19–24.

7. Janicak PG, Davis JM, Preskorn SH, Ayd FJ Jr. *Principles and Practice of Psychopharmacotherapy.* 2nd ed. Baltimore, MD: Williams & Wilkins; 1997.

8. Maggs R. Treatment of manic illness with lithium carbonate. *Br J Psychiatry.* 1963;109:562–565.

9. Stokes PE, Stoll PM, Shamoian CH. Efficacy of lithium as acute treatment of manic-depressive illness. *Lancet.* 1971;1:1319–1325.

10. Stokes P, Kocsis J, Arcuni O. Relationship of lithium chloride dose to treatment response in acute mania. *Arch Gen Psychiatry.* 1976;33:1080–1085.

11. Bowden CL, Brugger AM, Swann AC, et al. Efficacy of divalproex vs lithium and placebo in the treatment of mania. *JAMA.* 1994;271:918–924.

12. Souza FGM, Goodwin GM. Lithium treatment and prophylaxis in unipolar depression: a meta-analysis. *Br J Psychiatry.* 1991;158:666–675.

13. Coryell W, Endicott J, Master JD, et al. The likelihood of recurrence in bipolar affective disorder: the importance of episode recency. *J Affect Disord.* 1995;33:201–206.

14. Ebert D, Jaspert A, Mwiata H, Kaschka W. Initial lithium augmentation improves the antidepressant effect of standard TCA treatment in non-resistant depressed patients. *Psychobiology.* 1995;118:223–225.

15. Nilsson A. Mortality in recurrent mood disorders during periods on and off lithium. *Pharmacopsychiatry.* 1995;28:8–13.

16. Ahrens B, Muller-Oerlinghausen B, Schou M, et al. Excess cardiovascular and suicide mortality of affective disorders may be reduced by lithium prophylaxis. *J. Affect Disord.* 1995;33:67–75.

17. Guze SB, Robins E. Suicide and primary effective disorders. *Br J Psychiatry.* 1970;17:437–438.

18. Weeke A. Causes of death in manic-depressives. In: Schou M, Stromgen E, eds. *Origin, Prevention and Treatment of Affective Disorders.* New York: Academic Press; 1979:289–299.

19. Coppen A, Baily J, Houston G, Silcocks P. Lithium and mortality: a 15 year follow-up. *Clin Neuropharmacol.* 1992;15(suppl 1, pt A);448A–449A.

20. Lenz G. Increased mortality after drop-out from lithium clinic. *Neuropsychopharmacology.* 1994;10(suppl 3, pt 1):623S.

21. Muller-Oerlinghausen B, Wolf T, Ahrens B, et al. Mortality during initial and during later lithium treatment: a collaborative study by the International Group for the Study of Lithium-Treated Patients. *Acta Psychiatr Scand.* 1994;90:295–297.

22. Nilsson A. Mortality in recurrent mood disorders during periods on and off lithium. *Pharmacopsychiatry.* 1995;28:8–13.

23. Kocsis JH, Shaw E, Stokes PE, et al. Neuropsychologic effects of lithium discontinuation. *J Clin Psychopharmacol.* 1993;13:268–275.

24. Gelenberg AJ, Jefferson JW. Lithium tremor. *J Clin Psychiatry.* 1995;56:283–287.

25. Schou M. Effects of long-term lithium treatment on kidney function: an overview. *J Psychiatr Res.* 1988;22:287–296.

26. Waller DG, Edwards JG. Lithium and the kidney: an update. *Psychol Med.* 1989;19:825–831.

27. Gitlin MJ. Lithium-induced renal insufficiency. *J Clin Psychopharmacol.* 1993;13:276–279.

28. Rosenquist M, Bergfeldt L, Aili H, Mathe AA. Sinus node dysfunction during long-term lithium treatment. *Br Heart J.* 1993;70:371–375.

29. Jacobsen SJ, Jones K, Johnson K, et al. Prospective multicentre study of pregnancy outcome after lithium exposure during first trimester. *Lancet.* 1992;339(8792):530–533.

30. Bowden CL, McElroy SL. Introduction: history of the development of valproate for treatment of bipolar disorder. *J Clin Psychiatry.* 1995;6(suppl 3):3–5.

31. Pope HG, McElroy SL, Keck PE, Hudson JI. Valproate in the treatment of acute mania. *Arch Gen Psychiatry.* 1991;48:62–68.

32. McElroy SL, Keck PE, Pope HG, et al. Correlates of antimanic response to valproate. *Psychopharmacol Bull.* 1991;27:127–133.

33. Calabrese JR. Woyshville MJ, Kimmel SE, Rapport DJ. Predictors of valproate response in bipolar rapid cycling. *J Clin Psychopharmacol.* 1993;13:280–283.

34. Calabrese JR, Markovitz, Kemmel SE, Wagner SC. Spectrum of efficacy of valproate in 78 rapid-cycling bipolar patients. *J Clin Psychopharmacol.* 1992;12(suppl 1):53S–56S(B).

35. Papatheodorou G, Kutcher SP. Divalproex treatment in late adolescent and young adult acute mania. *Psychopharmacol Bull.* 1993;29:213–219.

36. Papatheodorou G, Kutcher SP, Katic M, Szalai JP. The efficacy and safety of divalproex in the treatment of acute mania in adolescents and young adults: an open clinical trial. *J Clin Psychopharmacol.* 1995;15:110–116.

37. Risinger RC, Risby ED, Risch SC. Safety and efficacy of divalproex in elderly bipolar patients (letter). *J Clin Psychiatry.* 1994;55:215.

38. Stall AL, Banov M, Kollerener M, et al. Neurologic factors predict a favorable valproate response in bipolar and schizoaffective disorders. *J Clin Psychopharmacol.* 1994;14:311–313.

39. Calabrese JC, Markovitz, Kenmel SE, Wagner SC. Spectrum of efficacy of valproate in 78 rapid cycling bipolar patients. *J Clin Psychopharmacol.* 1992;12(suppl 1):53S–56S(B).

40. Bowden CL, Janicak PG, Orsulak P, et al. Relation of serum valproate concentration to response in mania. *Am J Psychiatry.* 1996;153:765–770.

41. Keck PE, McElroy SL, Tugrul KC, Bennet JA. Valproate oral loading in the treatment of acute mania. *J Clin Psychiatry*. 1993;54:305–308.

42. Tohen M, Castillo J, Baldessarini RJ, et al. Blood Dyscrasias with carbamazepine and valproate: a pharmaco-epidemiological study of 2,228 patients at risk. *Am J Psychiatry*. 1995;152:413–418.

43. Miller LJ. Psychiatric medication during pregnancy: understanding and minimizing risks. *Psychiatric Annals*. 1994;24:69–75.

44. Janicak PG. The relevance of clinical pharmacokinetics and therapeutic drug monitoring: anticonvulsant mood stabilizers and antipsychotics. *J Clin Psychiatry*. 1993;54(suppl):35–41.

45. Ballenger JC, Post RM. Carbamazepine in manic-depressive illness: a new treatment. *Am J Psychiatry*. 1980;137:782–790.

46. Post RM, Unde TW, Ballenger JC, et al. Carbamazepine and its -10,11-epoxide metabolite in plasma and CSF: relationship to AD response. *Arch Gen Psychiatry*. 1983;40:673–676.

47. Kramlinger KG, Post RM. The addition of lithium to carbamazepine. *Arch Gen Psychiatry*. 1983;46:794–800.

48. Ahrens B, Reduced mortality, the ultimate indicator of treatment efficacy. Review and perspectives. *Pharmacopysychiatry*. 1994;27(suppl):37–40.

49. Hojer J, Malmlund HO, Berg A. Clinical features in 28 consecutive cases of laboratory confirmed massive poisoning with carbamazepine alone. *Clin Toxicol*. 1993;31:449–458.

50. Tibballs J. Acute toxic reaction to carbamazepine. *Pediatric Pharmacology and Therapeutics*. 1992;121:295–299.

51. Kale P, Thompson P, Provenzaro R, Higgins M. Evaluation of plasmapheresis in the treatment of acute overdose of carbamazepine. *Ann Pharmacother*. 1993;24:866-868.

52. Pollock BG. Recent developments in drug metabolism of relevance to psychiatrists. *Harv Rev Psychiatry*. 1994;2:204–213.

53. Mukherjee S, Sackheim HA, Schnur DB. Electroconvulsive therapy of acute manic episodes: a review of 50 years' experience. *Am J Psychiatry*. 1994;151:169–176.

54. Schnur DB, Mukherjee S, Sackeim HA, Lee C, Roth SD. Symptomatic predictors of ECT response in medication-nonresponsive manic patients. *J Clin Psychiatry*. 1992;53:63–66.

55. McCabe MS. ECT in the treatment of mania: a controlled study. *Am J Psychiatry*. 1976;133:688–691.

56. Black DW, Winokur G, Nasrallah H. Treatment of mania: a naturalistic study of ECT versus lithium in 438 patients. *J Clin Psychiatry*. 1987;48:132–139.

57. Small JG, Klapper MH, Kellams JJ, et al. ECT compared with lithium in the management of manic states. *Arch Gen Psychiatry*. 1988;45:727–732.

58. Mukherjee S, Sackeim HA, Lee C. Unilateral ECT in the treatment of manic episodes. *Convuls Ther*. 1988;4:74–80.

59. Milstein V, Small JG, Klapper MH, et al. Unilateral versus bilateral ECT in the treatment of mania. *Convuls Ther*. 1987;3:1–9.

60. Masiar SJ, Johns CA. ECT following clozapine. *Br J Psychiatry*. 1991;158:135–136.

61. Calabrese JR, Woyshville MH, McElroy S, et al. *Spectrum of efficacy of lamotrigine in treatment refractory manic depression.* Presented at the Second International Conference on Affective Disorders; September, 1995, Jerusalem, Israel.

62. Weisler R, Risner M, Ascher J, et al. Use of lamotrigine in the treatment of bipolar disorder. APA New Research Program and Abstracts, Annual Meeting. 1994;NR611:216.

63. Sporn J, Sachs G. The anticonvulsant lamotrigine in treatment-resistant manic-depressive illness. *J Clin Psychopharmacol.* 1997;17:185–189.

64. Levy RH, Matson RH, Mildrum BB, eds. *Antiepileptic Drugs, 4th ed.* New York: Raven; 1995.

65. Schaffer CB, Schaffer LC. Gabapentin in the treatment of bipolar disorder (letter to the editor). *Am J Psychiatry.* 1997;154:291–292.

66. Bennett J, Goldman WT, Suppes T. Gabapentin for treatment of bipolar and schizoaffective disorders (letter). *J Clin Psychopharmacol.* 1997;17:141–142.

67. Stanton SP, Keck PE Jr, McElroy SL. Treatment of acute mania with gabapentin (letter to the editor). *Am J Psychiatry.* 1997;154:287.

68. McElroy S, Weller SL. Psychopharmocological treatment of bipolar disorder across the life span. In: Dickstein LJ, Riba MB, Olham JM. *Review of Psychiatry 1997.* Washington, DC: APPI Press;1997;IV-7–IV-30.

69. Johnson G, Gershon S, Hekimian LJ. Controlled evaluation of lithium and chlorpromazine in the treatment of manic states: an interim report. *Compr Psychiatry.* 1968;9:563.

70. Johnson G, Gershon S, Burdock EI. Comparative effects of lithium and chlorpromazine in the treatment of acute manic states. *Br J Psychiatry.* 1971;119:267.

71. Spring G, Schweid D, Gray L. A double-blind comparison of lithium and chlorpromazine in the treatment of manic states. *Am J Psychiatry.* 1970;126:1306–1310.

72. Takahashi R, Sakuma A, Itoh K. Comparison of efficacy of lithium carbonate and chlorpromazine in mania. *Arch Gen Psychiatry.* 1975;32:1310–1318.

73. Shopsin B, Kim SS, Gershon S. A controlled study of lithium vs chlorpromazine in acute schizophrenia. *Br J Psychiatry.* 1971;119:435–440.

74. Rifkin A, Doddi, S, Karajgi B, Borenstein M, Munne R. Dosage of haloperidol for mania. *Br J Psychiatry.* 1994;165:113–116.

75. Janicak PG, Bresnahan DB, Sharma RP, et al. A comparison of thiothixene with chlorpromazine in the treatment of mania. *J Clin Psychopharmacol.* 1988;8:33–37.

76. Cookson J, Silverstone T, Wells B. Double-blind comparative clinical trial of pimozide and chlorpromazine in mania. *Acta Psychiatr Scand.* 1981;64:381–397.

77. Janicak PG, Javaid JI, Sharma RP, et al. A two-phase double-blind randomized study of three haloperidol plasma levels for acute psychosis with reassignment of initial non-responders. *Acta Psychiatr Scand.* 1997;95:343–350.

78. Sernyak MJ, Griffin RA, Johnson RM, et al. Neuroleptic exposure following inpatient treatment of acute mania with lithium and neuroleptic. *Am J Psychiatry.* 1994;151:133–135.

79. Cohen WS, Cohen NH. Lithium carbonate, haloperidol, and irreversible brain damage. *JAMA.* 1974;230:1283–1287.

80. Geoff DC, Baldessarini RJ. Drug interactions with antipsychotic agents. *J Clin Psychopharmacol.* 1993;13:57–67.

81. Suppes T, Phillips KA, Judd CR. Clozapine treatment of nonpsychotic rapid cycling bipolar disorder: a report of three cases. *Biol Psychiatry*. 1994;36:338–340.

82. Hillert A, Maier W, Wetzel H, et al. Risperidone in the treatment of disorders with a combined psychotic and depressive syndrome: a functional approach. *Pharmacopsychiatry*. 1992;25:213–217.

83. Suppes T, McElroy SL, Gilbert J, Dessain EC, Cole JO. Clozapine in the treatment of dysphoric mania. *Biol Psychiatry*. 1992;32:270–280.

84. Nowlin-Finch NL, Altshuler LL, Szuba MP, Mintz J. Rapid resolution of first episodes of mania: sleep related? *J Clin Psychiatry*. 1994;55:26–29.

85. Chouinard G, Annable L, Turnier L, Holobow N, Skrumelak J. Double-blind randomized clinical trial of rapid tranquilization with I.M. clonazepam and I.M. haloperidol in agitated psychotic patients with manic symptoms. *Can J Psychiatry*. 1993;38(suppl 4):S114–S120.

86. Bradwejn J, Shriqui C, Koszycki D, Meterissian G. Double-blind comparison of the effects of clonazepam and lorazepam in acute mania. *J Clin Psychopharmacol*. 1990;10:403–408.

87. Cohen LS, Rosenbaum JS. Clonazepam: new uses and potential problems. *J Clin Psychiatry*. 1987;48(suppl 10):50–55.

88. Kusalic M. Grade II and grade III hypothyroidism in rapid-cycling bipolar patients. *Neuropsychobiology*. 1992;25:177–181.

89. Bauer MS, Whybrow PC. Rapid cycling bipolar affective disorder II: treatment of refractory rapid cycling with high dose levothyroxine. *Arch Gen Psychiatry*. 1990;47:435–440.

90. Hurowitz GI, Liebowitz MR. Antidepressant-induced rapid cycling: six case reports. *J Clin Psychopharmacol*. 1993;13:52–56.

91. Altshuler LL, Post RM, Leverich GS, et al. Antidepressant-induced mania and cycle acceleration: a controversy revisited. *Am J Psychiatry*. 1995;152:1130–1138.

92. Nurnberg HG, Martin GA, Karaggi BM, Raskin JK, Lonshore CT. Response to anticonvulsant substitution among refractory bipolar manic patients. *J Clin Psychopharmacol*. 1994:14:207–209

7 Pharmacoeconomics of Lithium and Divalproex Sodium in the Treatment of Bipolar Disorder

Joseph F. Goldberg, MD, Lori L. Altshuler, MD, Mark Frye, MD, and Paul E. Keck, Jr., MD

Dr. Goldberg is Assistant Professor of Psychiatry, Payne Whitney Clinic, New York Hospital, Cornell University Medical College, New York, New York.

Dr. Altshuler is Associate Professor of Psychiatry, University of California, Los Angeles; Neuropsychiatric Institute, Los Angeles, California.

Dr. Frye is Senior Staff Fellow, Biological Psychiatry Branch, National Institute of Mental Health, Bethesda, Maryland.

Dr. Keck is Associate Professor of Psychiatry and Pharmacology, and Vice-Chairman for Research, University of Cincinnati College of Medicine, Cincinnati, Ohio.

Supported, in part, by a research grant from the Pritzker Depression Network and by funds established in the New York Community Trust by DeWitt-Wallace (Dr. Goldberg); and the Theodore and Vada Stanley Foundation, a program of the NAMI Research Institute (Drs. Altshuler and Keck).

Editor's Note

In 1990, the overall annual cost of bipolar illness was estimated to be about $27.8 billion in lost productivity, $7.7 billion in direct treatment costs, and another $7.5 billion attributed to mortality due to suicide, for a total of approximately $43 billion. In this chapter the authors present an analysis of the cost effectiveness of treating patients with bipolar disorder with lithium, and compare this approach with the cost of using divalproex sodium instead. The parameters of calculating costs within the model used are described.

The clinical efficacy of divalproex sodium appears to be comparable to that of lithium. But efficacy for any drug reflects optimal outcome among highly select patient samples and is often not the same as effectiveness, which reflects "real world" outcome among nonselect patients, many of whom are excluded from controlled clinical trials. In the author's study, the annual cost savings associated with divalproex sodium over lithium was approximately $4,000 per patient. A major clinical and pharmacoeconomic advantage of divalproex sodium involves the rapidity with which therapeutic levels can be achieved during an acute manic episode, in contrast to lithium, the dosage of which must be built up more gradually. The total direct costs of treating classical, mixed/dysphoric, or rapidly cycling bipolar disorder for one year with lithium were approximately 60% higher for bipolar patients who initially presented with mixed/dysphoric manic episodes as compared with classical or rapidly cycling presentations. Treatment with divalproex sodium allowed the cost of treating mixed dysphoric or rapidly cycling illness to be only about 30% higher than the cost of treating the classical form. Costs associated with patients on divalproex sodium were 15% lower in those with mixed/dysphoric episodes at intake, and approximately 66% lower for those with rapidly cycling index episodes, as compared to similar cases receiving lithium.

In psychiatry, the many variables which influence outcome make such studies exceedingly complex, particularly when psychosocial factors are considered. As managed care focuses on the most cost-effective ways to treat patients, more studies of this type will emerge to help us select treatment approaches that are both economical and effective.

Introduction

The introduction of anticonvulsant mood stabilizers has dramatically changed the acute management and prevention of affective episodes in bipolar disorder. In much the same way lithium revolutionized the treatment of mania and depression a generation ago, anticonvulsants, such as divalproex sodium (Depakote) and carbamazepine (Tegretol), are increasingly being used for the acute management of mania, for maintenance pharmacotherapy, and for otherwise treatment-resistant cases. Furthermore, a number of studies have identified subgroups of bipolar patients for which lithium provides only modest protection from manic or depressive recurrences. Although lithium remains a mainstay of both acute and long-term therapy for bipolar illness (it is the only medication currently approved by the Food and Drug Administration for the long-term prophylaxis of bipolar illness), treatment outcome is often suboptimal under ordinary clinical conditions.[1-5] **Even when lithium successfully reduces morbidity from bipolar illness, treatment is often limited due to its side effects, overdosing, noncompliance, residual symptoms, or comorbid conditions.** Bipolar disorder continues to produce substantial clinical, emotional, social, and financial hardship for patients; consequently, new and more effective treatment strategies are urgently needed. Anticonvulsants, such as divalproex sodium offer an important advance toward better pharmacologic management of bipolar disorder. **Notably, treatment with divalproex sodium has been associated with better efficacy than treatment with lithium for nonclassical and complex forms of mania, such as mixed states, rapid cycling, or comorbid presentations of the illness.**[6-11] Moreover, unlike lithium's effects in acute mania, divalproex sodium has a clinical onset of action as early as one week when administered via oral loading,[12] a time course comparable to that of haloperidol (Haldol).[13] **Divalproex sodium is associated with fewer side effects compared to lithium, and poses a lesser potential risk for treatment noncompliance.**[14,15] **Lithium-associated side effects, such as cognitive impairment,**[16] **also have been shown to remit when a treatment regimen is changed from lithium to divalproex sodium.**[17] These observations have created interest not only in the possible clinical benefits of divalproex sodium, but also in its potential efficiency and economic advantages.

Disability and Costs of Bipolar Illness

Ranked among the leading causes of disability worldwide,[18,19] **bipolar disorder is associated with frequent use of medical and psychiatric services, extensive vocational and social impairment,**[20-24] **and markedly elevated risk for additional disorders, such as comorbid substance abuse.**[10,25,26] **Even with treatment, most patients experience multiple recurrent manic or depressive episodes.**[27-30] **Recent follow-up studies have further shown that subsyndromal symptoms and impaired psychosocial functioning between episodes are common for**

many bipolar patients.[20–24,31,32]

Data from the NIMH Collaborative Depression Study revealed that at 2-year follow-up, 28% of patients with mixed mania had not yet recovered from an index episode (as contrasted with only 4% of patients who had pure mania at index); at five years, 17% of the mixed mania cohort remained unrecovered.[31] Other follow-up studies have reported that many patients who achieve symptomatic remission may have persistently impaired psychosocial functioning and may fail to regain premorbid levels of work performance.[20–24,32]

Greenberg and colleagues[33] estimated that **in 1990, bipolar illness and depression resulted in approximately 289 million days of patients being off work, a loss equivalent to $27.8 billion due to absenteeism and diminished work productivity; an additional $7.7 billion was associated with direct treatment costs; and $7.5 billion was attributed to mortality due to suicide. These figures total to a yearly deficit of approximately $43 billion.** In a similar 1991 economic survey by Wyatt and Henter, total treatment costs for bipolar disorder were estimated to be $45.2 billion.[34] Of this amount, only $7.5 billion (17%) was attributed to direct costs such as expenditures for inpatient/outpatient treatment and nontreatment-related expenditures, which included criminal justice system costs. An indirect cost of $37.6 billion (83%) was estimated as the lost productivity of: wage-earners, homemakers, individuals who were in institutions or committed suicide, and caregivers of family members with bipolar disorder.

Direct Expenses:

Direct expenses related to bipolar illness include costs of hospitalization and medications (including adjunctive medications and medications needed to counteract side effects), laboratory testing, and costs related to adverse treatment events (such as emergency room visits or medical intensive care admissions due to overdose or toxicity). Wyatt and Henter[34] categorized the major portion of direct costs as relating to housing and domiciliary needs ($3.1 billion); followed by inpatient costs ($2.4 billion); crime ($2.3 billion); substance use comorbidity ($720 million); outpatient services ($300 million); and medications ($130 million).

Similarly, in estimating total treatment-related costs during the first year following an initial manic episode, **Keck and colleagues**[35] estimated that the majority of expenses derive from initial hospitalization costs (57%–60% of total annual cost), followed by inpatient and outpatient expenses related to relapse (approximately 35% of 1-year costs). Drug acquisition and maintenance treatment (i.e., physician fees, laboratory tests, and concomitant medications for symptoms or side effects) accounted for the remaining 5%–8% of treatment expenses.

Indirect Expenses:

Indirect expenses of bipolar disorder include days lost from work or diminished work productivity and suicide. In economic analyses by Wyatt and Henter,[34] this amounted to $29.8 billion from lost work productivity and an additional $8 billion due to suicide. Lost earnings due to premature death constitute further devastation for patients, families, and society; completed suicide occurs in up to 20% of bipolar patients, making the risk for suicide in bipolar illness among the highest of any major psychiatric disorder.[36] Moreover, almost half of all bipolar patients attempt suicide at least once, making morbidity or death from uncompleted suicide attempts a substantial factor in both the suffering and cost of bipolar illness. Federal estimates suggest that a 25-year-old woman with untreated bipolar disorder will lose, on average, 9 years of life expectancy and 14 years in work productivity; with appropriate treatment, 6.5 years of life expectancy may be recaptured along with the equivalent of 10 years of work productivity.[37]

Comorbid Psychopathology or Medical Conditions:

Comorbid psychopathology or medical conditions account for a further source of treatment needs and health care costs of bipolar illness. According to data from the Epidemiological Catchment Area (ECA) Study, the prevalence of alcoholism or other substance abuse ranges from 30%–60% among patients with bipolar disorder, making substance abuse more likely to coexist with bipolar illness than with any other Axis I disorder.[38] In addition to substance abuse, a number of other medical and/or psychopathologic conditions are more frequent among bipolar patients than in the general population.[26] These include: panic disorder,[39] eating disorders,[40] obsessive-compulsive disorder,[41] and personality disorders.[42] Among children and adolescents, increasing attention has been paid to a possible diagnostic overlap or comorbidity between attention deficit-hyperactivity disorder and mania in half or more of adolescent bipolar patients.[43,44] Comorbid illness has been cited in connection with a substantial proportion of poor treatment outcomes during lithium prophylaxis.[25] Thus, treatment costs for bipolar disorder often entail the need for additional resources, medications, and psychosocial interventions for common secondary conditions.

Although complex or comorbid presentations of mania appear to be linked with a poorer disease course, several studies have observed that concurrent substance abuse does not result in greater treatment costs.[45–47] Bauer and colleagues[47] note that **bipolar patients with substance abuse may be less inclined to *seek* treatment, suggesting that *indirect* illness costs may be higher for complex bipolar patients even when service use is not elevated.** Bipolar patients who report a history of childhood physical abuse have been reported to use psychiatric services more intensively, an observation which could support the view that developmental psychosocial insults may impede coping and illness management skills.[47]

The Economic Impact of Lithium on Bipolar Disorder

Lithium carbonate has been credited with a dramatic reduction in the economic and psychosocial burden of bipolar disorder. Reifman and Wyatt[48] reviewed average inpatient and outpatient costs for bipolar disorder during the first decade following the introduction of lithium in the United States. **From 1970–1980, the use of lithium was linked with a reduction in treatment costs** (including medication, psychotherapy, laboratory monitoring, and hospitalization expenses) **estimated to be $2.88 billion; an additional $1.28 billion gain was estimated in increased work productivity, leading to a net gain of $4.16 billion.**[48]

Data have been mixed on trends in hospitalization for mania since the availability of lithium. Morrison and McCreadie[49] and McCreadie[50] observed a substantial decrease in the number and length of hospital stays for acute mania in Scotland from before lithium (average 25 days per year) to after (average 11 days per year), estimating the net savings in hospitalization costs to be $34 million (adjusted). On the other hand, Dickson and Kendell[1] found that the introduction of

Table 7.1
Comparative One-Year Treatment Costs For Bipolar Illness, By Initial Treatment (Mean Overall Costs)*

Component of Cost	Lithium	Divalproex Sodium
Total Cost, mean over all patients	$43,400	$39,643
Initial Hospitalization	$25,916	$22,531
Room, services, fees	$25,865	$22,467
Drug (either treatment)	$50	$65
Prophylactic Treatment	$1862	$1832
Physician fees	$876	$870
Lab tests, procedures	$802	$827
Side effects	$72	$51
Concomitant medications	$77	$82
Drug Acquisition	$727	$1086
Divalproex sodium	$604	$1021
Lithium	$124	$66
Treatment of Relapse	$14,931	$14,193
Inpatient costs	$14,493	$13,775
Outpatient costs	$343	$328
Drugs (either treatment)	$95	$90

*Negligible costs not included.

Keck PE Jr., Nabulsi AA, Taylor JL, Henke CJ, Chmiel JJ, Stanton SP, Bennett JA. A pharmacoeconomic model of divalproex sodium vs. lithium in the acute and prophylactic treatment of bipolar I disorder. *J Clin Psychiatry*. 1996;57:213–222. Physicians Postgraduate Press. Adapted with permission.

lithium was *not* associated with a significant decrease in the number of psychiatric hospitalizations for manic-depressive illness in Edinburgh during a comparable time period. In another study, **Mander**[51] noted an *increase* in admissions for mania during the 1970s and 1980s in Great Britain, despite the increased use of lithium—a finding which could not be fully accounted for by changes from diagnoses of schizophrenia to those of mania in some patients. Studies comparing the number of hospital admissions or length of hospital stay among different patient cohorts or different time periods may be skewed by nonpharmacologic factors, such as: changing trends in making the diagnosis of bipolar disorder; changes in the epidemiology of comorbid conditions (e.g., substance abuse); the growth of intensive outpatient programs and alternatives to hospitalization; and the increasing influence of managed care over inpatient treatment in the United States.

Table 7.2
Total Estimated Direct Costs of Bipolar Disorder During One Year of Treatment*

Bipolar Subtype	Lithium	Divalproex Sodium
Classical mania	$31,426	$33,139
Mixed/dysphoric mania	$50,856	$43,672
Rapid cycling	$49,078	$42,792

Data derived from Keck et al.[86]

In recent years, unexpectedly poor outcome has been described for a substantial number of bipolar patients who receive lithium under ordinary conditions.[1,2,4,27,28,52] Claims that lithium may be only moderately effective in actual practice derive from arguments **that studies of lithium's *efficacy*** (reflecting optimal outcome among highly select patients samples) **are not generalizable to its *effectiveness*** (reflecting "real world" outcome among non-select patients, those who are often excluded from controlled clinical trials). Indeed, Bowden and colleagues[53] noted that up to 90% of patients who are diagnosed as bipolar within the community fail to meet inclusion criteria for randomized clinical trials, suggesting that efficacy-based treatment studies too often represent treatment outcome for a small, nonrepresentative minority of bipolar patients. **Reasons for excluding bipolar patients from efficacy-based treatment studies typically involve comorbid psychopathology, medical conditions, or substance abuse disorders; such comorbidities are evident in over half of most patients with bipolar illness.**[26] Patients who are too severely ill to follow the demands of complying with a treatment protocol also may seldom enter and/or complete a rigorous treatment study.

Specialized lithium clinics, which promote close observation and psychosocial engagement, may lessen the gap between lithium efficacy and effectiveness for some bipolar patients.[54] Naturalistic follow-up studies have identified a number of *shortcomings* associated with

Table 7.3
**Total Estimated Annual Direct Costs Among Bipolar
Responders Who Do Not Relapse After One Year***

Bipolar Subtype	Lithium	Divalproex Sodium
Classical mania	$20,348	$19,721
Mixed/dysphoric mania	$26,714	$22,575
Rapid cycling	$24,708	$16,268

Data derived from Keck et al.[″]

lithium treatment, with implications for clinical outcome, as well as pharmacoeconomics and treatment cost. These shortcomings include the following:

- **High relapse rates.** Affective relapse rates, despite ongoing treatment with lithium, range from 40%–80%.[5,21,22,27,30]

- **Poor efficacy in nonclassical bipolar subtypes.** The efficacy of lithium appears to be diminished in presentations involving rapid cycling,[55] mixed mania,[6,7,56,57] comorbid substance abuse,[10] or the depressed phase of bipolar illness.[58-60]

- **High illness burden may diminish lithium responsivity.** Several investigators have observed that if multiple affective episodes elapse before lithium is begun, the likelihood of a favorable treatment outcome with lithium is poor.[5,54,61-63]

- **Need for additional medications.** During both acute and maintenance phases of treatment, most bipolar patients (approximately 80%) are not stabilized on lithium alone and require the use of one or more adjunctive medications.[35,63] These most often include benzodiazepines, antipsychotics, or anticonvulsant mood stabilizers. Only a small minority of patients who are stabilized on lithium monotherapy appear to have good outcome.[5,63]

- **Rapid titration of lithium dosing may be poorly tolerated.** It is possible that rapid loading of lithium may produce faster clinical improvement than a more gradual dosing titration for acute mania.[64,65] However, a higher incidence of gastrointestinal and other side effects may occur when patients are dosed aggressively with lithium.[66]

- **Lithium has a narrow therapeutic safety index.** The dosing range at which toxic levels may develop is not far beyond the therapeutic range, making the need for close monitoring of blood levels essential.

- **High noncompliance rates lead to relapse.** Goodwin and Jamison estimated that 50% or more of bipolar patients become noncompliant with lithium prophylaxis, contributing to a significant proportion of relapses and rehospitalizations for bipolar disorder.[36] Even among initial responders to lithium, up to 40% discontinue their own lithium prophylaxis after two years.[27] Noncompliance, in and of itself, has been associated with the use of *multiple psychotropic drugs* in the long-term treatment of bipolar disorder, thus contributing further to overall costs related to psychiatric care.[67]

- **Side effects.** Side effects of ongoing lithium treatment include: weight gain, mental slowing, urinary frequency, hypothyroidism, ataxia, gastrointestinal disturbances, and other features.[36] A survey by Gitlin and colleagues[16] *identified side effects, particularly cognitive blunting and lack of coordination, as a major source of noncompliance and patient dissatisfaction with lithium.*

- **Discontinuation-induced refractoriness.** Several reports in the literature have suggested that when bipolar patients abruptly discontinue lithium, they are more likely to relapse faster, as well as become *resistant* to subsequent retrials of lithium.[68–70]

The Impact of Divalproex Sodium

Divalproex sodium was approved for use as an anticonvulsant in the United States in 1978; it received subsequent approval for use in the treatment of mania from the Food and Drug Administration in 1995. **Two randomized, double-blind clinical trials have demonstrated its** superior efficacy to placebo and comparable efficacy to lithium for acute mania.[6,56] Subsequent analysis of the multi-center study of Bowden and colleagues[6] by Swann and colleagues[7] indicated that divalproex sodium was superior to lithium among acutely manic patients with concurrent depressive features. According to Expert Consensus Guidelines for the Treatment of Bipolar Disorder,[11] divalproex sodium is considered the treatment of choice for mixed/dysphoric mania or for patients with a rapidly cycling course.

At present, data are more plentiful regarding the acute, rather than long-term or maintenance, treatment of bipolar illness with divalproex sodium, especially as monotherapy. However, a recent pilot study by Solomon and colleagues[71] found that *augmentation* of lithium with divalproex sodium was associated with fewer relapses during a 1-year follow-up period, as compared to lithium plus placebo. Another preliminary report by Denicoff and colleagues[72] found moderate to marked clinical improvement over a one year period when divalproex sodium was added to lithium (6 of 18 subjects, or 33%) or to triple therapy with divalproex sodium, lithium and carbamazepine (3 of 7 patients, or 43%).

Divalproex sodium has been studied and shown to be **well-tolerated in special populations, including: bipolar adolescents;**[73] **patients with geriatric mania;**[74,75] **refractory bipolar patients with rapid cycling;**[9,76] **and medically ill bipolar patients, including those with AIDS-related mania.**[77]

Attaining Rapid Therapeutic Effects

Several lines of evidence suggest that **a major clinical and pharmacoeconomic advantage of divalproex sodium involves the rapidity with which therapeutic levels can be achieved during an acute manic episode.** Keck and colleagues[12] have described **the strategy of orally loading divalproex sodium dosed at 20 mg/kg body weight, a generally well-tolerated technique which can significantly reduce the extent and severity of manic symptoms within 3–5 days.** McElroy and colleagues[13] found that **when acute manic patients underwent oral loading with divalproex sodium, a 50% reduction in mania rating scores was evident in less than one week, and antipsychotic response was comparable to that of haloperidol** (Haldol). Moreover, **anti-manic thera-**

peutic blood levels of valproic acid[78] are measurable within 24 hours of oral loading; this suggests less variability and delay in reaching steady state levels of divalproex sodium as compared with lithium.

It is possible to infer, at least in part, that the speed of clinical improvement with divalproex sodium over other mood stabilizers involves the relatively short time in which a therapeutic level of medication is achieved.[79] Consistent with this hypothesis, Goldberg and colleagues[64] recently found that **the time required to achieve a therapeutic blood level of lithium, divalproex sodium, or carbamazepine was the strongest factor associated with remission in acute manic inpatients at the Payne Whitney Clinic of Cornell Medical Center.** Delays in reaching therapeutic blood levels predicted nonremission while controlling for: choice of mood stabilizer, mixed or pure manic subtype, baseline severity, lifetime duration of illness, or substance abuse history. **The probability of achieving remission declined by 27% for every week needed to attain a therapeutic blood level of either lithium, divalproex sodium, or carbamazepine.**

Conceivably, lithium loading for acute mania may produce remission at rates similar to that of divalproex.[65,80,81] Swift improvement from mixed or pure manic episodes may be strongly tied to the speed and aggressiveness of undertaking any mood-stabilizer. However, **because a rapid dosing titration of either lithium or carbamazepine is often less well tolerated than divalproex sodium,**[80,82] **routine clinical outcome may be less successful when oral loading strategies are attempted with agents other than divalproex sodium.**

Length of Hospital Stay

Frye and colleagues,[83] conducting a retrospective study of mixed and dysphoric manic inpatients at the UCLA Medical Center, found that **hospital discharge occurred significantly sooner among patients treated nonrandomly with either divalproex sodium** (mean 10.2 days) **or lithium plus carbamazepine** (mean 11.7 days), **as compared to lithium alone** (mean 17.6 days). Therapeutic blood levels were reached in most patients who received divalproex sodium within 5 days of beginning treatment, as compared with only about one-quarter of those who had received lithium.[82] Findings from the Cornell database,[64] on the equivalent outcome of rapidly-dosed lithium or divalproex sodium, are also consistent with data from the UCLA cohort by Frye and colleagues,[83] in that subtherapeutic blood levels of either agent were uncommon among patients with short-length hospitalizations.

Keck and colleagues[84] extrapolated total hospitalization costs for the differential lengths of stay from the UCLA database, using medication and hospitalization costs from the University of Cincinnati Hospital. **Using these cost parameters, patients who had been prescribed divalproex sodium rather than lithium had an associated cost savings of $4,693.45 per patient.** *However, published data on length of hospital stay and comparative response rates to lithium versus divalproex sodium are derived from only a small number of studies, focusing on patient cohorts from only several clinical settings; such limitations do not allow broad generalizability of these data.*[85]

Small sample sizes and the nonrandomization of treatment groups further limit definitive interpretations about the relationship between length of hospital stay and the choice of drug regimen in these studies. Nonetheless, **findings in this area suggest that** *some* **bipolar patients may fare better clinically and incur lower treatment costs with pharmacotherapies other than lithium.**

The impetus for pharmacoeconomic analyses of treating bipolar illness with divalproex sodium versus lithium stems in part from differences in the treatment response of mixed, rapidly cycling, or pure manic bipolar patients. Because mixed/dysphoric manic episodes resolve more slowly with lithium treatment than classical or pure manic episodes do,[31] **the likelihood for greater morbidity and expense in** *nonclassical* **mania is high. Even though the daily pill cost is at least twice as high for therapeutically-dosed divalproex sodium as for therapeutically-dosed lithium** (compare $6.88 for 2000 mg/day divalproex sodium versus $3.60 for 1200 mg/day of lithium according to data reported by Keck and colleagues[84]**), total treatment expenses become heavily influenced by an array of additional factors. These include: the prevalence of mixed states; the comparative risk for relapse; the need for additional medications; and the need for prolonged, ancillary, or adjunctive psychosocial treatments.** Furthermore, features often linked with disability and poor outcome with lithium may be associated with *less* disability and a *better* treatment outcome with divalproex sodium.[84]

Pharmacoeconomic Models of Divalproex Sodium in Bipolar Illness

Keck and colleagues[86] developed a decision-analytic model to estimate the comparative costs of treatment for one year regarding divalproex sodium versus lithium. Data for the model were pooled from two published studies,[83,84] the University of Cincinnati Mania Project database,[24] and a consensus panel of five senior psychiatrists. For lithium and divalproex **sodium, the parameters of calculating costs within the model included: length of hospital stay; response rates; relapse rates; probabilities of hospitalization at first presentation; side effect treatment costs; prophylactic treatment costs; ratios of reimbursement under Medicare; and prevalence rates of mixed mania, classical mania, and rapid cycling.** As illustrated in Figure 7.1, the model is weighted by coefficients derived from expert consensus panelists and from the University of Cincinnati database. The system allows the clinician to estimate the total projected costs with either lithium or divalproex sodium treatment for one year.

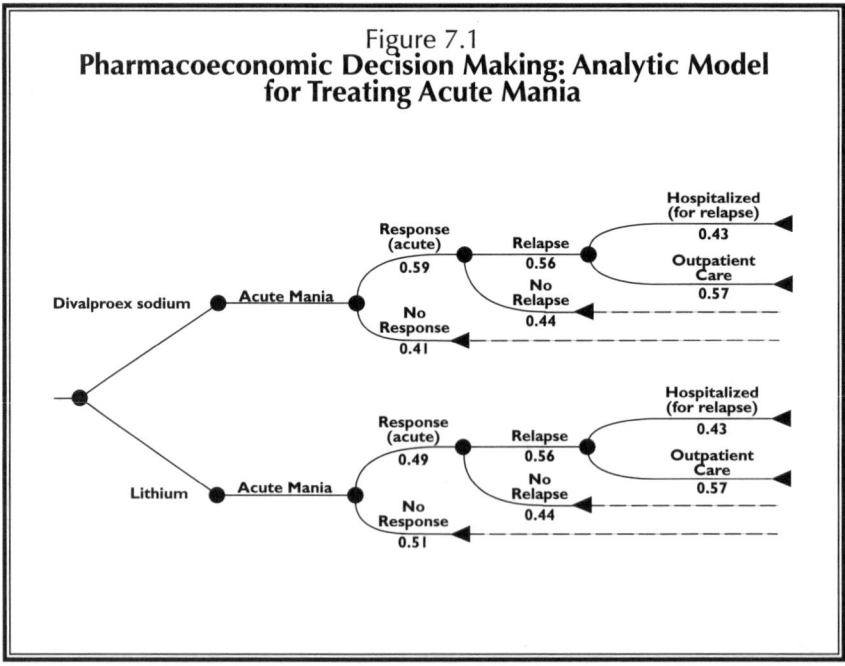

Figure 7.1
Pharmacoeconomic Decision Making: Analytic Model for Treating Acute Mania

Mean component treatment costs for one year of treatment with either lithium or divalproex sodium are summarized in Table 7.1. **In this model, the total annual cost savings associated with divalproex sodium over lithium was nearly $4,000 per patient.**

Stratification by bipolar subtypes further clarifies the relative costs associated with divalproex sodium or lithium. As outlined in Table 7.2, **the total direct costs of treating classical, mixed/dysphoric, or rapidly cycling bipolar disorder for one year with lithium were approximately 60% higher for bipolar patients who initially presented with mixed/dysphoric manic episodes, as compared with classical or rapidly cycling manic episodes. In contrast, treatment with divalproex sodium allowed the comparative direct cost of treatment for mixed/dysphoric or rapidly cycling bipolar illness to be only about 30% higher than the cost of treating classical mania.**

Breakdowns of treatment costs in most economic studies of bipolar illness suggest that a substantial proportion of expenses in the first year of aftercare derive from expenses related to relapse. Keck and colleagues[86] separately analyzed treatment costs for each bipolar subtype, focusing on patients who were initially medication-responsive, but who *remained euthymic* in the year following an initial bipolar episode. As shown in Table 7.3, **even among bipolar patients for whom no relapse occurred during the first year of ongoing treatment, costs for patients who received divalproex sodium rather than lithium were approximately 15% lower among those with mixed/dysphoric episodes at intake, and approximately 66% lower for those with rapidly cycling index episodes.**

Collectively, for all forms of bipolar illness weighted by the relative prevalence of each of these 3 diagnostic subtypes, treatment with divalproex sodium was associated with an overall cost savings of 9%. *For classical mania, however, illness costs were consistently lower (or nearly equivalent) with lithium than with divalproex sodium*

Implications of these data become more striking when one considers the relative prevalence of mixed versus pure mania among contemporary bipolar patients. Modern epidemiologic studies suggest that **mixed manic and depressive features may be evident in half or more of bipolar patients during an acute episode.**[64,87] **DSM-IV criteria for a mixed state require the presence of a full manic and full major depressive episode. However, a number of investigators have called** for broader definitions of mixed mania, citing a high prevalence of subsyndromal depressive features during acute mania.[87-90] Because suicidality and dysphoria may be evident in half or more of acutely ill manic patients[36,91] a careful distinction between pure/classical and mixed/dysphoric states is vital to forecast both prognosis and differential treatment costs.

Limitations of Current Pharmacoeconomic Models

Potential limitations have been described concerning the decision-analytic model proposed by Keck and colleagues,[86] as well as broader issues regarding estimates of illness cost in bipolar disorder. One factor concerns the high degree of variability associated with decisions about length of hospitalization for acute affective episodes. In the current healthcare climate, decisions about whether to hospitalize an acutely ill manic patient (rather than devise alternative stabilization strategies, such as intensive outpatient care or extended brief Emergency Department visits) are often multideterminate and involve nonclinical constraints.

Keck and colleagues[86] subanalyzed the sensitivity for each of the component variables in the decision analytic model, comparing the cost impact for changes in any single factor by **changes of one standard deviation. Hospital length of stay was considered to be a variable of high uncertainty, inasmuch as any change by one standard deviation resulted in marked changes in total costs. Nonclinical factors which may prolong acute psychiatric hospitalization commonly include: homelessness or the need to procure residential placement; access to intensive outpatient treatment or similar alternative levels of care; family support; vocational constraints; and the existence of an effective therapeutic alliance with a case manager or outpatient clinician.** "Experienced" bipolar patients who learn better skills for managing a chronic illness may also show greater adaptability and coping, which could further influence the trajectory of an affective recurrence and possible rehospitalization.[92]

Theoretically, **a potential advantage of divalproex sodium over other anti-manic treatments involves the capacity to stabilize even floridly ill manic patients using oral loading strategies and, conceivably, avert hospitalization altogether if intensive outpatient resources can be mobilized following extended (e.g., 72-hour) treatment within**

an Emergency Department. The longitudinal outcome for bipolar patients treated for acute mania through such a program has not yet been studied.

The decision-analytic model has also been criticized for assumptions it makes regarding the prophylactic efficacy of divalproex sodium, which has not yet been demonstrated in controlled clinical trials.[85]

Existing models also fail to account for the potential need for sequential treatment trials at the beginning of treatment for a presenting episode. **With the availability of multiple pharmacologic options for acute mania, stabilization of an acute episode may further depend on at least four factors: how far into a manic episode a treatment delay extends; how willing patients are to take a prescribed medication; whether medication interruptions** (e.g., noncompliance) **are frequent; and how likely it is that the first medication prescribed will prove successful. Among patients with refractory mania,** in ways similar to treatment-resistant unipolar depression,[93] **the need for multiple medication trials and potential augmentation strategies with second- or third-agent drugs may be significant.** Both the time course and treatment costs involved in such efforts may be disproportionately high relative to bipolar patients for whom a first-line agent requires only modest adjustment.

The need for adjunctive medications, both acutely and during long-term treatment, appears to be common in bipolar illness. Bipolar outpatients are significantly more likely than other psychiatric outpatients to receive multiple psychotropic agents.[94] **In the acute setting, almost all of the manic inpatients who received divalproex sodium in the studies by Frye and colleagues,**[83] **and by Goldberg and colleagues**[64] **received concomitant antipsychotics and/or benzodiazepines,** irrespective of treatment with divalproex sodium, lithium, or carbamazepine. **In the case of lithium maintenance, Sachs and colleagues**[63] **found that 80% of patients received two or more psychotropic agents; of patients on lithium monotherapy, 70% remained symptomatic.** Similarly, Sernyak and colleagues[95] and Keck and colleagues[35] found that long-term neuroleptic use was common in a substantial proportion of bipolar patients at follow-up.

Moreover, **little is known from controlled studies about the safety implications and possible toxic interactions when multiple mood stabilizers are combined.**[96,97] For example, **since lithium and divalproex** sodium may have clinical synergy, it is possible that their combination may produce additive side effects, leading to increased treatment costs. Given the popular practice of combining divalproex sodium or other anticonvulsants with lithium, maintenance studies with large bipolar samples are needed to further determine safety and cost, as well as whether adjunctive medications are less often needed with divalproex sodium than with other mood stabilizers.

Systematic studies have not, as yet, compared acute or prophylactic treatment outcome for divalproex sodium and other putative mood-stabilizing anticonvulsants, including carbamazepine,[98] lamotrigine (Lamictal),[99] and gabapentin (Neurontin).[100,101] It is currently unknown which anticonvulsants (with or without lithium) may provide the greatest synergy, clinical improvement, and cost-effectiveness. Especially among bipolar patients who respond poorly to lithium, such as those with rapid cycling and mixed states, the comparative efficacy and relative total costs associated with different anticonvulsants remains to be demonstrated. Preliminary data for a sample of 372 bipolar patients who received one year of double-blind maintenance treatment with divalproex sodium suggest superior prophylactic efficacy to placebo, and possibly to lithium, for some bipolar patients.[102]

The impact of pure depressed-phase episodes in bipolar illness also is not fully reflected in current models, and may represent a further source of high variation in costs with any current treatment. Bipolar depressive episodes are often less responsive to pharmacotherapy than are manic episodes,[60] and involve added complexities, such as the risk for either switches into mania[103] or accelerated cyclicity[104] induced by the use of antidepressants. Estimates of the risk for inducing mania in a depressed patient with no known history of bipolar illness have ranged from 10%-50%;[36] among known bipolar patients, the risk for accelerated cycling becomes even higher. While divalproex sodium appears superior to lithium among rapidly cycling bipolar patients, little data exist which specifically address the outcome of increased cycling or manias induced by treatment itself. Treatment costs also have not been compared for currently ill patients as a function of their past treatments; it is possible that bipolar patients who have been chronically exposed to antidepressants may have greater treatment needs or ultimately develop more refractory forms of illness. Whether or not divalproex sodium confers a pharmacologic advantage (and possible cost savings) **in such instances remains a matter for future study. In addition, little is known about whether divalproex sodium** (or other putative mood stabilizers) **effectively prevents both depressions and manias, or resolves episodes of bipolar-depression as readily as episodes of mania.**

Quitkin and colleagues[105] have noted that some patients with bipolar disorder may be more prone to manias or to depressions, suggesting that greater variability may arise depending on an individual's proclivity toward manias, depressions, or mixed states. Added costs related to the use (or avoidance) of antidepressants for bipolar depressions may drastically alter the overall cost of treatment. **In cases of severe or complex bipolar depression, as when suicidality, psychosis, or pregnancy are involved, many clinicians advocate electroconvulsive therapy (ECT) as the treatment of first choice.** Bipolar patients with especially severe or treatment-resistant depressions may require inpatient ECT, and therefore, may encounter prolonged hospitalizations and greater treatment costs.

The possible protective effect of divalproex sodium, specifically against suicide, in bipolar disorder has not yet been studied. Lithium treatment *has* been associated with a diminished incidence of suicide among bipolar patients.[106,107] ***Presumably*, since suicidality appears strongly linked with mixed manic states,**[90,108] **rates of attempted or completed suicide may be no greater** (and possibly lower) **with divalproex sodium than with lithium, although this remains to be demonstrated empirically.**

Cost-Effectiveness of Divalproex Sodium in Geriatric Samples

Bipolar disorder is common in the elderly,[109] **but the potential for drug sensitivities and adverse reactions to lithium, antipsychotics, or benzodiazepines can be high. Neuropsychological impairment is also common during lithium treatment and may aggravate underlying cognitive deficits in some elderly patients. Added costs for treating bipolar disorder in the elderly involve: morbidity due to medication intolerances; cognitive or other side effects; and the need for closer medical supervision than in younger bipolar patients** (e.g., lithium levels may readily become toxic due to malnutrition or underlying renal disease). In addition, other unique treatment costs in geriatric bipolar patients can stem from supportive living arrangements or homecare assistance, the impact of poorly-treated bipolar disorder on treatment compliance, and the course of concomitant medical illnesses.

Preliminary data support the efficacy and tolerability of divalproex sodium in the elderly.[74] **Recently, a retrospective study by Chen and Altshuler**[75] **found that lithium** (at levels >0.8 ug/mL) **and valproic acid** (at levels between 0.65–0.90 ug/mL) **were equally effective in treating acute mania** (both mixed and classical) **in elderly bipolar patients** when the outcome variable was a Clinical Global Impressions (CGI) score on discharge. While elderly patients required lithium serum levels comparable to those ordinarily needed among nonelderly patients for optimal antimanic response (i.e., >0.8mEq/L), a more narrow window for the serum level was observed for therapeutic response to valproic acid; patients with an optimal response (CGI score reflecting "much" or "very much" improvement) at discharge had valproic acid levels between 65-90 ug/mL. Only 20% of those elderly manic patients with valproic acid levels between 45-65 ug/mL had a CGI of marked or moderate improvement at discharge.

Cognitive deficits related to lithium have been shown to diminish by patient self-report when divalproex sodium is substituted for lithium during maintenance pharmacotherapy, as reported by Stoll and colleagues.[17] **Because divalproex sodium appears as effective as lithium in geriatric mania and may induce fewer cognitive side effects, the medical/psychiatric complications and costs associated with divalproex sodium in elderly bipolar patients may be significantly less.**

Summary

Divalproex sodium is an effective treatment for all phases of acute mania; it may also be effective in the maintenance treatment of bipolar disorder. Among bipolar patients with mixed or rapidly cycling episodes, divalproex sodium use is associated with an annual cost-savings of approximately $4000 per patient as compared with lithium, based on currently published treatment findings. In contrast, bipolar patients with pure/classical presentations of mania appear to have a comparable, if not better, clinical response and an overall greater cost savings when lithium is used as the primary mood stabilizer. Preliminary data further suggest that treatment with divalproex sodium is a safe and useful augmentation strategy when combined with other mood stabilizers for treating resistant forms of bipolar illness.

Clinical advantages of divalproex sodium may stem from the potential for rapidly achieving therapeutic dosages through oral loading, as well as a lower incidence of side effects and subsequent risks for non-compliance.

References

1. Dickson WE, Kendell RE. Does maintenance lithium therapy prevent recurrences of mania under ordinary clinical conditions? *Psychol Med.* 1986;16:521–530.

2. Markar HR, Mander AJ. Efficacy of lithium prophylaxis in clinical practice. *Br J Psychiatry.* 1989;155:496–500.

3. O'Connell RA, Mayo JA, Flatow L, Cuthbertson B, O'Brien BE. Outcome of bipolar disorder on long-term treatment with lithium. *Br J Psychiatry.* 1991;159:123–129.

4. Guscott R, Taylor L. Lithium prophylaxis in recurrent affective illness: efficacy, effectiveness and efficiency. *Br J Psychiatry.* 1994;164:741–746.

5. Goldberg JF, Harrow M, Leon AC. Lithium treatment of bipolar affective disorders under naturalistic followup conditions. *Psychopharmacol Bull.* 1996;32:47–54.

6. Bowden CL, Brugger AM, Swann AC,et al. Efficacy of divalproex sodium vs. lithium and placebo in the treatment of mania. *JAMA.* 1994;271:918–924.

7. Swann AC, Bowden CL, Morris D, et al. Depression during mania: treatment response to lithium or divalproex. *Arch Gen Psychiatry.* 1997;54:37–42.

8. Freeman TW, Clothier JL, Pazzaglia P, Lesem MD, Swann AC. A double-blind comparison of valproate and lithium in the treatment of acute mania. *Am J Psychiatry.* 1992;149:108–111.

9. Calabrese J. Spectrum of efficacy of valproate in 78 rapid-cycling bipolar patients. *J Clin Psychopharmacol.* 1992;12:53S–56S.

10. Brady KT, Sonne SC. The relationship between substance abuse and bipolar disorder. *J Clin Psychiatry.* 1995;56:19–24.

11. Frances A, Docherty JP, Kahn DA. The expert consensus guideline series: treatment of bipolar disorder. *J Clin Psychiatry.* 1996;57(suppl 12A):1–88.

12. Keck PE Jr., McElroy SL, Tugrul KC, Bennett JA. Valproate oral loading in the treatment of acute mania. *J Clin Psychiatry.* 1993;54:305–308.

13. McElroy SL, Keck PE Jr., Stanton SP, et al. A randomized comparison of divalproex sodium oral loading versus haloperidol in the initial treatment of acute psychotic mania. *J Clin Psychiatry.* 1996;57:142–146.

14. Tohen M. The adverse effect profile and safety of divalproex. *Rev Contemp Pharmacotherapy.* 1995;6:587–595.

15. Emilien G, Maloteaux JM, Seghers A, Charles G. Lithium compared to valproic acid and carbamazepine in the treatment of mania: a statistical meta-analysis. *European Neuropsychopharmacology*. 1996;6:245–252.

16. Gitlin MJ, Cochran SD, Jamison KR. Maintenance lithium treatment: side effects and compliance. *J Clin Psychiatry*. 1989;50:127–131.

17. Stoll AL, Locke CA, Vuckovic A, Mayer PV. Lithium-associated cognitive and functional deficits reduced by a switch to divalproex sodium sodium: a case series. *J Clin Psychiatry*. 1996;57:356–359.

18. Murray CJL, Lopez AD. Global mortality, disability and the contribution of risk factors: global burden of disease study. *Lancet*. 1997;349:1436–1442.

19. Jenkins R. Reducing the burden of mental illness. *Lancet*.1997;349:1340.

20. Dion GL, Tohen M, Anthony WA, Waternaux CS. Symptoms and functioning of patients with bipolar disorder six months after hospitalization. *Hosp Community Psychiatry*. 1988;39:652–657.

21. Gitlin MJ, Swendsen J, Heller T, Hammen C. Relapse and impairment in bipolar disorder. *Am J Psychiatry*. 1995;152:1635–1640.

22. Goldberg JF, Harrow M, Grossman LS. Course and outcome in bipolar affective disorder: a longitudinal follow-up study. *Am J Psychiatry*. 1995;152:379–384.

23. Strakowski SM, Keck PE Jr., McElroy SL, et al. Twelve-month outcome following hospitalization for affective psychosis. *Arch Gen Psychiatry*. 1998;55:49–55.

24. Keck PE Jr., McElroy SL, Strakowski SM, et al. Twelve-month outcome of bipolar patients following hospitalization for a manic or mixed episode. *Am J Psychiatry*. In Press.

25. Black DW, Winokur G, Hulbert J, Nasrallah A. Predictors of immediate response in the treatment of mania: the importance of comorbidity. *Biol Psychiatry*. 1988;24:191–198.

26. Strakowski SM, McElroy SL, Keck PE Jr, West SA. The co-occurrence of mania with medical and other psychiatric disorders. *Int J Med*. 1994;24:305–328.

27. Maj M, Pirozzi R, Kemali D. Long-term outcome of lithium prophylaxis in patients initially classified as complete responders. *Psychopharmacology*. 1989;98:521–530.

28. Harrow M, Goldberg JF, Grossman LS, Meltzer HY. Outcome in manic disorders: a naturalistic follow-up study. *Arch Gen Psychiatry*. 1990;47:665–671.

29. Tohen M, Waternaux CM, Tsuang MT. Outcome in mania: a 4-year prospective follow-up of 75 patients utilizing sirvival analysis. *Arch Gen Psychiatry*. 1990;47:1106–1111.

30. Coryell W, Winokur G, Solomon D, et al. Lithium and recurrence in a long-term follow-up of bipolar affective disorder. *Psychol Med*. 1997;27:281–289.

31. Keller MB, Lavori PW, Coryell W, Endicott J, Mueller TI. Bipolar I: a five-year prospective follow-up. *J Nerv Ment Dis*. 1993;140:689–694.

32. Coryell W, Scheftner W, Keller M, et al. The enduring psychosocial consequences of mania and depression. *Am J Psychiatry*. 1993;150:720–727.

33. Greenberg PE, Stiglin LE, Finkelstein SN, Berndt ER. The economic burden of depression in 1990. *J Clin Psychiatry*. 1993;54:405–418.

34. Wyatt RJ, Henter I. An economic evaluation of manic-depressive illness. *Soc Psychiatry Psychiatric Epidemiol.* 1995;30:213–219.

35. Keck PE Jr., McElroy SL, Strakowski SM, et al. Factors associated with maintenance neuroleptic treatment of patients with bipolar disorder. *J Clin Psychiatry.* 1996;57:147–151.

36. Goodwin FK, Jamison KR. *Manic-Depressive Illness.* New York: Oxford University Press;1990.

37. United States Department of Health, Education and Welfare. *Medical Practice Project: A State of the Science Report for the Office of the Assistant Secretary for the US Department of Health, Education and Welfare.* Baltimore, MD: Policy Research;1979.

38. Regier DA, Farmer ME, Rae DS, et al. Comorbidity of mental disorders with alcohol and other drug abuse: results from the Epidemiologic Catchment Area (ECA) Study. *JAMA.* 1990;264:2511–2518.

39. Chen W-W, Dilsaver SC. Comorbidity of panic disorder in bipolar illness: evidence from the Epidemiologic Catchment Area Survey. *Am J Psychiatry.* 1995;152:280–282.

40. Kruger S, Shugar G, Cooke RG. Comorbidity of binge eating disorder and the partial binge eating syndrome with bipolar disorder. *Int J Eating Disord.* 1996;19:45–52.

41. Kruger S, Cooke RG, Hasey GM, Jorna T, Persad E. Comorbidity of obsessive-compulsive disorder in bipolar disorder. *J Affect Disord.* 1995;34:117–120.

42. Akiskal HS. The prevalent clinical spectrum of bipolar disorders: beyond DSM-IV. *J Clin Psychopharmacol.* 1996;16:4–14.

43. West SA, McElroy SL, Strakowski SM, Keck PE Jr., McConville BJ. Attention deficit hyperactivity disorder in adolescent mania. *Am J Psychiatry.* 1995;152:271–273.

44. McElroy SL, Strakowski SM, West SA, Keck PE Jr, McConville BJ. A comparison of the phenomenology of adolescent versus adult mania in hospitalized patients with bipolar disorder. *Am J Psychiatry.* 1997;154:44–49.

45. Fogel B, Bauer M, Kendall S, Holden F. Psychiatric comorbidities and hospitalization for mania. *Biol Psychiatry.* 1994;35:421A.

46. Bradley C, Zarkin G. In-patient stays for patients diagnosed with severe psychiatric disorders and substance abuse. *Health Services Research.* 1996;31:387–409.

47. Bauer MS, Shea N, McBride L, Gavin C. Predictors of service utilization in veterans with bipolar disorder: a prospective study. *J Affect Disord.* 1997;44:159–168.

48. Reifman A, Wyatt RD. Lithium: a brake in the rising cost of mental illness. *Arch Gen Psychiatry.* 1980;37:385–388.

49. Morrison DP, McCreadie RG. The impact of lithium in South-West Scotland: II. a longitudinal study. *Br J Psychiatry.* 1985;146:74–77.

50. McCreadie RG. The economics of lithium therapy. In: Johnson FN, ed. *Depression and Mania: Modern Lithium Therapy.* Oxford: IRL Press;1987:257–259.

51. Mander AJ. Diagnosis change, lithium use and admissions for mania in Edinburgh. *Acta Psychiatr Scand.* 1989;80:434–436.

52. Goldberg JF, Harrow M, eds. *Bipolar Disorders: Clinical Course and Outcome.* Washington, DC: American Psychiatric Press;In Press.

53. Bowden CL, Calabrese JR, Wallin BA, et al. Illness characteristics of patients in clinical drug studies of mania. *Psychopharmacol Bull.* 1995;31:103–109.

54. Maj M, Pirozzi R, Magliano L, Bartoli L. Long-term outcome of lithium prophylaxis in bipolar disorder: A 5-year prospective study of 402 patients at a lithium clinic. *Am J Psychiatry.* 1998;155:30–35.

55. Dunner DL, Fieve RR. Clinical factors in lithium carbonate prophylaxis failure. *Arch Gen Psychiatry.* 1974;30:229–233.

56. Pope HG Jr, McElroy SL, Keck PE Jr, Hudson JI. Valproate in the treatment of acute mania: A placebo-controlled study. *Arch Gen Psychiatry.* 1991;68:62–68.

57. Prien RF, Himmelhoch JM, Kupfer DJ. Treatment of mixed mania. *J Affect Disord.* 1988;15:9–15.

58. Kane JM, Quitkin FM, Rifkin A, et al. Prophylactic lithium with and without imipramine for bipolar patients: A double-blind study. *Psychopharmacol Bull.* 1981;17:144–145.

59. Prien RF, Kupfer DJ, Mansky PA, et al. Drug therapy in the prevention of recurrences in unipolar and bipolar affective disorders: Report of the NIMH Colaborative Study Group comparing lithium carbonate, imipramine, and a lithium carbonate-imipramine combination. *Arch Gen Psychiatry.* 1983;41:1096–1104.

60. Sachs GS. Treatment-resistant bipolar depression. *Psychiatric Clinics of North America.* 1996;19:215–236.

61. Gelenberg AJ, Kane JM, Keller MB, et al. Comparison of standard and low serum levels of lithium for maintenance treatment of bipolar disorder. *NEJM.* 1989;332:1489–1493.

62. Post RM, Rubinow DR, Ballenger JC. Conditioning and sensitization in the longitudinal course of affective illness. *Br J Psychiatry.* 1986;149:191–201.

63. Sachs GS, Lafer B, Truman CJ,et al. Lithium monotherapy: Miracle, myth and misunderstanding. *Psychiatric Annals.* 1994;24:299–306.

64. Goldberg JF, Garno JL, Leon AC, Kocsis JH, Portera L. Rapid titration of mood stabilizers predicts remission from mixed or pure mania. *J Clin Psychiatry.* 1998;59:151–158.

65. Moscovich DG, Shapira B, Lerer B, Belmaker RH. Rapid lithiumization in acute manic patients. *Human Psychopharmacol.* 1992;7:343–345.

66. Keck PE Jr, Bennett JA, Stanton SP. Reply to Baker et al. (letter). *J Clin Psychiatry.* 1997;58:364.

67. Keck PE Jr., McElroy SL, Strakowski SM, et al. Factors associated with pharmacologic noncompliance in patients with mania. *J Clin Psychiatry.* 1996;57:292–297.

68. Suppes T, Balessarini RJ, Faedda GL, Tohen M. Risk of recurrence following discontinuation of lithium treatment in bipolar disorder. *Arch Gen Psychiatry.* 1991;48:1082–1088.

69. Post RM, Leverich GS, Altshuler L, Mikalauskas K. Lithium-discontinuation-induced refractoriness: preliminary observations. *Am J Psychiatry.* 1992;149:1727–1729.

70. Faedda GL, Tondo L, Baldessarini RJ, Suppes T, Tohen M. Outcome after rapid vs. gradual discontinuation of lithium treatment in bipolar disorders. *Arch Gen Psychiatry.* 1993;50:448–455.

71. Solomon DA, Ryan CE, Keitner GI, et al. A pilot study of lithium carbonate plus divalproex sodium for the continuation and maintenance treatment of patients with bipolar I disorder. *J Clin Psychiatry*. 1997;58:95–99.

72. Denicoff KD, Smith-Jackson EE, Bryan AL, Ali SO, Post RM. Valproate prophylaxis in a prospective clinical trial of refractory bipolar disorder. *Am J Psychiatry*. 1997;154:1456–1458.

73. Papatheodorou G, Kutcher SP. Divalproex sodium treatment in late adolescent and young adult mania. *Psychopharmacology Bull*. 1993;29:213–219.

74. McFarland BH, Miller MR, Straumfjord AA. Valproate use in the older manic patient. *J Clin Psychiatry*. 1990;51:479–481.

75. Chen S, Altshuler LL. *Efficacy of lithium versus valproic acid in the treatment of acute mania in the elderly*. Manuscript in preparation.

76. Schaff MR, Fawcett J, Zajecka JM. Divalproex sodium in the treatment of refractory affective disorders. *J Clin Psychiatry*. 1993;54:380–384.

77. RachBeisel JA, Weintraub E. Valproic acid treatment of AIDS-related mania (letter). *J Clin Psychiatry*. 1997;58:406–407.

78. Bowden CL, Janicak PG, Orsulak P, et al. Relation of serum valproate concentration to response in mania. *Am J Psychiatry*. 1996;153:765–770.

79. Baker CB, Woods SW, Sernyak MJ. Cost-effectiveness of divalproex sodium versus lithium (letter). *J Clin Psychiatry*. 1997;58:363.

80. Bowden CL. Dosing strategies and time course of response to antimanic drugs. *J Clin Psychiatry*. 1996;57(suppl 13):4–9.

81. Townes P, Swartz CM. Comparison of valproic acid and lithium in mania (letter). *J Clin Psychiatry*. 1997;58:273.

82. Altshuler LL, Frye MA. Reply to Townes and Swartz (letter). *J Clin Psychiatry*. 1997;58:273–274.

83. Frye MA, Altshuler LL, Szuba MP, Finch NN, Mintz J. The relationship between antimanic agent for treatment of classic or dysphoric mania and length of hospital stay. *J Clin Psychiatry*. 1996;57:17–21.

84. Keck PE Jr., Bennett JA, Stanton SP. Health-economic aspects of the treatment of manic-depressive illness with divalproex. *Rev Contemp Pharmacother*. 1995;6:597–604.

85. Dardennes RM, Even C. Is divalproex sodium a cost-effective alternative in the acute and prophylactic treatment of bipolar I disorder? (letter) *J Clin Psychiatry*. 1997;58:495–496.

86. Keck PE Jr., Nabulsi AA, Taylor JL, Henke CJ, Chmiel JJ, Stanton SP, Bennett JA. A pharmacoeconomic model of divalproex sodium vs. lithium in the acute and prophylactic treatment of bipolar I disorder. *J Clin Psychiatry*. 1996;57:213–222.

87. McElroy SL, Keck PE Jr., Pope HG, et al. Clinical and research implications of the diagnosis of dysphoric or mixed mania or hypomania. *Am J Psychiatry*. 1992;149:1633–1644.

88. Hantouche EG, Akiskal HS. Clinical assessment of affective temperaments. *Encephale*. 1997;23:27–34.

89. Bauer MS, Whybrow PC, Gyulai L, Gonnel J, Yeh H-S. Testing definitions of dysphoric mania and hypomania: prevalence, clinical characteristics, and inter-episode stability. *J Affect Disord.* 1994;32:201–211.

90. McElroy SL, Strakowski SM, Keck PE Jr., et al. Differences and similarities in mixed and pure mania. *Compr Psychiatry.* 1995;36:187–194.

91. Strakowski SM, McElroy SL, Keck PE Jr., West SA. Suicidality in mixed and manic bipolar disorder. *Am J Psychiatry.* 1996;153:674–676.

92. Bauer MS, McBride L. *Structured Group Psychotherapy for Bipolar Disorder: The Life Goals Program.* New York: Springer-Verlag;1996.

93. Thase ME, Rush AJ. Treatment-resistant depression. In: Bloom FE, Kupfer DJ, eds. *Psychopharmacology: The Fourth Generation of Progress.* New York: Raven Press;1995:1081–1097.

94. Nichols NB, Stimmel GL, Lange SC. Factors predicting the use of multiple psychotropic medications. *J Clin Psychiatry.* 1995;56:60–66.

95. Sernyak MJ, Woods SW. Chronic neuroleptic use in manic-depressive illness. *Psychopharmacol Bull.* 1993;29:375–381.

96. Frye MA. The increasing use of polypharmacy for refractory mood disorders: twenty-five years of study. New Research poster presentation at the 149th Annual Meeting of the American Psychiatric Association, New York, N.Y. May 7, 1996.

97. Freeman MP, Stoll AL. Mood stabilizer combinations: A review of safety and efficacy. *Am J Psychiatry.* 1998;155:12–21.

98. Denicoff KD, Smith-Jackson EE, Disney ER, et al. Comparative prophylactic efficacy of lithium, carbamazepine, and the combination in bipolar disorder. *J Clin Psychiatry.* 1997;58:470–478.

99. Sporn J, Sachs G. The anticonvulsant lamotrigine in treatment-resistant manic-depressive illness. *J Clin Psychopharmacol.* 1997;17:185–189.

100. Schaffer CB, Schaffer LC. Gabapentin in the treatment of bipolar disorder (letter). *Am J Psychiatry.* 1997;154:291–292.

101. Stanton SP, Keck PE Jr, McElroy SL. Treatment of acute mania with gabapentin (letter). *Am J Psychiatry.* 1997;154:287.

102. Bowden CL. Long-term prophylactic treatment priorities in bipolar disorder. Abstracts of the 20th Collegium International Neuropsychopharmacologicum Congress, Vienna, Austria, September, 1997. *European Neuropsychopharmacology.* 1997;7(suppl 2):S123.

103. Altshuler LL, Post RM, Leverich GS, Mikalauskas K, Rosoff A, Ackerman L. Antidepressant-induced mania and cycle acceleration: a controversy revisited. *Am J Psychiatry.* 1995;152:1130–1138.

104. Wehr TA, Goodwin FK. Can antidepressants cause mania and worsen the course of affective illness? *Am J Psychiatry.* 1987;144:1403–1411.

105. Quitkin FM, Rabkin JG, Prien RF. Bipolar disorder: are there manic-prone and depressive-prone forms? *J Clin Psychopharmacology.* 1986;6:167–172.

106. Muller-Oerlinghausen B, Muser-Causemann B, Volk J. Suicides and parasuicides in a high-risk patient group on and off lithium long-term medication. *J Affect Disord.* 1992;25:261–269.

107. Ahrens B, Muller-Oeringhausen B, Schou M, et al. Excess cardiovascular and suicide mortality of affective disorders may be reduced by lithium prophylaxis. *J Affect Disord.* 1995;33:67–75.05.

108. Goldberg JF, Garno JL, Leon AC, Kocsis JH. Suicidality in mixed versus pure mania. Scientific Proc 150th Ann Meet Am Psychiatric Assoc. 1997:4–5.

109. Young RC, Klerman GL. Mania in late life: focus on age at onset. *Am J Psychiatry.* 1992;149:867–876.

8 Management of Treatment-Resistant Bipolar and Schizoaffective Disorders

Trisha Suppes, MD, PhD

Dr. Suppes is Assistant Professor of Psychiatry and Director of the Bipolar Disorders Clinic, University of Texas Southwestern Medical Center, Dallas, and Codirector, Stanley Foundation Bipolar Network, Dallas.

Supported, in part, by grants from a NARSAD Young Investigator Award, the Forrest C. Lattner Foundation, and the Stanley Foundation.

Thanks to Chris Claeson for secretarial support and to Andrew Webb for editorial assistance.

Editor's Note

Although treatment for bipolar disorder is improving, with studies showing the effectiveness of new medications, a substantial portion of patients remain treatment resistant. In this chapter, Dr. Suppes reviews recent advances in the pharmacotherapy of treatment-resistant patients.

Lithium remains the best studied treatment for bipolar disorder, both for acute mania and long-term maintenance therapy. Data support the use of valproic acid (Depakene) and carbamazepine (Tegretol) for acute treatment, but neither has been well studied for long-term maintenance treatment. When treatment with a single mood stabilizer fails, combination treatment is indicated. In the absence of rigorous studies comparing outcomes with each possible combination, clinicians must proceed through trial and error, carefully monitoring target symptoms and side effects.

In addition to combinations of lithium and the anticonvulsants, other agents may be useful. Several open studies support the effectiveness of clozapine (Clozaril), an atypical antipsychotic agent, for treatment-resistant patients. Data on the usefulness of risperidone (Risperdal) and olanzapine (Zyprexa), two newer atypical antipsychotics, are more preliminary.

169

Also under investigation for treatment of bipolar disorder are two newer anticonvulsants, lamotrigine (Lamictal) and gabapentin (Neurontin). Both have been approved by the Food and Drug Administration for the treatment of epilepsy. Early experience suggests that each may be useful as mood stabilizers, although they may have different applications in the treatment of bipolar patients.

Introduction

The severe and persistent nature of bipolar disorder has been increasingly recognized in recent years, even in patients in whom primary symptoms are well controlled.[1,2] Awareness of the limitations of long-term lithium monotherapy parallels developing appreciation of the severity of this illness.[3-8] **A universally accepted definition of treatment-resistant bipolar disorder does not yet exist.** Some authors define it as failure of one mood stabilizer when used with a typical antipsychotic.[9] Others view treatment resistance as the failure of two mood stabilizers when used simultaneously and, if the patient is psychotic, the failure of an antipsychotic medication.[10] However, relatively few controlled trials on the maintenance treatment and management of patients with bipolar disorder or schizoaffective illness exist.[11-13]

Long-term follow-up studies of patients receiving lithium support that effective maintenance treatment may occur in approximately only one third to one half of patients initially responding to lithium.[3-6,8,14] The causes of symptom recurrences, whether because of medication failure or lack of treatment compliance, are unresolved.[5,7]

Treatment guidelines or algorithms have sought to develop treatment plans for patients with a history of mania. None of these guidelines has focused on treatment-resistant conditions specifically but has included possible options after the first treatment fails. In addition, treatment recommendations do not come from randomized control trial data after the first monotherapy line (because there are none) but are based on opinion or clinical consensus.[15-19]

This chapter briefly reviews the current state of knowledge and consensus on treating patients with bipolar disorder and schizoaffective illness. It examines some newer medications currently available such as the anticonvulsants (e.g., gabapentin [Neurontin] and lamotrigine

[Lamictal]). Before discussing treatment options, basic principles important to treating patients with a history of mania are outlined.

Principles of Managing Medications in Patients with a History of Mania

Three principles are critical for managing patients with a history of mania: (a) how medication changes are made, (b) the use of combinations of medications, and (c) the need for patient education (Table 8.1). These principles apply to all patients with bipolar-type disorders, from the mildest bipolar II to the most severe bipolar I or schizoaffective bipolar-type patient.

The first principle is that all medication changes should be done in an overlap and taper fashion. Accumulated naturalistic data suggest that how medication changes are made influences the rate of recurrence.[20–23] Traditionally, patients with major depressive disorder have been "switched" from one antidepressant to another with no overlap. However, this is highly contraindicated in patients with a history of mania. In fact, a distinguishing characteristic of patients with bipolar versus unipolar mood disorder may be that patients with bipolar disorders are susceptible to destabilization when changes are made too quickly.[21–24] A common strategy among physicians treating bipolar patients is to add on (i.e., overlap) and later begin tapering partially effective or ineffective medication once the patient is well stabilized.

Given that the rate of medication discontinuation may affect rates of recurrence for patients with a history of mania, one implication of making rapid changes is the difficulty of evaluating the relative effectiveness of a new medication. For example, assume lithium was abruptly stopped and an anticonvulsant mood stabilizer started in its place. Three weeks later, the patient is within therapeutic levels for the anticonvulsant but decompensates. One possibility is the anticonvulsant was ineffective. However, based on the accumulated studies of lithium discontinuation for bipolar patients, an equally viable hypothesis is that the decompensation is because of abrupt lithium discontinuation. Based on the naturalistic data cited above, any taper of 2 weeks or less is considered rapid. Very little information exists on the impact of discontinuing mood stabilizers other than lithium.

In sum, regardless of the patient's illness severity when changes are necessary, the recommendation is to overlap and gradually taper medications, except in cases of medical necessity. This implies medication changes will be a long-term process, but this approach to medication changes is crucial to treating these patients. Furthermore, patients need to know how limited the information on combining medications is if monotherapy proves ineffective. Because it often will take 4–6 months to find an effective combination of medications, it is crucial that the patient develop a long-term perspective.

Table 8.1
Principles in Treatment of Bipolar Patients

- Overlap and gradually taper all medications.
- More than one medication may be needed for fully efficacious treatment.
- Treatment is empiric because of limited understanding of the pathophyisiology of the illness.
- Do not be afraid to carefully mix and match possible medication choices.
- Treat subsyndromal or residual symptoms of the illness.
- Patient (and family) education about the illness and medications is crucial.

The second principle is that many patients with bipolar or schizoaffective disorder will need more than one medication to manage the symptoms of their illness. One likely reason is that mood stabilizers may work through different mechanisms. For example, different effects on intracellular second messenger systems have been postulated for different mood stabilizers.[25] Thus, lack of response to carbamazepine (Tegretol), for example, does not necessarily predict lack of response to divalproex sodium (Depakote).

The clinical syndromes defined as schizoaffective illness, bipolar I, II, or not otherwise specified, likely arise from a range of specific causes. Although we describe bipolar disorder as an illness, it is more accurate to define bipolar disorder as a syndrome characterized by pathophysiology, course, genetic contribution, and comorbid conditions.[26] For example, a bipolar I disorder developed after a severe closed head trauma versus a spontaneous onset of the disorder at age 12 likely represent different pathophysiologic pathways. **Given our limited under-**

standing of the changes in brain function leading to bipolar disorder, the treatment is purely empiric. Information on mixing and matching among the different mood stabilizers is limited. Failure of one does not predict response to a second. **Thus, patients must be educated about the importance of methodically trying different mono- and polypharmacy combinations.**

An additional chapter in combining medications comes from neurology, a field that has produced a number of studies finding the combination of two anticonvulsants to be more effective than monotherapy in treatment-resistant epilepsy.[27] Thus, the decision between ongoing polypharmacy over periodic need for adjunctive medication, such as an antidepressant added to a mood stabilizer, needs to be individually based. The fundamental principle of overlap and then taper gradually continues to apply whether using one or more medications.

Whether all mood stabilizers are equally efficacious or if more specific functions will be identified within a category of medications, such as anticonvulsants, is unknown. Lamotrigine, a new anticonvulsant currently in clinical trials for treatment of bipolar depression, may be one such possibility, providing mood stabilization and consistent antidepressant effects. **The clinical point is the importance of using trial, error, and combination of mood stabilizers to dampen not only primary syndromal symptoms but also residual symptoms, such as irritability, difficulty concentrating, and tendency to become overstimulated.**

The third principle is the need for patient education. In bipolar-type disorders, patients may experience symptomatic change during the course of illness or in response to medication. Without education about the illness, patients may abuse substances or stop and start their medication multiple times without seeking appropriate medication changes. **Substance abuse and frequent discontinuation of medication have been associated with a worsened course of illness and, possibly, diminished treatment response.**[28-31] As with all chronic illnesses that require lifetime medication, it is critical to find the best combination with the fewest side effects to enhance compliance.[32] **Unlike classic psychotherapy modalities, which exclude the family, inclusion of family members whenever possible is preferred.**

Treatment Options

This section discusses current medications used to treat schizoaffective and bipolar disorder and how those medications may be combined in more treatment-resistant patients. Two new anticonvulsants undergoing clinical trials are briefly mentioned along with newer atypical antipsychotics, including clozapine (Clozaril) and olanzapine (Zyprexa). The section closes discussing two special cases in the treatment and management of this illness: the depressive phase and the rapid cycling patient.

The subtypes of bipolar disorder, such as rapid cycling and mixed mania, are unique to bipolar disorder in terms of range of presentations and varied approaches needed for medication management. In fact, a recent consensus guideline by the Tri-University group on treatment of bipolar disorder required over 80 questions, whereas the schizophrenia guidelines needed only about 40 questions.[15]

One complicating factor addressing treatment for patients with schizoaffective or bipolar disorder is the wide distribution of medication responsivity across the patient population. Some patients respond to one medication for decades; others show minimal response despite combination treatments.

Promising new medications are available to treat bipolar-type illnesses. Clearly, this is good news because there are more treatment options. Patients who have lost responsivity or need different medication may be helped by these new medications (i.e., new anticonvulsants). Interestingly, although various anticonvulsants have different physiologic actions, they are also physiologically distinct from atypical antipsychotics, some of which have apparent mood-stabilizing properties. Unfortunately, figuring out how to mix, match, and change medications (all with somewhat different mechanisms, risks, and benefits) has become more complicated with the appearance of these new medications. Adding to this dilemma is the large number of combinations possible with the newer and older medications. The likelihood of controlled trials being completed on all combinations is remote.

Combination Therapy with Mood Stabilizers:

Little scientific information addresses the combined use and appropriate combinations of mood stabilizers to treat patients who respond inadequately to one mood stabilizer.[27,33] A few studies have examined the use and safety of combining medications.[34-36] **A number of treatment guidelines now recommend a combination of mood stabilizers, although recommendations are based on consensus rather than controlled treatment trials.**[15,17,18] Because the future likelihood of controlled trials on all various combinations is remote, the application of these consensually based treatment guidelines may provide a mechanism to collect broad-based treatment response data in the future.[37]

Established mood stabilizers for acute treat-ment include lithium, valproic acid (Depakene), and carbamazepine. Both lithium and divalproex sodium (the enteric-coated form of valproic acid) **have Food and Drug Administration approval for treatment of acute mania.**[38] **However, only lithium has been well studied and validated as efficacious in the long-term treatment and management of this illness.**[22] Debate continues over the impact of noncompliance, course of illness, treatment discontinuation, and other factors contributing to the limited success of lithium monotherapy.[5,7,8,11,30,31,39]

Controlled and uncontrolled study data support the use of anticonvulsants over lithium in certain cases. Anticonvulsants are more likely to be effective for patients having more than three episodes of mania, a history of substance abuse or neurologic insult (including head injury), manic episodes characterized by noneuphoric or mixed mania, and mood incongruent psychosis.[29,40-45] However, no controlled published studies exist examining anticonvulsants for long-term maintenance treatment, or, in particular, as monotherapy maintenance treatment.

The likelihood of using monotherapy with treatment-resistant patients is, by definition, very low. The majority of those patients who fall into this category have failed one or more of the first-line medications. The literature on controlled pharmacologic treatment of schizoaffective disorder has been reviewed by Keck and colleagues.[12] **This review states that patients with schizoaffective illness may respond to a single medication, although often combinations of a single mood stabilizer and an antipsychotic are used.** The advent of clozapine increases the possibility of using a single medication for treatment-resistant patients with both bipolar disorder and schizoaffective illness.[9,10,46,47]

In one small prospective, open-label study, the addition of a second mood stabilizer allowed 35% of the study group to improve

enough to return to the clinic (N = 28). **Approximately 45% of the sample improved somewhat but continued to be significantly ill.**[48,49] **In this study, divalproex sodium was added to ongoing lithium treatment.** The clinical improvement was rapid (less than a month) and, in most cases, sustained. Interestingly, the majority completed the 6-month study on more medications without change in somatic complaints. The addition of more medications was associated with improved psychiatric status but not decreased somatic complaints.

A majority of tertiary care psychiatrists are using multiple medications to help patients stabilize, as suggested by various consensually based treatment guidelines. This is clearly affected by the population likely to go to academic centers. However, long-term naturalistic data also support a tendency for monotherapy to be inadequate over longer time periods.

We are sadly lacking information on how to pharmacologically manage patients who respond poorly to the simple medication regimes. There is little guid-ance considering differences between anticonvulsants themselves in terms of clinical utility. There are no controlled randomized studies examining whether different spectrums and efficacies exist among the anticonvulsants, or whether they are as interchangeable as (appears for) neuroleptics in the treatment of schizophrenia.

At this time, the treatment of bipolar disorder and schizoaffective illness must proceed with careful trial-and-error using multiple medications, starting with single medication and progressing toward two mood stabilizers. Because of symptom severity or poor toleration, the use of three mood stabilizers, and the potential addition of an atypical antipsychotic such as clozapine (usually in combination with mood stabilizers) or the newer anticonvulsants, may be warranted. **Potential for drug interactions and side effects must be considered when combining medications.** Figure 8.1 illustrates a detailed algorithm for the treatment of refractory cases of bipolar disorder and schizoaffective illness.

Two new anticonvulsants, lamotrigine (Lamictal) and gabapentin (Neorontin), are undergoing clinical trials for bipolar disorder treatment. Lamotrigine and gabapentin are FDA-approved treatment agents for epilepsy. Early anecdotal experience suggests that lamotrigine may be particularly useful in treating bipolar depression.[50–52] **Treatment of patients in a depressive phase of bipolar disorder often requires two medications because no established mood-stabilizer has**

shown consistent antidepressant efficacy. Gabapentin appears to have mood-stabilizing properties for patients with significant mood lability as well as antianxiety effects. **Additionally, gabapentin is somewhat unique for its lack of drug interactions, limited drug metabolism by the liver, and low toxicity at high doses, thus allowing it to be combined with other drugs and used in patients with liver disease.** Both gabapentin and lamotrigine have different side-effect profiles and drug interactions. Importantly, these newer medications may for the first time fill specialized niches in the treatment and management of bipolar disorder. Randomized, double-blind, placebo-controlled trials are currently underway to evaluate this possibility.

Accumulating evidence indicates that the atypical antipsychotic clozapine may be effective in patients with treatment-resistant affective illness. Most open trials from Europe and the United States, during the compassionate-use period of clozapine, when it was tried on the most severely ill, supported its likely effectiveness for affectively ill patients.[46,47,53] Its use has broadened since being approved for schizophrenia. Additional uncontrolled studies indicate that clozapine is likely to be an effective medication for patients with treatment-resistent affective illness.[9,10,54-56] **A controlled, randomized, open 1-year study, comparing clozapine to treatment as usual, associated clozapine with significant clinical improvement in patients with treatment-resistant bipolar disorder and schizoaffective illness.[10] In this recent study, "treatment resistance" was defined as failure to achieve mood stabilization with the use of two concurrent mood stabilizers and, if the patient was psychotic, an antipsychotic.**

Other atypical antipsychotics are, or soon will be, on the market. Atypical antipsychotics are often defined as medications with an antipsychotic efficacy and broader receptor affinities than typical antipsychotics, including interaction with the serotonergic, a-adrenergic, histaminic, and muscarinic receptor systems. **Clinical evidence with risperidone** (Risperdal) **for mood stabilization has been equivocal. Early reports suggested that risperidone could worsen acute manic episodes when used for monotherapy.[57] More recent findings suggest it may be useful for bipolar disorder and schizoaffective illness if combined with other mood stabilizers.[58]** A second atypical agent, olanzapine, has just been released on the market. Preliminary data have been positive, and the manufacturer is launching controlled studies on

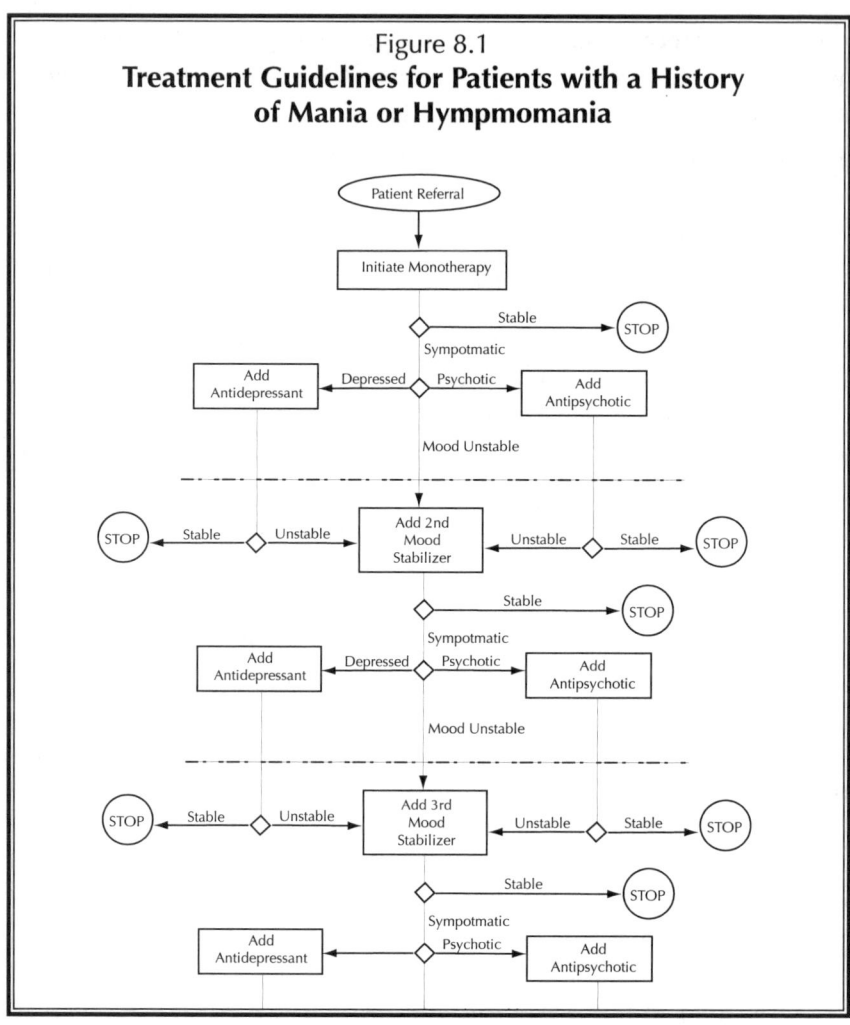

Figure 8.1
Treatment Guidelines for Patients with a History of Mania or Hympmomania

Generally, it is reasonable to add (change) medication if the patient is nonresponsive by weeks 1 or 2, or only partially responsive by weeks 2 or 3. Antipsychotics are treated as adjunctive agents in this treatment guideline. However, tapering once the patient is stabilized should always be considered. If an antipsychotic agent is used, the possibilities of the agent providing additive mood stabilization should be considered, especially for clozapine. Benzodiazepines are treated as purely adjunctive agents because the evidence for primary mood-stabilizing properties is limited. Caution should be exercised in the use of benzodiazepines because of the potential for tolerance, dependence, and addiction.

Mood stabilizers for lines 1-3 include the relatively well-established treatments of lithium, valproate, or carbamazepine (see line 4, also).

Line 1: If the patient is in a mixed phase or is cycling rapidly, you may start with an anticonvulsant. Antidepressants should not be used as an early treatment if the patient is experiencing a mixed episode. Until mood lability is decreased, it is not

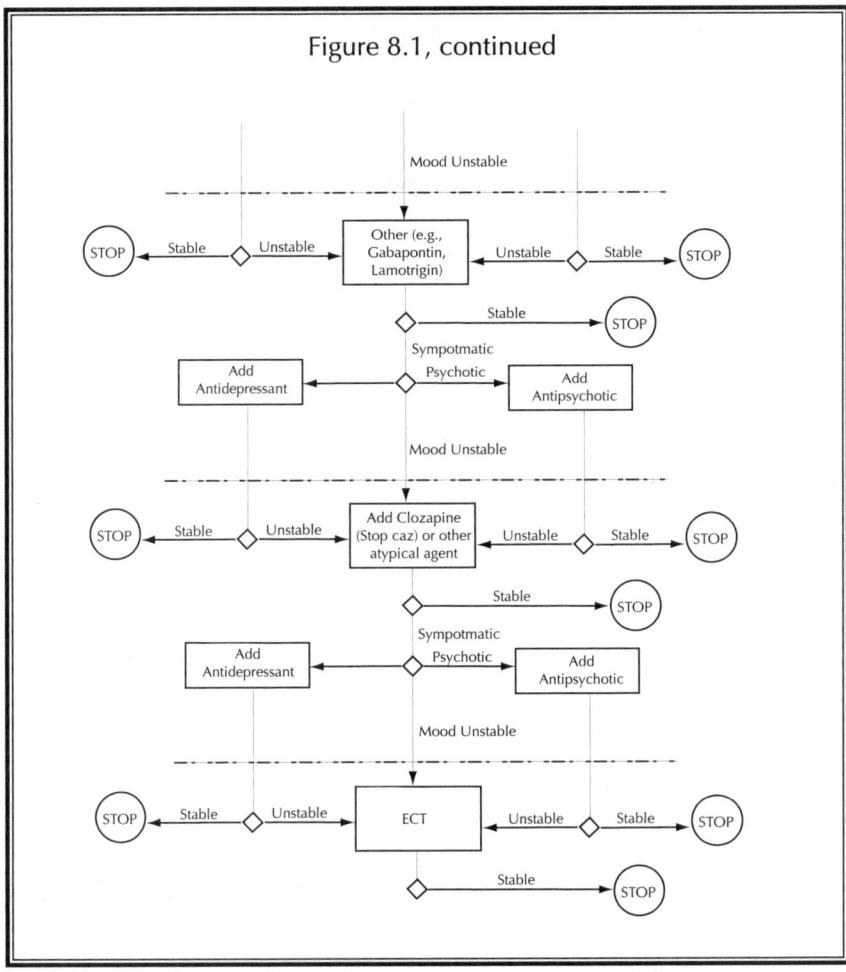

Figure 8.1, continued

predictable how severe the residual depressive symptoms will be. If a patient presents as depressed, be sure to rule out the presence of dysphoric hypomanic symptoms intermixed with depressive symptoms, as well as medical causes such as clinical or subclinical hypothyroidism.

Line 2: As above. Be aware of possible drug interactions and changes in blood levels with the use of multiple medications.

Line 3: Many patients will not tolerate these three mood stabilizers in combination. If this is the case, moving to line 4 and combining newer possibilities for treatment with established mood stabilizers is reasonable.

Line 4: Included in this box, besides the newer anticonvulsants, might be calcium channel blockers or high-dose thyroid medication.

Line 5: To date, there are reasonable data supporting mood-stabilizing properties only for clozapine. Information will soon be available on other atypical agents.

Line 6: Depending on symptoms, past medication response and so on, electroconvulsive therapy also could be considered at an earlier step.

its efficacy as a treatment of acute mania. **Although olanzapine has the closest receptor profile to clozapine, it is not associated with agranulocytosis; therefore, no weekly blood work is required.** It is unknown whether its side-effect profile and clinical efficacy will compare with those of clozapine in long-term treatment. Additional atypical antipsychotics expected in the near future include quetiapine, sertindole (Serlect), and ziprasidone. Little is known about the potential of these medications for treating affective disorders or patients with a history of mania.

Special Cases:

To conclude the discussion on treatment options, the special cases of bipolar depression and patients with rapid cycling or significant mood lability are reviewed.

Bipolar Depression

Patients with schizoaffective disorder and bipolar disorder are vulnerable to depression. **Moreover, some researchers believe that patients with bipolar disorder are more prone to atypical depression symptoms, including hypersomnia and hyperphagia.**[59] Early naturalistic longitudinal data indicate that women have a greater lifetime history of depression than men.[11]

Treatment of bipolar depression is complex for a number of reasons. Many psychiatrists believe, as is now reflected in the fourth edition of the *Diagnostic and Statistical Manual of Mental Disorders (DSM-IV)*,[60] that antidepressants can precipitate a switch into mania for patients with a history of mania.[61] In addition, many psychiatrists, particularly those in Europe, believe antidepressants can affect the long-term course of illness, causing continued rapid cycling perhaps even after the antidepressant is withdrawn.[62-64]

A complicating factor is that although most mood stabilizers are reasonably effective antimanic medications, they may inadvertently contribute to the development of depressive symptomatology; that is, the patient's mania remits, but instead of developing euthymia, the patient develops mild to moderate depressive symptoms. **This possibility suggests that lowering the dosage of the mood stabilizer and evaluating depressive symptomatology before initiating antidepressant pharmacotherapy is a reasonable strategy.** Another option is to increase the dosage of lithium because of its moderate efficacy as an antidepressant.

Some case reports suggest that carbamazepine and valproate offer effective treatment of bipolar depression. **However, in many cases, it may be necessary to use an antidepressant with a mood-stabilizing agent to ensure a return to euthymic status because of persistent or worsening depressive symptoms. These recommendations assume the depressive symptoms are not secondary to a medical condition such as clinical or subclinical hypothyroidism. Recent studies on suicide in bipolar patients affirm that current and, in particular, past severe depression is associated with a high risk of suicidal acts.**[65–68]

To date, nearly all antidepressants appear to have some potential to cause mania, but tricyclic antidepressants may have a somewhat greater propensity. The general recommendation is to use antidepressants at the lowest dosage possible to relieve bipolar depressive symptoms. However, in clinical practice, the dose needed is often similar to that required with major depression. Clozapine may be an option for patients with persistent bipolar depression because its profound mood-stabilizing properties allow antidepressants to be used at higher doses without causing hypomania or mania (Suppes, unpublished data, 1997).

One early, double-blind study comparing bupropion (Wellbutrin) to desipramine (Norpramin) in a small number of patients (N = 15) indicated that bupropion is less likely to cause a switch into mania.[69] Other open trials report the risk of switches into hypomania or mania with bupropion to be similar to other antidepressants.[70,71]

A number of newer antidepressants may be helpful to manage and treat patients with this illness, including venlafaxine (Effexor), nefazodone (Serzone), and mirtazipine (Remeron). These medications appear clinically efficacious in bipolar patients but, like all such medications, have the potential to cause patients to become hypomanic or manic.[61] Finally, early case reports indicate that lamotrigine may be useful, particularly in rapid-cycling patients who are depressed.[52]

Virtually no information is currently available on how long antidepressants should be continued for patients suffering from bipolar disorder or schizoaffective disorder once depressive symptoms remit. The rule of thumb is to continue for 2–6 months following remission of symptoms, with a gradual taper to minimize the risk of recurrence. However, some centers taper and stop antidepressants within a few weeks of decreased symptoms. No consensus or scientific studies exist that deal with this point. Early naturalistic studies suggest that the average bipolar depressive episode will last a total of 4–6 months.[11,72]

The overall scientific literature involving placebo-controlled trials on the appropriate treatment and management of the depressive phase of bipolar and schizoaffective disorder is limited.[73]

Rapid Cycling

Although rapid cycling formally refers to patients with four or more full episodes per year,[60] the term is often used to describe patients with ongoing mood lability and subsyndromal symptoms of hypomania or mild to moderate depression. These patients are characterized by significant mood changes over days or even hours, not necessarily meeting full criteria for mania or depression (especially not the duration criteria). These patients are often irritable and unstable and complain about the unpredictable nature of their mood. Some of these patients will be labeled as sufferers of personality disorders or treatment-resistant depression, when they are actually suffering from dysphoric hypomanic episodes of less than 4 days' duration.[74] One practical tactic to distinguish bipolar rapid cyclers or bipolar disorder not otherwise specified from Axis II or other disorders is to treat such patients with mood stabilizers.

For many rapid-cycling patients, it may be necessary to prescribe anticonvulsants or multiple medications.[14,48,49,56,75] The need for multiple medications reflects our limited understanding of the pathophysiology of the illness. Once the patient is off the first line of treatment, lithium or divalproex sodium, physicians are essentially working from limited or no controlled information. Although clinical experience and consensually based treatment algorithms guide treatment development,[15,19] the current limitations in the field are apparant. In particular, practitioners not in academic settings may be hesitant to use multiple medications with treatment-resistant patients. Nevertheless, this is a common practice among virtually all tertiary care and academic physicians. Academic psychiatrists are just beginning to publish results based on large clinical practices.[14]

Cumulative work with rapid-cycling patients supports that anticonvulsants may be the best first-line treatment.[42,75–77] **If one anticonvulsant does not effectively treat symptoms, it is reasonable** (using overlap and taper) **to try a second one as a monotherapy agent. If, during the switching process, the patient stabilizes on two medications, it would be prudent to continue both, gradually tapering the one with the lesser efficacy or more severe side effects.** Additional treatments with clinical promise for management of difficult-to-treat patients include clozapine,[56,78] calcium channel blockers,[79,80] and high-dose tri-iodothyronine (T3).[81] **Treating rapid-cycling patients entails an ongoing trial-and-error process to achieve the best single or combination treatment. It is important to continue medication trials until both physician and patient are satisfied symptoms are minimized as much as possible.**

Summary

The strategies presented in this chapter on management of treatment-resistant bipolar and schizoaffective disorders include the importance of making all medication changes in an overlap and taper fashion. Many patients will need more than one medication to treat their symptoms effectively. It is critical to educate patients about their illness and the significant periods needed to achieve the best treatment response through trying different medications. When possible, family members should be included in this education process.

A number of treatment options are available to manage the clinical symptoms of mania, depression, and psychosis. Cumulative data and clinical experience support the use of anticonvulsants as first-line treatment agents, particularly data on the use of divalproex sodium for acute mania—the only anticonvulsant approved for this indication. Frequently, more than one medication is needed for treatment-resistant patients. Recent studies support that clozapine may be effective for the severely ill. It is hoped that other atypical agents will share similar utility, but studies are still pending. Moreover, two new anticonvulsants, gabapentin and lamotrigine, may be useful in treatment-resistant patients. Results from ongoing studies will be available in the next year.

References

1. Mintz J, Mintz LI, Arruda MJ, Hwang SS. Treatments of depression and the functional capacity to work. *Arch Gen Psychiatry.* 1992;49:761–768.

2. Coryell W, Scheftner W, Keller M, et al. The enduring psychosocial consequences of mania and depression. *Am J Psychiatry.* 1993; 150:720 –727.

3. Page C, Benaim S, Lappin F. A long-term retrospective follow-up study of patients treated with prophylactic lithium carbonate. *Br J Psychiatry.* 1987;150:175 –179.

4. Maj M, Pirozzi R, Kemali D. Long-term outcome of lithium prophylaxis in patients initially classified as complete responders. *Psychopharmacology.* 1989;98:535 –538.

5. Markar HR, Mander AJ. Efficacy of lithium prophylaxis in clinical practice. *Br J Psychiatry.* 1989;155:496 –500.

6. Harrow M, Goldberg JF, Grossman LS, Meltzer HY. Outcome in manic disorders: a naturalistic follow-up study. *Arch Gen Psychiatry.* 1990;47:665 – 671.

7. Guscott R, Taylor L. Lithium prophylaxis in recurrent affective illness. Efficacy, effectiveness, and efficiency. *Br J Psychiatry.* 1994; 164:741–746.

8. Dickson WE, Kendell RE. Does maintenance lithium therapy prevent recurrences of mania under ordinary clinical conditions? *Psychol Med.* 1986;16:521–530.

9. Calabrese JR, Kimmel SE, Woyshville MJ, et al. Clozapine for treatment-refractory mania. *Am J Psychiatry.* 1996;153:759 –764.

10. Suppes T, Rush AJ, Webb A, Carmody T, Kraemer H. *A One-Year Randomized Trial of Clozapine vs Usual Care in Bipolar I Patients.* Paper presented at Society of Biological Psychiatry Annual Meeting; New York; 1996.

11. Goodwin FK, Jamison KR. *Manic-Depressive Illness.* New York: Oxford University Press; 1990.

12. Keck PE Jr, McElroy SL, Strakowski SM, West SA. Pharmacologic treatment of schizoaffective disorder. *Psychopharmacology.* 1994; 14:529–538.

13. Bowden CL. Role of newer medications for bipolar disorder. *J Clin Psychopharmacol.* 1996;16(1):48S –55S.

14. Peselow ED, Fieve RR, Difiglia C, Sanfilpo MP. Lithium prophylaxis of bipolar illness: the value of combination treatment. *BMJ.* 1994;164:208–214.

15. Frances A, Docherty JP, Kahn DA. The expert consensus guidelines series: treatment of bipolar disorder. *J Clin Psychiatry.* 1996; 57(12a):1– 88.

16. Sachs GS. Bipolar mood disorder: practical strategies for acute and maintenance phase treatment. *J Clin Psychopharmacol.* 1996; 16(1): 32S– 47S.

17. Suppes T, Calabrese JR, Mitchell PB, et al. B. Algorithms for the treatment of bipolar, manic-depressive illness. Psychopharmacol Bull. 1995;31:469 – 474.

18. American Psychiatric Association. Practice guideline for the treatment of patients with bipolar disorder. *Am J Psychiatry.* 1994; 151:1–36.

19. Calabrese JR, Woyshville MJ. A medication algorithm for treatment of bipolar rapid cycling? *J Clin Psychiatry.* 1995;56(suppl 3): 11–18.

20. Suppes T, Baldessarini RJ, Faedda GL, Tohen M. Risk of recurrence following discontinuation of lithium treatment in bipolar disorder. *Arch Gen Psychiatry.* 1991;48:1082–1088.

21. Faedda GL, Tondo L, Baldessarini RJ, Suppes T, Tohen M. Outcome after rapid vs gradual discontinuation of lithium treatment in bipolar disorders. *Arch Gen Psychiatry.* 1993;50:448–455.

22. Suppes T, Baldessarini RJ, Faedda GL, Tondo L, Tohen M. Discontinuing maintenance treatment in bipolar manic-depressive disorders: risks and implications. *Harvard Rev Psychiatry.* 1993;1:131–144.

23. Baldessarini RJ, Tondo L, Faedda GL, et al. Effects of the rate of discontinuing lithium maintenance treatment in bipolar disorders. *J Clin Psychiatry.* 1996;57:441– 448.

24. Montgomery SA, Dufour H, Brion S, et al. The prophylactic efficacy of fluoxetine in unipolar depression. *Br J Psychiatry.* 1988; 153:69 –76.

25. Stoll AL, Severus WE. Mood stabilizers: shared mechanisms of action at postsynaptic signal-transduction and kindling processes. *Harvard Rev Psychiatry.* 1996;4:77– 89.

26. Suppes T, Rush AJ. Evolving clinical characteristics or distinct disorders? In: Shulman K, Tohen M, Kutcher S, eds. *Mood Disorder Throughout the Life Span.* New York: John Wiley & Sons; 1996: 3 –16.

27. Ketter TA, Pazzaglia PJ, Post RM. Synergy of carbamazepine and valproic acid in affective illness: case report and review of the literature. *J Clin Psychopharmacol.* 1992;12:276 –281.

28. Himmelhoch JM, Mulla D, Neil JF, Detre TP, Kupfer DJ. Incidence and significance of mixed affective states in a bipolar population. Arch Gen Psychiatry. 1976;33:1062–1066.

29. Himmelhoch JM, Garfinkel ME. Sources of lithium resistance in mixed mania. *Psychopharmacology.* 1986;22:613 – 620.

30. Post RM, Leverich GS, Altshuler L, Mikalauskas K. Lithium-discontinuation–induced refractoriness: preliminary observations. *Am J Psychiatry.* 1992;149:1727–1729.

31. Maj M, Pirozzi R, Magliano L. Nonresponse to reinstituted lithium prophylaxis in previously responsive bipolar patients: prevalence and predictors. *Am J Psychiatry.* 1995;152:1810 –1811.

32. Basco MR, Rush AJ. *Cognitive-Behavioral Therapy for Bipolar Disorder.* New York: Guilford Press; 1996.

33. Sharma V, Persad E, Mazmanian D, Karunaratne K. Treatment of rapid-cycling bipolar disorder with combination therapy of valproate and lithium. *Can J Psychiatry.* 1993; 38:137–139.

34. Tohen M, Castillo J, Pope HG Jr, Herbstein J. Concomitant use of valproate and carbamazepine in bipolar and schizoaffective disorders. *J Clin Psychopharmacol.* 1994;14:67–70.

35. Keck PE, McElroy SL, Vuckovic A, Friedman L. Combined valproate and carbamazepine treatment of bipolar disorder. *J Neuropsychiatry Clin Neurosci.* 1992;4:319–22.

36. Ketter TA, Pazzaglia PJ, Post RM. Synergy of carbamazepine and valproic acid in affective illness: case report and review of the literature. *J Clin Psychopharmacol.* 1992;12:276 –281.

37. Suppes T, Swan A, Crismon ML, et al. *Will medication algorithms provide adequate information on treatment response in bipolar disorder?* Abstract submitted for the New Clinical Drug Evaluation Unit Annual Meeting; 1997.

38. Bowden CL, Brugger AM, Swann AC, et al. Efficacy of divalproex sodium vs lithium and placebo in the treatment of mania. *JAMA.* 1994;271:918–924.

39. Baldessarini RJ, Tondo L, Suppes T, Faedda GL, Tohen M. Pharmacological treatment of bipolar disorder throughout the life cycle. In: Shulman K, Tohen M, Kutcher S, eds. *Mood Disorder Throughout the Life Span.* New York: John Wiley & Sons; 1996: 299 –338.

40. Bowden CL. Predictors of response to divalproex sodium and lithium. *J Clin Psychiatry*. 1995;3(56S):25–30.

41. Pope HG Jr, McElroy SL, Keck PE Jr, Hudson JI. Valproate in the treatment of acute mania: a placebo-controlled study. *Arch Gen Psychiatry*. 1991;48:62– 68.

42. Calabrese JR, Woyshville MJ, Kimmel SE. Rapport DJ. Predictors of valproate response in bipolar rapid cycling. *J Clin Psychopharmacol*. 1993;13:280–283.

43. Gelenberg AJ, Kane JM, Keller MB, et al. Comparison of standard and low serum levels of lithium for maintenance treatment of bipolar disorder. *N Engl J Med*. 1989;321:1489–1493.

44. McElroy SL, Keck PE Jr, Pope HR Jr, et al. Clinical and research implications of the diagnosis of dysphoric or mixed mania or hypomania. *Am J Psychiatry*. 1992; 49:1633 –1644.

45. Solomon DA, Keitner GI, Miller IW, Shea MT, Keller MB. Course of illness and maintenance treatments for patients with bipolar disorder. *J Clin Psychiatry*. 1995; 6:5 –13.

46. McElroy SL, Dessain EC, Pope HG Jr, et al. Clozapine in the treatment of psychotic mood disorders, schizoaffective disorder, and schizophrenia. *J Clin Psychiatry*. 1991;52:411– 414.

47. Suppes T, McElroy SL, Gilbert J, Dessain EC, Cole JO. Clozapine in the treatment of dysphoric mania. *Biol Psychiatry*. 1992; 32:270 –280.

48. Suppes T, Rush AJ, Kraemer H, Webb A. Treatment optimization of symptomatic patients with a history of mania using a treatment algorithm. *J Clin Psychiatry*. Submitted for publication.

49. Suppes T, Rush AJ, Harrison S, Webb A, Paul B. *Treatment Algorithm Project for Bipolar Disorder*. Paper presented at New Clinical Drug Evaluation Unit Program (NCDEU) Annual Meeting; 1994; Marco Island, FL.

50. Bowden CL. *New concepts in mood stabilization: evidence for the effectiveness of valproate and lamotrigine* [abstract]. XXth Collegium Internationale Neuro-Psychopharmacologicum Congress; June 1996; Melbourne, Australia.

51. Calabrese J, Bowden C, McElroy S, et al. *Lamotrigine in treatment refractory manic depression*. Second International Conference on New Directions in Affective Disorders; September 1995; Jerusalem; Israel. Abstract.

52. Calabrese JR, Fatemi SH, Woyshville MJ. Antidepressant effects of lamotrigine in rapid-cycling bipolar disorder. *Am J Psychiatry*. 1996;153:1236. Letter.

53. Naber D, Hippius H. The European experience with use of clozapine. *Hosp Commun Psychiatry*. 1990;41:886 –890.

54. Banov MD, Zarate CA, Tohen M, et al. Clozapine therapy in refractory affective disorders: polarity predicts response in long-term follow-up. *J Clin Psychiatry*. 1994;55:295–300.

55. Zarate CA, Tohen M, Baldessarini RJ. Clozapine in severe mood disorders. *J Clin Psychiatry*. 1995;56:411– 417.

56. Suppes T, Phillips K, Judd C. Clozapine treatment of non-psychotic rapid-cycling bipolar disorder: a report of three cases. *Biol Psychiatry*. 1994; 6:338–340.

57. Dwight MM, Keck PE Jr, Stanton SP, Strakowski SM, McElroy SL. Antidepressant activity and mania associated with risperidone treat-ment of schizoaffective disorder. *Lancet*; 1994(Aug 20):554 –555.

58. Tohen M, Zarate CA Jr, Centorrino F, et al. Risperidone in the treatment of mania. *J Clin Psychiatry.* 1996;57:249–253.

59. Himmelhoch JM, Thase ME, Mallinger AG, Houck P. Tranylcypromine vs imipramine in anergic bipolar depression. *Am J Psychiatry.* 1991;148:910–916.

60. American Psychiatric Association. *Diagnostic and Statistical Manual of Mental Disorders.* 4th ed. Washington, DC: Author; 1994.

61. Stoll AL, Mayer PV, Kolbrener M, et al. Antidepressant-associated mania: a controlled comparison with spontaneous mania. *Am J Psychiatry.* 1994;151:1642–1645.

62. Kukopulos A, Reginaldi D, Laddomada P, Floris G, et al. Course of the manic-depressive cycle and changes caused by treatments. *Neuropsychopharmakologie.* 1980;13:156–167.

63. Altshuler LL, Post RM, Leverich GS, et al. Antidepressant-induced mania and cycle acceleration: a controversy revisited. *Am J Psychiatry.* 152:1130–1138.

64. Wehr TA, Goodwin FK. Can antidepressants cause mania and worsen the course of affective illness? *Am J Psychiatry.* 1987; 144: 1403–1411.

65. Tondo L, Baldessarini RJ, Floris G, et al. Lithium treatment reduces risk of suicidal behavior in bipolar disorder patients. *Arch Gen Psychiatry.* In press.

66. Jamison K, Baldessarini RJ, Tondo L. *Antisuicide effects of lithium.* Ann N Y Acad Sci. In press.

67. Tondo L, Baldessarini RJ, Floris G, Silvetti F, Rudas N. *Lithium maintenance treatment reduces risk of suicidal behavior in bipolar disorder patients.* In: Gallicchio VS, Birch NJ, eds. Lithium: Biochemical and Clinical Advances: Proceedings of a 1995 Malta Lithium Symposium. Cheshire, C T: Weidner Publishing Group; 1996: 161–171.

68. Dilsaver SC, Chen Y-W, Swann AC, Shoaib AM, Krajewski KJ. Suicidality in patients with pure and depressive mania. *Am J Psychiatry.* 1994;151:1312–1315.

69. Sachs GS, Lafer B, Stoll AL, et al. *Bupropion vs Desipramine for Bipolar Depression.* American Psychiatric Association Annual Meeting; 1993; San Francisco.

70. Wright G, Galloway L, Kim J, et al. Bupropion in the long-term treatment of cyclic mood disorders: mood stabilizing effects. *J Clin Psychiatry.* 1985;46:22–25.

71. Fogelson DL, Bystritsky A, Pasnau R. Bupropion in the treatment of bipolar disorders: the same old story? *J Clin Psychiatry.* 1992; 53:443–446.

72. Angst J. The course of affective disorders, II: typology of bipolar manic-depressive illness. *Arch Psychiatr Nervenkr.* 1978;226:65–73.

73. Zornberg GL, Pope HG Jr. Treatment of depression in bipolar disorder: new directions for research. *J Clin Psychopharmacol.* 1993; 13:397–408.

74. Akiskal HS. The prevalent clinical spectrum of bipolar disorders: beyond DSM-IV. *J Clin Psychopharmacol.* 1996;16(suppl 2):4S–14S. Review.

75. Calabrese JR, Rapport DJ, Kimmel SE, Reece B, Woyshville MJ. Rapid-cycling bipolar disorder and its treatment with valproate. *Can J Psychiatry.* 1993;38(suppl 3):57S–61S. Review.

76. Calabrese JR, Markovitz PJ, Kimmel SE, Wagner SC. Spectrum of efficacy of valproate in 78 rapid-cycling bipolar patients. *J Clin Psychopharmacol.* 1992;12:53–56.

77. Ananth J, Wohl, Ranganath V, Beshay M. Rapid cycling patients: Conceptual and etiological factors. *Neuropsychobiology*. 1993;27: 193 –198.

78. Frye MA, Altshuler LL, Bitran JA. Clozapine in rapid-cycling bi-polar disorder. *J Clin Psychopharmacol*. 1996;16:87–90. Letter.

79. Goodnick PJ. Nimodipine treatment of rapid-cycling bipolar disorder. *J Clin Psychiatry*. 1995;56:330. Letter.

80. Pazzaglia PJ, Post RM, Ketter TA, George MS, Marangell LB. Preliminary controlled trial of nimodipine in ultra-rapid cycling affective dysregulation. *Psychiatry Res*. 1993;49:257–272.

81. Whybrow PC. The therapeutic use of triiodothyronine and high-dose thyroxine in psychiatric disorder. *Acta Medica Austriaca*. 1994; 21:47–52. Review.

9   Atypical Antipsychotics in Schizophrenia

William C. Wirshing, MD, Donna A. Wirshing, MD,
Brad Spellberg, and Ted Amanios

Dr. William Wirshing is Professor of Psychiatry, UCLA School of Medicine and Chief of the Psychiatric Treatment Unit at the West Los Angeles Veterans Affairs Medical Center, Los Angeles, CA.

Dr. Donna Wirshing is Assistant Professor of Psychiatry, UCLA School of Medicine, Co-Chief of the Scizophrenia and Patient Treatment Unit at the West Los Angeles Veterans Affairs Medical Center, and also Co-Chief of the Scizophrenia and Research Outpatients Clinic in Los Angeles.

Brad Spellburg and Ted Amanios attend UCLA School of Medicine.

Editor's Note

Schizophrenia remains the most pressing problem in clinical psychiatry. A third of patients show either no or inadequate response toreatment. Recently, a series of atypical antipsychotic drugs have been introduced. They hold out the promise of both better efficacy and an improved side effect profile.

In this chapter, Dr. Wirshing and his colleagues list the newer drugs which have become available, as well as a few which are not yet approved in the U.S. but may be in the near future. These drugs—clozapine, risperidone, sertindole, olanzapine, quetiapine, and ziprasidone—constitute the latest therapeutic armament against schizophrenia. In their comprehensive chapter, copiously referenced, the authors give an account of each new drug in terms directly related to their use in everyday practice (i.e., pharmacologic mechanism of action, dosing strategies, adverse side effects). The efficacy of each drug is noted to be still unclear except for clozapine, which undoubtedly improved efficacy, especially in the treatment of the refractory group. A common factor in these compounds is a low and almost absent likelihood of inducing extrapyramidal symptoms, and their overall safety compared to older agents is noteworthy.

Introduction

The dawn of modern antipsychotic pharmacotherapy occurred in 1952, when Delay et al. described the use of chlorpromazine (Thorazine) to treat hallucinations and delusions in hospitalized patients.[1] The discovery of this therapeutic modality was entirely fortuitous, as chlorpromazine had been utilized initially as a sedative based upon the previous experience with promethazine. It was the French anesthesiologist, Henri Laborit, who recommended the drug to his psychiatric colleagues based upon observations gleaned from anesthetizing patients.

When chlorpromazine began to be used by the psychiatric community, it was noted that the efficacy of the drug was coincident with a curious parkinsonism, phenomenologically indistinguishable from idiopathic Parkinsons Disease. These observations led to the use of the term *neuroleptic*, meaning seize the neuron, to describe this class of medications. The link between the movement disorders, which came to be known as extrapyramidal side effects (EPS), and the drugs' efficacy was so strong that new neuroleptics were screened for by their ability to produce EPS-like effects in laboratory animals. For three decades after the discovery of chlorpromazine, it was assumed that dopaminergic blockade in the central nervous system was responsible for both the efficacy and side effect profile of neuroleptics.

Recently, however, a new class of atypical antipsychotics have been developed. These drugs possess equivalent, and in some cases superior, efficacy to neuroleptics, and induce minimal to no EPS. Several of these drugs exert minimal activity at dopamine$_2$ (D_2) receptors, demonstrating that antipsychotic efficacy is not related entirely and solely to blockade at these sites. These drugs are novel enough that their full potential for antipsychotic therapy has only begun to be explored. **Unlike in the previous pharmacologic era, when random molecules were screened in lab animals for induction of EPS, these new drugs have been target-designed based upon their three-dimensional molecular structures.** The advent of the atypical antipsychotics bears the promise of ushering in a new era in the pharmacotherapeutic care of schizophrenic patients.

Atypical Drugs

Clozapine:

Pharmacology

Clozapine (Clozaril), a *dibenzodiazepine* compound, was the first atypical antipsychotic to be developed and marketed, and thus has served as a pharmacodynamic prototype after which other molecules have recently been designed. Clozapine owes its atypical status to both its **enhanced efficacy in refractory populations and its lack of associated EPS.**

Prior to the advent of clozapine, neuroleptics were selected, either directly or indirectly, based upon their ability to antagonize D_2 receptors. Unlike the typical antipsychotics, **clozapine demonstrates very little binding at D_2 sites.** In fact, it has the lowest affinity for D_2 receptors of any antipsychotic agent currently available, typical or atypical.[2] Instead, it acts as **a potent antagonist of 5-$HT_{2A/C}$ sites.**[3] Its in vivo ratio of 5-HT_{2A}/D_2 affinity is 4:8.[4] The drug's antagonism of 5-HT_2 sites has been hypothesized to explain its efficacy in treating schizophrenia.[5] However, **clozapine also binds with high affinity at 5-HT_6 and D_4 sites, and antagonism of both of these receptor subtypes may also mediate antipsychotic effect.**[6-9] **Finally, clozapine binds to muscarinic$_1$ (M_1), histamine$_1$ (H_1), and α_1-adrenergic receptors with high affinity.**[2] **Binding at these receptors has been linked to the drug's side effects** (see next table).

Clozapine is **metabolized by cytochrome P450 1A2, 2D6, and 3A3/4 (CYP1A2, CYP2D6, CYP3A3/4) isoenzymes.**[10] This indicates that clozapine **may interact with other psychotropic medications, including tricyclic antidepressants (TCAs) such as imipramine (Tofranil), selective serotonin reuptake inhibitors (SSRIs) such as fluvoxamine (Luvox), monoamine oxidase inhibitors (MAOIs), and other neuroleptics,** all of which are also metabolized by these P450 subtypes.[11-13] **Concomitant administration of fluvoxamine has been shown to elevate serum levels of clozapine from 20%–60% above baseline,** due to inhibition of CYP1A2 metabolism of the drug.[14] **Fluoxetine (Prozac) and sertraline (Zoloft) also elevate serum clozapine levels, although their effect is much weaker than that of fluvoxamine.**[15-17] The atypical neuroleptic risperidone (Risperdal)[18-21] also ele-

Table 9.1
Summary of Clinical Pharmacology of Atypical Antipsychotics

Drug	Starting Dose	Titration	Target Range(mg/day)	Common Adverse Effects	Notes
Clozapine	12.5 mg b.i.d.	$\geq$ 50 mg/2 days	200–600	Sedation, orthostatic hypotension, weight gain, constipation, siezures	Weekly CBCs required due to 1% incidence of agranulocytosis. Beware of potential for diabetes in patients with risk factors. Minimal EPS is seen.
Olanzapine*	5 mg q.i.d.	5 mg/4–6 days	5–25	Weight gain, sedation, xerostomia	Beware of potential for diabetes in patients. Prolactin elevations are mild and EPS is minimal.
Quetiapine[a]	25 mg t.i.d.	unclear	150–750	Sedation, insomnia, headache xerostomia, weight gain, agitation	Transient elevations in ALT have been reported. Minimal EPS and prolactin elevation.
Risperidone	1 mg b.i.d.	1–2 mg/week	2–8	Sedation, orthostatic hypotension, weight gain, erectile dysfunction, increased prolactin	Onset of EPS indicates that therapeutic window has been exceeded. Treatment is to lower dose until EPS dissipates
Sertindole	4 mg q.i.d.	4 mg/4–6 days	12–24	Orthostatic hypotension, nasal congestion, reflect tachycardia decreased ejaculatory volume, weight gain	QTc prolongation occurs in 2%–5% of patients, but no serious adverse effect has thus far been reported. Prolactin elevation is mild. Minimal EPS is seen.
Ziprasidone[o]	20–80 mg b.i.d.	unclear	40–200	Transient prolactin elevation	Minimal EPS, sedation, orthostatic hypotension

* Some patients, particularly the elderly, cannot tolerate the sedation and/or akathisia at this dose. We have successfully treated such patients at 2.5 mg q.i.d.

[a] Further studies are needed to clarify the titration schedule. 25 mg t.i.d. has been shown to be a safe starting dose.[145]

[o] Further studies are needed to clarify the titration schedule. 20–80 mg b.i.d. has been shown to be safe and efficacious.[139,140]

vates serum clozapine levels. Finally, case reports have described reversible clozapine-related toxicity secondary to elevated serum clozapine levels in patients taking either erythromycin[22] or cimetidine,[23] both of which are well known competitors of P450 metabolism.

Tobacco smoke induces CYP1A2, which can lead to decreased tissue clozapine levels,[11,24] which is a concern due to the high prevalence of smoking among psychotic patients. The anti-seizure medications phenytoin (Dilantin) and carbamazepine (Tegretol) induce P450 isoenzymes and have been shown to cause a drop in serum clozapine levels.[16,25,26] Of greater concern, one study found that concurrent administration of carbamazepine and clozapine raised the relative risk for development of neutropenia by 5- to 6-fold as compared to clozapine therapy alone.[27] Therefore, carbamazepine is contraindicated for patients receiving clozapine. The neutropenia risk associated with carbamazepine is perhaps not surprising, because it is known to pose a risk of blood dyscrasias when administered by itself.

Valproate, which has been used both for therapy of clozapine-induced seizures as well as for adjunctive therapy for schizoaffective disorder, has been variably reported to increase or decrease clozapine levels.[16,25,28,29] It has been suggested that valproate may somehow antagonize the antipsychotic effects of clozapine.[30] Since few adverse patient outcomes have been reported secondary to concurrent valproate and clozapine therapy,[31] valproate remains a clinically acceptable modality with which to treat clozapine-induced seizures.

Lithium and benzodiazepines also appear to interact with clozapine. One case report found that the addition of lithium to a regimen of clozapine led to clinically significant neurotoxicity in one patient.[32] There are also case reports of benzodiazepines exacerbating clozapine-related sedation, as well as inducing ataxia and even respiratory arrest in patients taking clozapine.[33-35]

Finally, several nonpharmacologic forces act upon the efficiency of the P450 system. Age is positively correlated with a decrease in CYP efficiency, and a decrease in clozapine metabolism has been found in elderly patients.[36,37] There are also genetic components to P450 metabolism. Considerable polymorphism has been found in the CYP2D6 system, and 7% of caucasions are considered slow metabolizers.[38] Recently polymorphism has been suggested to exist in the CYP1A2 system as well.[11-13] Although of questionable clinical significance, because patients are not routinely typed for their P450 alleles, the CYP1A2 findings may help explain the varying efficacy of clozapine at a wide range of doses in different people.

Clinical Indications and Efficacy

Clozapine has become the standard of care for patients with treat-ment-refractory schizophrenia or schizoaffective disorder.[39] Several studies have shown that clozapine is highly effective in such patients compared to typical antipsychotics. The first study to examine this topic was a European multicenter trial that compared clozapine to stan-dard antipsychotics.[40] Clozapine was most beneficial to those patients who were most psychotic, as well as to those with a history of poor responses to typical neuroleptics.

In a double-blind, multicenter study of 268 patients refractory to at least three neuroleptics, 30% of patients randomized to receive clozap-ine met stringent improvement criteria for both positive and negative symptoms,[41] whereas only 4% of the patients randomized to receive chlorpromazine improved. Subsequent double-blind studies suggested that the 30% rate of improvement might well have been significantly higher had the trial lasted for longer than six weeks. A 16-week placebo-controlled, cross-over trial comparing clozapine to fluphenazine found a 38% response in 21 treatment-refractory patients treated with clozapine.[42] Recently, Marder et al. reported on a 29-week trial of treatment-refractory patients in which clozapine demonstrated a 60% improvement rate compared to a 12% improvement rate for haloperidol.[43]

Further evidence for clozapine's efficacy in refractory patients can be derived from trials examining its effect on rehospitalization rates. Essock et al. randomized patients who had failed at least two 6-week trials of conventional neuroleptics to one year of either clozapine or typical antipsychotic therapy.[44] Although no difference was noted in the discharge rates of patients in the two arms, the investigators found that after one year only 17% of the clozapine patients had been rehos-pitalized as compared to 31% of the standard neuroleptic patients. This suggests that subpopulations of schizophrenics exist who are more responsive to clozapine than to the more "pure" D_2 antagonists, while other subpopulations are refractory to both.

Prior reports have indicated that childhood-onset schizophrenic patients are more refractory to treatment with antipsychotics than are patients with an average age at onset.[45–47] Kumra et al. examined the effect of clozapine in 20 patients with childhood-onset schizophrenia (mean age 14 years old) in a 6-week, double-blind trial of flexible dose clozapine versus haloperidol (Haldol). They found that clozapine induced significantly greater improvement than haloperidol in both positive and negative symptoms, as measured by multiple behavioral rating scales, including the Brief Psychiatric Rating Scale (BPRS) and Clinical Global Impression (CGI).

The evidence that clozapine is effective in treatment-refractory psychosis is compelling. In addition, clozapine is apparently more effective at treating the negative symptoms of schizophrenia than are typical agents. The superior efficacy of clozapine at treating negative symptoms has been reported in several double-blind, placebo-controlled studies, including those by Kane et al.[41] and Breier et al.[49] However, in the latter study, negative symptoms that responded well to therapy seemed to represent secondary negative symptoms (those due to positive symptoms, EPS, dysphoria, or an impoverished environment[39]) rather than true primary negative symptoms.

Recently, investigators have examined other potential therapeutic indications for clozapine. **Several studies have found that it is an effective alternative therapy for mania,[50] even in patients who are refractory to first line agents.[51,52] In addition, a retrospective chart review found that 76% of patients treated with clozapine for psychosis secondary to Parkinson's disease demonstrated significant improvement within three months initiation.[53] Further, clozapine was found to be as efficacious as benztropine (Cogentin) in treating the tremor of Parkinson's patients.** Finally, studies have found that **clozapine improved behavioral symptoms in mentally retarded patients[55,56] as well as in people who suffered from neurobehavioral conditions secondary to trauma, Alzheimer's disease, and Parkinson's disease.[57]**

It is well established that clozapine is effective in treatment-resistant schizophrenia. The drug has also been found to aid in the treatment of psychosis, mania, and behavioral symptoms secondary to disorders other than schizophrenia.

Dosing and Adverse Effects

The usual dose range for clozapine is 400–700 mg per day, and it is generally given in a divided dose schedule. It is worth noting that the average European dose range is approximately one-half that of the U.S. range. This more than likely reflects the U.S. practice of reserving clozapine for the most unresponsive patients. Such subjects typically, and predictably, require higher doses than more responsive patients. **Because of clozapine's pronounced α_1 blockade** (which induces a marked decrease in peripheral vascular resistance with a reflex increase in cardiac output and possibly clinically significant orthostatic hypotension) **and H_1 blockade** (which induces sedation), **it must be titrated very slowly, over several weeks, to the target dose range.** In general, patients should be started at 12.5 mg b.i.d. with gradual titration to approximately 500 mg by no more than 50 mg increments every two days. In addition to the required weekly monitoring of white blood cell counts, patients should have vital signs (with orthostatic changes) taken on a daily basis during the first week of titration if possible. Subjects who demonstrate cardiovascular intolerance of the clozapine-induced decrease in peripheral vascular resistance (i.e., persistent, subjectively distressing orthostatic hypotension) should be titrated with extreme caution.[58] **The constipation** (occasionally severe) **that occurs in two thirds of patients taking clozapine should be anticipated.** Some clinicians prescribe lactulose or metamucil (i.e., psyllium husk fiber) prophylactically. Other common problems include **weight gain** (probably secondary to blockade of $5HT_{2C}$[59]), **sedation** (probably related to a combination of α_1 and H_1 blockade), and sialorrhea (secondary to increase in salivary output, the mediation of which is unclear). The sedation can often be managed by slowing the titration and shifting the bulk of the daily dose to bedtime. Weight gain should be anticipated, and appropriate behavioral strategies instituted before significant changes in weight occur. Once patients gain weight it is virtually impossible to get them to return to their baseline weight as long as the clozapine, or any other atypical antipsychotic, is continued. The sialorrhea, which is generally dealt with by using "pillow towels" or adding anticholinergics or even clonidine (Catapres), is most problematic at night.[60]

Unless contraindicated by adverse effects, the titration should be continued until either psychotic symptoms begin to remit, or a target

dose of 500 mg per day is reached. Once improvement is shown, several weeks of negligible clinical improvement should be tolerated before the dose is again increased. In the absence of clinical improvement once 500 mg per day has been reached, a trough plasma level for clozapine should be drawn. If possible, trough levels should be obtained on consecutive days because of the marked variability of this laboratory measure. Plasma levels of 250 ng/ml or higher are highly predictive of optimal clinical outcome.[61] A plasma level below this should prompt an increase in dose, while one above should signal the treating clinician to wait longer for clinical benefit to accrue.

Several other relatively mild adverse effects have commonly been reported. α_1-blockade can lead to the development of urinary incontinence in patients. This has been successfully treated with ephedrine (Quadrinal).[62] The drug's antagonism of muscarinic sites can lead to tachycardia and constipation, and may also be involved in the sialorrhea mentioned above. These findings have been taken as evidence that clozapine is a partial agonist at some muscarinic sites, rather than a strict antagonist. In fact, two studies have shown that clozapine does have agonist activity at M_4 receptors.[63,64]

Other side effects of the drug are more severe than the above. **Recently, there have been numerous reported cases of clozapine-induced neuroleptic malignant syndrome** (NMS).[65-68] This topic has been reviewed by Sachdev et al.,[69] who found four cases out of approximately 1,250 patients taking clozapine. They suggest that the rates of NMS in clozapine-treated patients may approach those seen with typical neuroleptics. In addition, we have recently reviewed **the published case reports of treatment-emergent diabetes mellitus in patients taking clozapine.**[70] There have been 12 such cases published since 1994, and it is becoming apparent that induction of diabetes should be a major concern in patients with positive risk factors, including a personal history of diabetes, glucose intolerance, obesity, and a positive family history.

The two most severe adverse effects reported in patients taking clozapine are seizures and agranulocytosis. The former have been shown to be dose-related, with a 1% incidence at 300 mg and below, a 2.7% incidence at 300–600 mg, and a 4.4% incidence at 600 mg and above.[71] The seizures can generally be alleviated by lowering the dose or, as mentioned earlier, by the co-administration of valproate.[72]

Idiosyncratic agranulocytosis has been reported in slightly less than 1% of patients taking clozapine.[73,74] Because of this potentially fatal side effect, patients in the U.S. who receive clozapine therapy must have weekly blood count checks. Further, additional checks are mandated if any significant drop in the white blood cell (WBC) count is noted, if the WBC count drops below 3500/mm, or if the WBC count drops for three consecutive weeks. Daily monitoring should be initiated if the WBC count falls below 3000/mm^3 or if the absolute neutrophil count drops below 1500/mm^3. If total and absolute neutrophil counts return above the 3000/mm^3 and 1500/mm^3 thresholds, respectively, therapy can be continued. If these counts fall below 2000/mm^3 and 1000/mm^3, clozapine should be immediately withdrawn. Any patient whose clozapine is withdrawn for agranulocytosis (defined as a neutrophil count $\leq$ 300/mm^3 should never be rechallenged with the drug.

Physicians should be aware that **the agranulocytosis is often preceded by a spike in total WBC counts.** Indeed, an increase of 15% in the total WBC count from one week to the next carries with it a threefold increase in relative risk (95% CI = 1.38-6.57) for the development of agranulocytosis in the subsequent 75 days.[73]

Recently, data have shown that the rate of agranulocytosis drops markedly after six months on medication, and investigators have considered the idea of decreasing the frequency of complete blood count (CBC) monitoring, or even halting it altogether after six months of therapy.[73-76] In Canada and Europe, CBCs are currently drawn biweekly after six months of therapy.[74,77,78] **An FDA advisory subcommittee has recently recommended that monitoring be decreased to biweekly after six months of therapy, and be discontinued completely after 18 months. The final FDA recommendations are forthcoming.**

Despite the wide spectrum of adverse effects outlined above, clozapine has a very favorable side effect profile for two reasons. First, it induces significantly fewer EPS than typical antipsychotics.[79,80] **Second, it is not associated with significant prolactin elevation.**[81] Thus, clozapine is indicated in patients who are intolerant of standard neuroleptics due either to severe EPS or amenorrhea and galactorrhea.

Risperidone:

Pharmacology

The *benzisoxazole-derivative* risperidone (Risperdal) has a high affinity for 5-HT$_2$ and D$_2$ receptors.[82] Risperidone also binds to and blocks α_1-adrenergic receptors significantly enough that tachycardia and orthostatic hypotension are sometimes observed. It has a low affinity for α_2-adrenergic and H$_1$ receptors and has essentially no activity at muscarinic receptors.

Risperidone is readily absorbed from the GI tract and peak plasma levels are reached approximately 0.8–1.4 hours after oral administration.[83-85] A steady-state is usually reached in one to seven days by risperidone and about five days by its equally active metabolite, 9-hydroxy risperidone.[85,86] This metabolite is of clinical significance because it has similar activity to its parent compound at D$_2$ and 5-HT$_2$ receptors, the sites thought to be responsible for the therapeutic effects of neuroleptics.[84,87]

Eighty percent of risperidone is cleared via non-renal routes, while the metabolite, 9-hydroxy risperidone, is removed by renal excretion. Thus, caution must be exercised in the administration of risperidone to patients with liver or renal problems; extensive liver disease may raise risperidone levels and extensive renal disease may increase 9-hydroxy risperidone levels. Although these problems have not been adequately studied, lower starting doses are recommended in patients whose organs are compromised.[88] Moreover, as CYP2D6 is the P450 enzyme system suspected of being the major metabolizer of risperidone,[89] the possibility of interactions with other CYP2D6 substrates exists and should also be considered during drug titration.

Clinical Indications and Efficacy

Early flexible dose studies established that risperidone is an effective antipsychotic that displays symptomatic efficacy equivalent to that seen with haloperidol.[90,91] These findings were corroborated by a large 8-week study of 1,362 patients with chronic schizophrenia randomly assigned to either risperidone (1,4,8,12, or 16 mg), or haloperidol (10 mg) group.[82] Results of this investigation clearly illustrated that the optimal response was found in the 4 mg and 8 mg risperidone groups with somewhat lower response rates found at the highest two doses.

Similar results were found in the Canadian portion of an 8-week, multicenter comparison of placebo, risperidone (2, 6, 10, and 16 mg), and haloperidol (20 mg) in the treatment of 135 patients with chronic schizophrenia.[92] All doses of risperidone except 2 mg were superior to placebo in improving CGI and Positive and Negative Symptoms Scale (PANSS) total scores. Furthermore, risperidone had an earlier onset of action than haloperidol with significant improvement occurring after the first week. Importantly, **only the patients receiving 6 mg of risperidone exhibited negative symptom improvement superior to placebo as measured on the PANSS negative symptoms subscale.** The 6 mg risperidone dose was also superior to haloperidol in improving PANSS, BPRS, and GPS scores. **These results suggest that treatment with risperidone follows a curvilinear "optimal dose" relationship in which efficacy falls off when the dose is increased beyond about 6 mg.**[93] **It was proposed that the fall in efficacy seen at higher doses was due to a higher number of parkinsonian side effects that could limit clinical improvement as measured by certain psychopathology scales.**[92] For example, **akinesia could produce depression and hostility while akathisia could produce excitability and hostility,** all of which could be measured on ratings scales (e.g., PANSS). Other authors have also suggested that EPS could manifest themselves on psychopathology rating scales.[94-96] While compelling and convenient, this explanation does not accord with findings that the vast majority of conventional agents fail to show a fall in efficacy with rising EPS toxicity.

In the U.S. portion of this multicenter study, the results were similar except that negative symptoms improved in both the 6 mg and 16 mg risperidone conditions.[97] The improvement at 16 mg stands out, as it contrasts with the findings of the above studies which found superior efficacy in the mid-dosage ranges (4–8 mg). In addition, even in the U.S. portion of the study, no statistically significant improvement was found in the 10 mg group. Efficacy at this intermediate dose might be expected if the 16 mg dose of risperidone were as effective as the 6 mg dose. Whether or not higher risperidone doses are effective, the authors of the U.S. study still preferred the 6 mg regimen because its rates of EPS were similar to placebo, while the rates of EPS with 10 mg and 16 mg of risperidone were significantly higher than placebo.

Dosing and Adverse Effects

The most important finding in the North American risperidone trials is **that risperidone should not be dosed to the neuroleptic threshold—the greatest benefit to cost ratio occurs at a dose below that necessary to induce clinical neurotoxicity.** Since it is impossible to predict the neuroleptic threshold in a given patient, **it is necessary to begin therapy at a low dose and slowly *titrate to efficacy, while remaining below toxic levels.*** A general guideline is to begin dosing at 1 mg b.i.d. (0.5 mg qd for the elderly) and to slowly titrate in 1 mg increments every five to seven days. Once target symptoms begin to show a therapeutic response, the titration should be halted. The dose should be increased further only if the ultimate therapeutic effect obtained is inadequate. **If demonstrable neurotoxicity** (either parkinsonism or akathisia) **emerges, the dose should be decreased. This is in marked distinction to the usual pattern of adding an anti-EPS medication like benztropine or trihexiphenidyl (Artane) to conventional medications.** The most commonly prescribed dose range for chronic schizophrenia is 4–6 mg. Some patients can be maintained on doses as low as 1 mg, while others will require as much as 20 mg. Regardless of the ultimate dose necessary, the clinician should be guided to dose to antipsychotic efficacy but below the neuroleptic threshold.

Side effects associated with risperidone that have at least a 5% prevalence include somnolence, dizziness, constipation, and tachycardia.[97] Statistically significant positive correlations have also been found between risperidone doses and fatigue, sedation, accommodation disturbances, orthostatic dizziness, palpitations or tachycardia, diminished sexual desire, weight gain, and erectile dysfunction.[82,90,92,97] Like other antipsychotics, **risperidone increases serum prolactin and may lead to galactorrhea or amenorrhea.**[82] **A much rarer but more serious side effect associated with risperidone use is neuroleptic malignant syndrome (NMS).** Several cases of NMS have been reported and are assumed to be an effect of risperidone's antidopaminergic activity.[42,98–100]

Sertindole:

The manufacturer has recently withdrawn the application for FDA approval due to the drug's prolongation of QT intervals (see below). Because QT prolongation is associated with induction of torsades de pointe ventricular arrhythmias, it was decided that more clinical experience was needed before approval. Although the rate of sertindole-induced QT prolongation was significantly greater than that caused by haloperidol, it is not yet clear that this QT prolongation increases the risk of sudden death. Since sertindole is marketed in other countries, information regarding the risk of sudden death will likely be forthcoming fairly soon.

Pharmacology

Sertindole is an *imidazolidinone* compound, somewhat structurally distinct from other atypical neuroleptics. Sertindole has not been approved yet by the U.S. Food and Drug Administration. However, it has been well tested in hundreds of patients and is approved in the United Kingdom and several other European countries. **Like clozapine, sertindole antagonizes serotonin and D$_4$ receptors. Sertindole binds 5-HT$_{2A}$ receptors 4 times more potently than does clozapine**[2] **and to D$_4$ sites twice as avidly as does clozapine.**[3] However, **unlike the atypical prototype, sertindole is also a potent antagonist of D$_2$ receptors. Sertindole also antagonizes α$_1$ receptors 20 times more potently than does phentolamine** (Regitine). **Sertindole exerts almost no activity at muscarinic and histaminergic sites.**

Sertindole is metabolized by CYP2D6 and CYP3A3/4, and thus has the potential for pharmacokinetic interactions with SSRIs and other antidepressants.[72] **CYP inducers such as carbamazepine, barbiturates, and phenytoin can decrease serum levels of sertindole.**[101] Therefore, sertindole doses may need to be higher if co-administered with such drugs.

Clinical Indications and Efficacy

Several double-blind, placebo-controlled studies have evaluated sertindole's efficacy in treating schizophrenia. McEvoy et al.[102] enrolled 38 patients in a flexible dose pilot study of sertindole, and found that the drug led to significant improvement in psychotic symptoms as compared to placebo. These findings were recently extended in a double-blind trial performed by van Kammen et al.[103] They utilized a fixed dose design, comparing 8, 12, and 20 mg of sertindole to placebo in 205 acutely ill schizophrenic patients. These investigators reported that **only the 20 mg dose was significantly more effective than placebo** as measured on the PANSS, BPRS, and CGI. However, there was a trend towards a dose response relationship between the 8 mg and 12 mg arms, suggesting that 12 mg should be considered the lower end of the therapeutic range.

Results from a third double-blind trial have been described by Zimbroff et al.[104] These investigators reported on an 8-week fixed dose trial involving nearly 500 chronic schizophrenics at 43 centers in the US and Canada. They compared low, medium, and high doses of sertindole (12, 20, and 24 mg) versus haloperidol (4, 8, and 16 mg) and placebo, and **found that all doses of both drugs were associated with improvement in PANSS and BPRS scores.** Only the 4 mg haloperidol arm failed to achieve significant improvement in CGI scores. **Although the 12 mg sertindole arm demonstrated some efficacy, the 20 mg and 24 mg sertindole arms were clearly superior to the lower dose for improvement of positive symptoms.**

The effect of sertindole on negative symptoms is more difficult to discern. Interestingly, **of all the arms of the multicenter trial, only 20 mg sertindole led to significant improvement in negative symptoms.** The effectiveness of the 12 mg and 24 mg doses on negative symptoms approached statistical significance, with the lower dose showing greater effect than the highest. However, **another sertindole study found that negative symptoms only improved significantly in a 24 mg group, and not in a 20 mg group, which just missed statistical significance.**[105] Zimbroff et al. point out that when the results of the two studies are combined, statistical significance is achieved at both the 20 mg and 24 mg doses. The authors further indicate that the sertindole-induced improvement in negative symptoms was still increasing at 8 weeks. **The implication is that negative symptom improvement becomes more significant after longer periods of time,** and that eight weeks may be too short a trial for an accurate analysis of the drug's efficacy on these highly refractory symptoms.

Dosing and Adverse Effects

Like risperidone, **sertindole has a very narrow therapeutic range. Most of the clinical trials suggest that the greatest improvement in positive and negative symptoms occur at the higher doses of 20 mg and 24 mg.** Sertindole does not appear to have linear pharmacokinetics, so an increase of 4 mg results in a substantially higher plasma level. Sertindole dosing should begin at 4 mg and be increased by 4 mg doses every 2 to 30 days until 20 mg is reached.

Sertindole metabolism does not appear to be affected by age, and **dosages do not need to be altered for the elderly**. However, gender does affect the drug's pharmacokinetics. Sertindole clearance is mildly decreased in females, necessitating dosages towards the lower end of the therapeutic range. The presence of liver disease mitigates for halving of normal dosages. However, renal disease is not an indication for dosage alterations.

Side effects commonly reported with sertindole are related to its α_1-blockade. These include orthostatic hypotension, which can limit the rate of dosage titration, nasal congestion secondary to vasodilation, reflex tachycardia, decreased ejaculatory volume, and weight gain.[102–104] Decreased ejaculatory volume has been reported to occur at a rate of 15%–20%.[59,103,104] It has not been associated with loss of libido or erectile dysfunction. This adverse effect is of some concern because it could lead to reduced compliance in sexually active males. Average weight gain ranged from 2.2 to 3.3 kg in the Zimbroff et al. trial,[104] and Wirshing et al. reported a mean weight gain of 5 kg.[59]

The most potentially serious adverse effect reported in patients taking sertindole is prolongation of the QT segment of the EKG.[103,106] In the Daniel et al. study, 2,700 EKGs were examined by blinded cardiologists who described a 2%–5% cumulative incidence of QT segment prolongation. The mean QTc time, equivalent to the QT corrected for heart rate, remained well within normal limits. However, 1% of the patients possessed QTc's that exceeded 500 msec, which is the accepted lower limit of clinical toxicity.[107] Despite concern about the development of *torsades de pointes*, an often fatal arrhythmia associated with prolonged QTc, no pathological arrhythmia or clinical symptom developed in any of the patients.

Two favorable aspects of sertindole's adverse effect profile are its effects on prolactin and EPS. **Most patients on sertindole show no increases in prolactin levels, and when elevations occur they are generally much milder than those seen in patients taking pure D$_2$ blockers.**[106] **Prolactin levels have not been reported to be elevated beyond the upper end of normal in such patients.**[103] The frequency and severity of EPS in sertindole patients has been reported to be equal to placebo,[103] and one study even reported EPS levels in sertindole patients which were lower than the placebo-treated patients.[106] It is unclear whether this finding represents a true palliative effect of sertindole on EPS, or a statistical artifact.[81] Sertindole's lack of EPS is interesting because, as mentioned above, the drug is a very potent antagonist of D_2 receptors. It has been hypothesized that sertindole's effects on serotonin receptors might protect against the EPS induction of its D_2 antagonism,[108] but this theory remains to be proven.

Olanzapine:

Pharmacology

Olanzapine (Zyprexa) is a *thienobenzodiazepine derivative* with activity at D_1, D_2, D_4, 5-HT$_{2A}$, 5-HT$_{2C}$, 5-HT$_6$, H_1, α_1-adrenergic, and muscarinic receptors.[3,109,110] As expected of an atypical antipsychotic, it has a characteristically higher affinity for 5-HT$_2$ receptors than for D_2 receptors, although its 5HT$_2$/D$_2$ of 2.7 is noticeably lower than that of clozapine.[2,3,111]

Olanzapine is readily absorbed and reaches steady-state concentrations in five to seven days.[112] It is actively metabolized by the liver with 40% of an oral dose never reaching systemic circulation. So far, ten inactive liver metabolites of olanzapine are known.[112] The CYP1A2 and CYP2D6 systems are thought to be responsible for olanzapine's oxidative metabolism.[113] In vivo, the latter appears to play a lesser role than the former in that subjects deficient in this enzyme do not have reduced clearance of olanzapine. Nevertheless, drug interactions with SSRIs and other antidepressants that use the CYP2D6 enzyme may exist.[72] **Coadministration of lithium and olanzapine** (olanzapine dosage: 10 mg, 8 days; lithium dosage: 32.4 mm one time) **does not seem to affect serum lithium concentrations or the pharmacokinetics of olanzapine.[114]**

Even though the liver is primarily responsible for olanzapine's metabolism, subjects with clinically significant cirrhosis showed no significant reduction in clearance of olanzapine. **Renal impairment also did not have any major impact on the pharmacokinetics of olanzapine.[112]**

Clinical Indications and Efficacy

Numerous studies have shown that **olanzapine can improve both the**

negative and positive symptoms of schizophrenia. A recent study, comparing the effects of two doses of olanzapine (1 mg and 10 mg) and placebo in 152 patients with schizophrenia, showed that the higher dose of olanzapine was clearly superior to placebo in improving BPRS and PANSS total scores.[115] In addition, the high dose of olanzapine was superior to placebo in improving positive symptoms (i.e., positive factors of the BPRS and PANSS). According to scores on the PANSS-negative subscale, **the harder to treat core negative symptoms were much more responsive to the 10 mg dose of olanzapine**. The lower dose of olanzapine was undoubtedly below the therapeutic level since 1 mg demonstrated no efficacy compared to placebo.

In another study, three dose ranges of olanzapine (2.5–7.5 mg, 7.5–12.5 mg, and 12.5–15.0 mg) were compared to haloperidol (10–20 mg) and placebo in 335 schizophrenic patients during an acute exacerbation of their illness.[116] Decreases in total BPRS scores and decreases on the positive factors of the BPRS from baseline were observed in the haloperidol group as well as in the medium and high dose olanzapine groups. The high dose olanzapine group, however, had the largest decrease (35.7%) in total BPRS scores. **The high olanzapine dose group displayed greater improvement in negative symptoms as measured on the SANS than did the haloperidol group and the lower olazapine dose groups.**

The results of this investigation were later reanalyzed to determine **what proportion of olanzapine's advantage in improving negative symptoms was due to its indirect effects** (i.e., less EPS or improved positive symptoms) **and what was due to its direct effects on core negative symptoms.**[117] Use of a path analysis technique revealed that **olanzapine's advantage over placebo in improving negative symptoms was partially due to its superior effects on positive symptoms (43%). The largest proportion of olanzapine's advantage (53%) was due to its direct effects on primary negative symptoms.** When the same analysis was applied to find the reason for olanzapine's superiority over haloperidol in negative symptom improvement, an even larger proportion (84%) was due to direct effects on negative symptoms.

The improvements noted by the previous studies were confirmed by a study of 1,996 schizophrenics that were randomized to either 5–20 mg of olanzapine (mean dose 13.2 mg) or 5–20 mg of haloperidol (mean dose 11.8 mg).[118] In addition to greater improvement on several measures of psychotic symptoms (BPRS total, CGI, PANSS total and negative), olanzapine seemed to be better tolerated in that 66.5% of the patients on olanzapine completed the 6 week trial compared to 46.8% of the haloperidol patients. The better side effect profile of olanzapine likely contributed to olanzapine's superior tolerability. Olazapine also produced improvement in depressive symptoms. Its effect was twice that of haloperidol as measured on the Montgomery-Asberg Depression Rating Scale.

Dosing and Adverse Effects

The current dosing recommendation for olanzapine is that **10 mg is a therapeutic dose and that no titration is necessary for the majority of patients. However, not all patients can tolerate 10 mg of olanzapine.** An elderly patient, for example, may find 10 mg too sedating, and patients with extreme sensitivity to EPS may actually experience some EPS (usually akathisia) at this dose. We have treated several patients (including one clozapine non-responder) who have done well on 5 mg per day. Similarly, careful examination of the large (1996 patients) study[118] reveals that patients were judged clinically improved on all four dose levels of the medication, and that the most commonly prescribed dose was 20 mg (31%). The average olanzapine dose in a trial comparing olanzapine to risperidone was 16.9 mg.[119] Examination of all of the available controlled studies involving multiple doses of olanzapine shows that in large part, higher doses are superior. The lack of a plateau in the dose response curves means that we have not yet found the maximum effective dose. It may ultimately be determined that higher doses of olanzapine (e.g., 30–50 mg per day) are superior to the dose ranges tested to date. However, in the absence of controlled safety data, such dose ranges cannot be currently recommended.

In aggregate, these data clearly demonstrate that **olanzapine has utility at doses well below and well above 10 mg. A prudent dosing strategy is to begin at 5 mg** (except in very fragile elderly patients, for whom 2.5 mg should be the starting dose) **and titrate up every four to six days in 5 mg increments. The titration should be terminated once clinical therapeusis can be demonstrated or significant toxicity has emerged.** While this strategy means that patients who ultimately require the higher dosages will be undertreated for some period of time, it does maximize safety, minimize toxicity, and perhaps ultimately give rise to the most compliant patient.

The most common problems reported with olanzapine use were **increased appetite, weight gain, slight drowsiness, and dry mouth.**[111,115] In two recent studies of patients on various doses of olanzapine, the average weight gains reported were 1.88 kg[118] and 4.8 kg.[59] The difference in the results could be due to differences in the study populations or use of different doses of olanzapine. In addition, **we have recently described two cases of treatment-emergent diabetes in patients taking olanzapine.**[70] This indicates that, **like clozapine, olanzapine should be used cautiously in patients with risk factors for diabetes.**

Elevations in prolactin were mild, transient, and similar to placebo.[115,116] When compared to haloperidol, the transient prolactin increases with olanzapine were significantly smaller in magnitude.[118] Liver transaminases were also found to be elevated in some patients (7.9% with alanine aminotransferase [ALT] elevation), although they were mild and not associated with any clinical symptoms. Most importantly, none of these elevations required discontinuation of olanzapine.

Olanzapine has consistently been shown to have **much milder effects on EPS than does haloperidol.** A recent meta-analysis of clinical trials with a total of 1796 patients on olanzapine and 810 patients on haloperidol clearly indicated that olanzapine had significantly lower rates of discontinuation due to EPS (3% vs. 2.7%) as well as lower incidence of treatment-emergent parkinsonism (defined as a total score of >3 on Simpson-Angus scale). Furthermore, olanzapine actually lowered patients' scores on the Simpson-Angus scale and Barnes Akathisia scale, while haloperidol increased these scores.[120] This phenomenon occurred despite a three-fold more frequent use of anticholinergic medication in the haloperidol group.

Quetiapine:

Pharmacology

Quetiapine (Seroquel), a *dibenzothiazepine* derivative, is a relatively new atypical antipsychotic that has **activity at a broad range of receptors including 5-HT$_{2A}$ receptors, H$_1$ receptors, and α_1 and α_2 adrener-**

gic receptors.[121] Its blockade of a_1 and H_1 receptors is significant enough to cause postural hypotension and drowsiness. It has minimal activity at D_1 and $5\text{-}HT_{1A}$ receptors and essentially no activity at benzodiazepine receptors.[122] Like clozapine and other atypical antipsychotics, it has activity at $5\text{-}HT_2$ and D_2 receptors. But it differs from clozapine because it has almost no activity at muscarinic receptors.[122] It binds to D_2 sites with markedly less affinity than do risperidone, sertindole, and ziprasidone,[123] which could be the reason that **quetiapine has not been shown to elevate prolactin.**

The amount of time required to achieve steady-state with quetiapine is relatively short and is estimated to range from one to two days. **The drug is metabolized in the liver by the CYP3A4 system** which indicates that interactions with other substrates of this system are possible and may require dosage adjustments. Possible interactions were tested by Wong et al. who showed that the mean clearance of quetiapine was increased by 5-fold in the presence of the specific CYP3A4 inducer, phenytoin.[124] Cimetidine did not, however, alter quetiapine's pharmacokinetics. A study in which quetiapine (250 mg, TID) was co-administered with lithium to 10 schizophrenic, schizoaffective, or bipolar patients, concluded that **quetiapine could safely be added to a lithium regimen since there was no statistically significant change in lithium C-min or area under the curve (AUC) values.**[125]

Clinical Indications and Efficacy

A multicenter international trial with 118 schizophrenic patients was one of the first studies to establish quetiapine's efficacy.[126] The patients were treated with 50 to 750 mg of quetiapine (mean dose 278 mg) for an average of 21 days. Significant improvement from baseline was seen in BPRS total scores and CGI-S item scores. Forty-one percent of the patients were responders (as indicated by ≥ 30% decreases in BPRS total scores), with two-thirds responding within two weeks. A similar study was done in which 100 patients received quetiapine in the same dosage range as the previous study but with a higher mean dose of 407 mg.[127] This study found an even higher response rate (65%) indicating that the optimum therapeutic dose had not been reached in the previous study.

Small et al. established that **higher doses of quetiapine were more** effective in a large (286 patients) **6-week comparison study of low quetiapine doses** (mean dose 209 mg), **high quetiapine doses** (mean dose 360 mg), **and placebo.**[128] The high dose quetiapine group was found to be superior to the placebo group on total BPRS scores from day 14 to endpoint, on CGI-S item scores from day 21 to endpoint, and on Scale for the Assessment of Negative Symptoms (SANS) summary scores from day 28 to endpoint. Furthermore, the high dose quetiapine group was superior to the low dose quetiapine group in mean changes in BPRS total scores from baseline as well as in SANS summary scores from day 28 to endpoint. These results indicate that **quetiapine's time to onset of action is approximately two weeks, although improvements in negative symptoms, as measured by SANS summary scores, may require about four weeks.**

The optimum quetiapine dose appears to be in the 150–750 mg range, as indicated by a fixed dose study of quetiapine (75 mg, 150 mg, 300 mg, 600 mg, and 750 mg), haloperidol (12 mg), and placebo in 361 patients.[129] At the end of this 6-week investigation, quetiapine improved symptoms (BPRS total, and CGI-S item scores) better than placebo in the 150 mg to 750 mg range with maximum clinical benefits observed at 300 mg. Improvements in BPRS positive cluster scores were similar to the BPRS total improvements, indicating that quetiapine is effective at relieving positive symptoms. Superior improvements in negative symptoms (i.e., SANS summary scores), relative to placebo, were seen in the quetiapine 300 mg group but not in any of the other groups.

Dosing and Adverse Effects

The average patient will probably require 300–600 mg per day of quetiapine. Predictably, younger, older, and recent onset patients will have their dose response curve shifted lower than their chronic counterparts, and **the refractory population very well may require substantially higher doses.**

The side effect profile of quetiapine is relatively mild when compared to other typical and atypical antipsychotics. The most common complaints include **somnolence, agitation, insomnia, headache, postural hypotension, and dry mouth.**[130,131] The agitation and insomnia, however, are very likely to be an expression of the underlying illness since these two symptoms had equal prevalence in the placebo group.[131]

Similar to other antipsychotics, **clinically significant weight gain, defined as $\geq$ 7% increase in body weight, was reported to occur in as many as 25% of patients on quetiapine.**[130] These patients' mean weight increase was 5.5 kg. In addition, **transient and clinically asymptomatic elevations of liver enzymes have consistently been reported, especially with ALT.** Some ALT elevations have been as high as 18 times the upper limit of normal,[128,132] but returned to normal after continued administration of quetiapine.

Quetiapine did not produce plasma elevations of prolactin in patients treated for six weeks.[128] In fact, many of the studies reported that **the prolactin levels, which were often on the high end of normal at baseline, decreased during quetiapine treatment.**[132] This implies that the patients' prior exposure to neuroleptics had caused mild elevations in prolactin which returned to near normal levels during the quetiapine trial. The incidence of EPS in quetiapine-treated patients was found to be similar to placebo, as evidenced by scores on standard tests of EPS (i.e., Neurologic Rating Scale [NRS], Barnes Akathisia Scale, AIMS) and less frequent use of adjunctive anticholinergic medication.[132]

Ziprasidone:

[Nota Bene—At the time of publication, FDA approval of ziprasidone has been indefinitely delayed in light of safety concerns related to the prolongation of the QT interval revealed in clinical trials.]

Pharmacology

Ziprasidone is the latest atypical antipsychotic to enter widespread clinical trials. It is a fairly non-specific drug, binding to numerous receptors with high affinity. It is seven times more avid for $5\text{-}HT_{2A}$ receptors than is clozapine, and in addition, possesses a high specificity for $5\text{-}HT_1$ and $5\text{-}HT_3$ receptors.[3] Interestingly, ziprasidone appears to serve as an agonist, not an antagonist, of $5\text{-}HT_1$ sites. It also binds to $D_{2,3,4}$ and H_1 receptors, and is twice as potent at α_1 sites as is clozapine. Its $5\text{-}HT_{2A}/D_2$ affinity ratio is approximately 10.[133] Ziprasidone does not bind appreciably to M_1 receptors.

The pharmacokinetics of ziprasidone have been worked out in detail. To date, there are no known active metabolites among the nine to twelve currently known.[134] Its half-life is four to five hours, and a serum assay has been developed and validated.[135] Serum levels are enhanced by food (probably due to the lipid component) so the BID dosing required by the half-life should be with meals.[136]

Clinical Indications and Efficacy

Although ziprasidone is the newest of the drugs reviewed here, several studies examining its efficacy in schizophrenia have already been published. Harrigan and Morrissey reported on a 4-week, double-blind, randomized trial in 76 patients with acute psychotic exacerbation.[137] They studied doses of 40 mg and 120 mg of ziprasidone and found that only the higher dose improved BPRS and CGI scores significantly above placebo. **A subsequent 6-week study, examining 80 mg and 160 mg doses of ziprasidone in 302 similar patients, found significant improvement in PANSS, BPRS, and CGI scores in both treatment arms.**[138] Importantly, both doses also improved PANSS negative symptom scores as compared to placebo.

Ziprasidone has also been studied for efficacy in conditions other than psychosis. **Early results from an ongoing Phase III trial suggest that ziprasidone can treat affective symptoms.**[139] Its agonism of 5-HT_1 receptors led Wilner et al. to perform a double-blind, placebo-controlled study comparing the anxiolytic effects of ziprasidone and diazepam.[140] The investigators chose to work with 90 patients undergoing dental surgery, presumably to ensure a high baseline anxiety level so that anxiolysis could be detected. One dose of drug (20 mg of ziprasidone, 20 mg diazepam, or placebo) was administered orally three hours prior to the surgery. Subjective evaluations filled out by each patient, as well as by the investigators, indicated that both drugs decreased anxiety 55% from baseline. However, while no difference in efficacy was seen, diazepam induced significantly more sedation than ziprasidone.

Ziprasidone has shown very promising results as a therapeutic modality in schizophrenia, improving both positive and negative symptoms of psychosis, and may be indicated for other uses as well.

Dosing and Adverse Effects

A dosing range of 40 mg–80 mg b.i.d. seems ideal based on known studies, but recommendations are currently uncertain because the drug is not approved at this time. Ziprasidone should be taken with

food to maximize its clinical effects.[136,141] Ziprasidone may also be available in the near future in a short-acting injectable form.

At doses up to 200 mg,[139] few adverse effects have been reported. Ziprasidone does appear to **elevate prolactin levels** as compared to placebo,[142] although this effect seems to be transient.[139] The drug has **minimal associated EPS, sedation, and orthostatic hypotension,**[139] and no severe adverse effects have been described in any of the trials thus far completed.[137,138]

The Clinical Choice—Is an Algorithm Possible?

Investigational studies leading to drug approval in the U.S. tend to involve narrowly defined and homogenous populations of schizophrenia subjects. The generalizeability of these data to other clinical subpopulations (e.g., women; the elderly; children; subjects with concomitant medical illness, co-morbid substance abuse, atypical psychotic syndromes, etc.) is questionable. Further, most of these trials use conventional antipsychotics in the control treatment arm of the experiment. This makes direct comparisons among the various newer medications of either their comparative efficacies or toxicities impossible. In spite of these methodologic shortcomings in the data base, some conclusions can be drawn, and a few reasonably certain predictions made.

It is clear that the newer medications (including clozapine) all possess lower extrapyramidal toxicity than their conventional counterparts. In fact, this is the characteristic that loosely defines the group. Therefore, clinical populations that have either known or predictable sensitivity to neurotoxic side effects (e.g., first break subjects, children, the elderly, non-schizophrenic psychotic conditions, etc.) would predictably derive the greatest benefit from this low EPS characteristic. Among the available novel agents, clozapine and quetiapine possess the lowest EPS toxicity, followed closely by olanzapine and then risperidone. When extrapyramidal toxicity is of clinical concern, clozapine or quetiapine would be the first choice. However, the other toxicities associated with clozapine (e.g., blood dyscrasias, seizures, sedation, cardiotoxicity, etc.) lower its appeal for clinical use, even in the cases of severe acute extrapyramidal toxicities.

The newer agents are also distinguishable themselves from conventional compounds along endocrinologic lines. **Clozapine and quetiapine do not elevate prolactin above the baseline level measuredduring placebo run-in and olanzapine generally induces only a mild, and usually transient, prolactin elevation. Risperidone, on the other hand, elevates prolactin at least as much as its conventional counterparts.** In subpopulations where prolactin elevation is of clinical concern (e.g., young or adolescent females, or patients with clinically pertinent intolerance of hyperprolactinemia (amenorrhea), galactorrhea, gynecomastia, testicular atrophy, erectile incompetence, etc.), clozapine, quetiapine, or olanzapine should be used. **Because of the other toxicities associated with clozapine, olanzapine and quetiapine would be superior first choices.**

Other toxicities of clinical significance that vary among the atypical antipsychotics include **sedation, weight gain liability, and cardiovascular toxicity due to the combination of antihistaminic, antiadrenergic, and antimuscarinic properties.** Sedation is most severe with clozapine, and is generally the titration-limiting characteristic of this compound. Olanzapine has somewhat more sedative potential than either risperidone or quetiapine but substantially less than clozapine.

Weight gain should be anticipated whenever most of the new compounds are given. Measures to avoid weight gain are consistently more effective than those employed to remove weight induced by antipsychotic treatment. In our experience, clozapine and olanzapine have the greatest liability with risperidone and quetiapine inducing measurably smaller increases in weight. All these compounds increase weight more than the high potency conventional medications.

Cardiovascular toxicity has recently become a more prominent clinical concern because sertindole has been associated with more QT prolongation than have conventional medications (see above). There may be differences in the rates at which these compounds induce **ventricular arrhythmias**, but a precise rank ordering is not known at this time. A reasonable estimate is that clozapine has somewhat more potential to cause this than any of the other compounds. **Orthostatic hypotension with reflex tachycardia is the other major cardiovascular toxicity induced by these drugs.** Again, clozapine is much more problematic than the other compounds.

Quetiapine's toxic profile, while favorable in most respects, includes a theoretical increased risk of cataracts. This risk is inferred from the observation that quetiapine use in certain animal models results in the development of cataracts.[147] This animal toxicity has prompted the manufacturer and the FDA to advise slip lamp examinations before and during quetiapine treatment. Phenathiazines have, for years, been associated with an increased risk for the development of lenticular cataracts. Chlorpromazine is most notorious in this regard. Because the time course to the development of clinically significant cataracts is very slow, it is not our clinical practice to obtain a slip lamp examination before treatment. Instead, we perform routine clinical ophthalmoscopy on all patients before treatment, and refer only chronically treated subjects for opthamologic (or optometric) consultation. This way, only those subjects who are successfully treated with quetiapine will have to undergo these more extensive, and expensive, examinations.

Another important clinical question concerns the relative efficacy of these compounds. **For the refractory individual,** (i.e., one who is resistant to the mechanism of action of conventional antipsychotic medications) **clozapine is clearly the most powerful medication. Among the other atypical compounds, only risperidone has shown superior therapeutic efficacy compared to conventional medications in such populations.**[144] In treatment-responsive populations, both risperidone and olanzapine (but not quetiapine) appear superior to conventional drugs. **Clozapine also performs remarkably better than conventional medications in moderately refractory individuals.**[145] A few studies have compared risperidone to olanzapine directly in heterogenous populations.[146] These data suggest that there is very little difference in efficacy between the two drugs, although, as mentioned above, they do have somewhat different side effect profiles.

In summary, **these compounds clearly have lower EPS liabilities than its conventional counterparts, though they all have other toxicities that distinguish them.** The clinical scenario for an individual patient may guide the clinician in choosing among these various toxicity profiles. While clozapine is without question more toxic than the other compounds, it is without question the most efficacious antipsychotic treatment available. Thus, when toxicity is a major concern, clozapine should be tried last, but when inefficacy is problematic, clozapine should be tried earlier in the algorithm. Among the other compounds, quetiapine has the lowest toxicity, but the available data suggest it also has the lowest efficacy. **Because risperidone and olanzapine** are similar in efficacy, the choice between them is usually based on their adverse effect profile. Olanzapine is accompanied by more sedation, weight gain, and hepatotoxicity, and is more expensive than risperidone. Risperidone produces more EPS and endocrinologic toxicities.

There are even fewer controlled studies to guide the treatment of disorders other than schizophrenia. Clozapine has shown some efficacy in treating schizoaffective and rapid cycling bipolar populations.[50-52,148,149] Studies are currently under way to determine whether olanzapine and risperidone effectively treat these disorders. In our clinical laboratory, neither risperidone nor olanzapine has been as powerful as clozapine at producing improvement in a mood-disordered population. Risperidone, but not olanzapine, has been demonstrated to induce improvement in psychotic and behavioral symptoms in agitated and demented elderly subjects.

As clinical and experimental experience with these compounds accrues, their comparative advantages for treating the various non-schizophrenic syndromes that require the use of antipsychotic pharmacotherapy should become more clear. Because non-schizophrenic psychotic diagnoses are associated with more sensitivity to extrapyramidal neurotoxicity than is schizophrenia, these lower EPS compounds may virtually replace conventional medications in such populations. Also, if these newer compounds are demonstrated to be safer than their predecessors for chronic use (i.e., to have lower liability to induce tardive dyskinesia), then these medications might reasonably be used to treat disorders that currently have an unacceptable risk benefit ratio (i.e., refractory anxiety disturbances, severe attention deficit disorder, developmental delay and interpersonal violence in adolescents, somatiform disorder syndromes, severe PTSD, etc.). These medications (especially risperidone) are being used for these nonschizophrenic syndromes based on the empirical evidence outlined here. These "nonclassic" uses are theoretically and medically defensible, but they should be resorted to more cautiously, and the dose ranges and the titration schedule should be lower and slower, than for use in schizophrenic syndromes.

Summary

The atypical antipsychotics offer substantial benefit over standard neuroleptics in several parameters of antipsychotic pharmacotherapy and should be used as first line interventions. Although only one drug, clozapine, has been definitively demonstrated to have efficacy in treatment-refractory patients, it is likely that future studies will find that others of this class of drugs work similarly in such patients. **The relative lack of associated EPS, the reduced impact on prolactin levels, and the improved efficacy on negative symptoms in schizophrenic patients, make these novel drugs attractive alternatives to standard antipsychotic therapy.** Future studies should help delineate differences amongst the atypical drugs, allowing clinicians to assign priority for use of the drugs based on the clinical circumstances.

References

1. Delay J, Deniker P, Harl JM. The treatment of excitation and agitation states by a method of medication derived from hibernotherapy. *Annals of Method Psychology.* 1952;110:267.

2. Richelson E. Preclinical pharmacology of neuroleptics: focus on new generation compounds. *J Clin Psychiatry.* 1996;57:4–11.

3. Schotte A, Janssen PFM, Gommeren W, et al. Risperidone compared with new and referenced antipsychotic drugs: in vitro and in vivo receptor binding. *Psychopharmacology.* 1996;124:57–73.

4. Casey DE. Clozapine: neuroleptic-induced EPS and tardive dyskinesia. *Psychopharmacology.* (Berl) 1989;99:47–53.

5. Meltzer HY, Matsubara S, Lee J. Classification of typical and atypical antipsychotic drugs on the basis of dopamine D-1, and D-2 and serotonin2 pKi values. *J Pharmacol Exp Ther.* 1989;251:238–246.

6. Van Tol HHM, Bunzow JR, Guan H-C, et al. Cloning of the gene for a human dopamine D4 receptor with high affinity for the antipsychotic clozapine. *Nature.* 1991;350:610–611.

7. Van Tol HHM, Wu CM, Guan HC, et al. Multiple dopamine-D4 receptor variants in the human population. *Nature.* 1992;358:149–152.

8. Glatt CE, Snowman AM, Sibley DR, et al. Clozapine: selective labelling of sites resembling 5HT(6) serotonin receptors may reflect psychoactive profile. *Mol Med.* 1995;1:398–406.

9. Seeman P, Guan HC, Van Tol HHM. Dopamine D4 receptors elevated in schizophrenia. *Nature.* 1993;365:441–445.

10. Meyer MC, Baldessarini RJ, Goff DC, Centorrino F. Clinically significant interactions of psychotropic agents with antipsychotic drugs. *Drug Experience.* 1996;15:333–346.

11. DeVane CL. Pharmacogenetics and drug metabolism of newer antidepressant agents. *J Clin Psychiatry.* 1994;55:38–45.

12. Pollock B. Recent developments in drug metabolism of relevance to psychiatrists. *Harvard Review of Psychiatry.* 1994;2:204–213.

13. Nemeroff C, DeVane C, Pollock B. Newer antidepressants and the cytochrome P450 system. *Am J Psychiatry.* 1996;153:311–320.

14. Hiemke C, Weigmann H, Hartter S, Dahmen N, Wetzel H, Muller H. Elevated levels of clozapine in serum after addition of fluvoxamine [Letter]. *J Clin Psychopharmacol.* 1994;14:279–281.

15. Brosen K, Skjelbo E, Rasmussen BB, Poulsen HE, Loft S. Fluvoxamine is a potent inhibitor of cytochrome P4501A2. *Biochem Pharmacol.* 1993;45:1211–1214.

16. Centorrino F, Baldessarini RJ, Kando J, et al. Serum concentrations of clozapine and its major metabolites: effects of cotreatment with fluoxetine or valproate. *Am J Psychiatry.* 1994;151:123–125.

17. Centorrino F, Baldessarini RJ, Frankenburg FR, et al. Serotonin reuptake inhibitors alter metabolism of clozapine. *Am J Psychiatry.* 1996;153:820–822.

18. Koreen AR, Liberman JA, Kronig M, et al. Cross-tapering clozapine and risperidone [letter]. *Am J Psychiatry.* 1995;152:1690.

19. McCarthy RH, Terkelsen KG. Risperidone augmentatino of clozapine. *Pharmacopsychiatry.* 1995;38:61-3.

20. Tyson SC, DeVane CL, Risch SC. Pharmakokinetic interaction between risperidone and clozapine. *Am J Psychiatry.* 1995;152:1401–1402.

21. Baldessarini RJ, Gardner DM, Garver DL. Conversions from clozapine to other antipsychotics. *Arch Gen Psychiatry.* 1995;52:1071–1072.

22. Funderburg LG, Vertrees JE, True JE, et al. Seizure after the addition of erythromycin to clozapine treatment. *Am J Psychiatry.* 1994;151:1840–1841.

23. Szymanski S, Lieberman A, Picou D, Masiar S, Cooper T. A case report of cimetidine-induced clozapine toxicity. *J Clin Psychiatry.* 1991;52:21–22.

24. Guengerich FP. Human cytochrome P450 enzymes. *Life Sciences.* 1992;50:1471–1478.

25. Centorrino F, Baldessarini RJ, Kando J, et al. Clozapine and metabolites: serum concentrations and clinical findings during treatment of chronically psychotic patients. *J Clin Psychopharmacol.* 1994;4:119–125.

26. Miller DD. Effect of phenytoin on plasma clozapine concentrations in two patients. *J Clin Psychiatry.* 1991;52:23–25.

27. Junghan U, Albers M, Woggon B. Increased risk of hematological side-effects in psychiatric patients treated with clozapine and carbamazepine [letter]. *Pharmacopsychiatry.* 1993;26:262.

28. Finley P, Warner D. Potential impact of valproic acid therapy on clozapine disposition. *Biol Psychiatry.* 1994;36:487–488.

29. Longo LP, Salzman C. Valproic acid effects on serum concentration of clozapine and norclozapine [letter]. *Am J Psychiatry.* 1995;152:650.

30. Wilson WH. Do anticonvulsants hinder clozapine treatment? *Biol Psychiatry.* 1995;37:132–133.

31. Wirshing WC, Ames D, Bisheff S, Pierre JM, Mendoza A, Sun A. Hepatic encephalopathy associated with combined clozapine and divalproex sodium treatment. *J Clin Psychopharmacol.* 1996;17:120–121.

32. Garcia G, Crismon ML, Dorson PG. Seizures in two patients after the addition of lithium to a clozapine regimen. *J Clin Psychopharmacol.* 1994;14:426–428.

33. Grohmann R, Ruther E, Sassim N, et al. Adverse effects of clozapine. *Psychopharmacology.* 1989;99:S101–S104.

34. Cobb CD. Possible interaction between clozapine and lorazepam. *Am J Pscyhiatry.* 1991;148:1606–1607.

35. Jackson CW, Mankowitz JS, Brewerton TD. Delirium associated with clozapine and benzo-diazepine combinations. *Ann Clin Psychiatry.* 1995;7:139–141.

36. Baker LA, Cheng LY, Amara IB. Withdrawal of benztropine mesylate in chronic schizo-phrenic patients. *Br J Psychiatry.* 1983;143:584–590.

37. Jann MW, Grimsley S, Gray E, et al. Pharmacokinetics and pharmacodynamics of clozap-ine. *Clin Pharmacokinet.* 1993;24:161–176.

38. Bertilsson L, Lou YQ, Du YL, et al. Pronounced differences between native Chinese and Swedish populations in the polymorphic hydroxylations of debrisoquine and S-mepheny-toin. *Clin Pharmacol Ther.* 1992;51:388–397.

39. Marder SR. Managment of treatment-resistant patients with schizophrenia. *J Clin Psychiatry.* 1996;57:26–30.

40. Fischer-Cornelssen KA, Ferner UJ. An example of European multicenter trials: multispec-tral analysis of clozapine. *Psychopharmacol Bull.* 1976;12:34–39.

41. Kane J, Honifeld G, Singer J, Meltzer H. Clozapine for the treatment-resistant schizo-phrenic: a double-blind comparison with chlorpromazine. *Arch Gen Psychiatry.* 1988;45:789–796.

42. Pickar D, Owen RR, Lutman RE, et al. Clinical and biologic response to clozapine in patients with schizophrenia: crossover comparison with fluphenazine. *Arch Gen Psychiatry.* 1992;49:345–353.

43. Marder SR, Kane JM, Schooler NR, et al. Clozapine and haloperidol for treatment resistant outpatients with schizophrenia. NCDEU Annual Meeting, Boca Raton, Florida, May, 1996.

44. Essock SM, Hargreaves WA, Covell NH, Goethe J. Antipsychotics in reseach and clinical settings. *Psychopharmacol Bull.* 1996;32:683–697.

45. Realmuto GM, Erickson WD, Yellin AM, Hopwood JH, Greenberg LM. Clinical compari-son of thiothixene and thioridazine in schizophrenic adolescents. *Am J Psychiatry.* 1984;141:440–442.

46. Green W, Gayol M, Hardesty A, Bassiri M. Schizophrenia with childhood onset: a phenom-enological study of 38 cases. *J Am Acad Child Adolesc Psychiatry.* 1992;31:968–976.

47. Campbell M, Spencer E. Psychopharmacology in child and adolescent psychiatry: a review of the past five years. *J Am Acad Child Adolesc Psychiatry.* 1988;27:269–279.

48. Kumra S, Frazier JA, Jacobsen LK, et al. Childhood-onset schizophrenia: a double-blind clozapine-haloperidol comparison. *Arch Gen Psychiatry.* 1996;53:1090–1097.

49. Breier A, Buchanan RW, Kirkpatrick B, et al. Effects of clozapine on positive and negative symptoms in outpatients with schizophrenia. *Am J Psychiatry.* 1994;151:20–26.

50. Zarate CAJ, Tohen M, Banov MD, Weiss MK, Cole JO. Is clozapine a mood stabilizer? *J Clin Psychiatry.* 1995;56:108–112.

51. Shulman RW, Singh A, Shulman KI. Treatment of elderly institutionalized bipolar patients with clozapine. *Pscyhopharmacol Bull.* 1997;33:13–118.

52. Calabrese JR, Kimmel SE, Woyshville MJ, et al. Clozapine for treatment-refractory mania. *Am J Psychiatry.* 1996;153:759–764.

53. Wagner ML, Defilippi JL, Menza MA, Sage JI. Clozapine for the treatment of psychosis in Parkinson's disease: chart review of 49 patients. *J Neuropsychiatry Clin Neurosci.* 1996;8:276–280.

54. Friedman JH, Koller WC, Lannon MC, Busenbark K, Swanson-Hyland E, Smith D. Benztropine versus clozapine for the treatment of tremor in parkinson's disease. *Neurology.* 1997;48:1077–1081.

55. Cohen SA, Underwood MT. The use of clozapine in a mentally retarded and aggressive population. *J Clin Psychiatry.* 1994;55:440–444.

56. Sajatovic M, Ramirez LF, Kenny JT, Meltzer HV. The use of clozapine in borderline intellectual functioning and mentally retarded schizophrenic patients. *Compr Psychiatry.* 1994;35:29–33.

57. Duffy JD, Kant R. Clinical utility of clozapine in 16 patients with neurological disease. *J Neuropsychiatry Clin Neurosci.* 1996;8:92–96.

58. Bredbacka PE, Paukkala E, Kinnunen E, Koponen H. Can severe cardiorespiratory dysregulation induced by clozapine monotherapy be predicted? *Int Clin Psychopharmacol.* 1993;8:205–206.

59. Wirshing DA, Wirshing WC, Marder SR, Harmon L, Pashdag J, Hwang SS. Novel antipsychotics: comparison of weight gain liabilities. *J Clin Psychiatry.* submitted.

60. Fritze J, Elliger T. Pirenzepine for clozapine-induced hypersalivation [letter]. *Lancet.* 1995;346:1034.

61. VanderZwaag C, McGee M, McEvoy JP, et al. Response of patients with treatment-refractory schizophrenia to clozapine within three serum level ranges. *Am J Psychiatry.* 1996;153:1579–1584.

62. Fuller MA, Borovicka MC, Jaskiw GE, Simon MR, Kwon K, Konicki PE. Clozapine-induced urinary incontinence: incidence and treatment with ephedrine. *J Clin Psychiatry.* 1996;57:514–518.

63. Zeng XP, Le F, Scarisbrick I, et al. Muscarinic m4 receptor agonism by atypical but not typical antipsychotics. *Society for Neuroscience Abstracts.* 1995;21:1707.

64. Zorn SH, Jones SB, Ward KM, et al. Clozapine is a potent and selective muscarining M(4) receptor agonist. *Eur J Pharmacol.* 1994; 269:R1–R2.

65. Dalkilic A, Grosch WN. Neuroleptic malignant syndrome following intiiation of clozapine therapy [letter]. *Am J Psychiatry.* 1997;154:881–881.

66. Chatterton R, Cardy S, Schramm TM. Neuroleptic malignant syndrome and clozapine monotherapy. *Aust N Z J Psychiatry.* 1996;30:692–693.

67. Tsai G, Crisostomo G, Rosenblatt ML, Stern TA. Neuroleptic malignant syndrome associaited with clozapine treatment. *Ann Clin Psychiatry.* 1995;7:91–95.

68. Thornberg SA, Ereshefsky L. Neuroleptic malignant syndrome assocaited with clozapine monotherapy. *Pharmacotherapy.* 1993;13:510–514.

69. Sachdev P, Kruk J, Kneebone M, Kissane D. Clozapine-induced neuroleptic malignant syndrome: review and report of new cases. *J Clin Psychopharmacol.* 1995;15:365–371.

70. Wirshing DA, Wirshing WC, Erhart SM, Marder SR. Adult onset diabetes mellitus: a possible consequence of treatment with novel antipsychotics. *Biol Psychiatry.* In press.

71. Devinsky O, Honigfeld G, Patin J. Clozapine-related seizures. *Neurology.* 1991;41:369–371.

72. Marder SR, Wirshing WC, Ames D. New antipsychotic drugs. *Psychiatr Clin North Am.* 1997;4:195–207.

73. Alvir JM, Liberman JA. Agranulocytosis: incidence and risk factors. *J Clin Psychiatry.* 1994;55:137–138.

74. Alvir JJ, Lieberman JA, Safferman AZ, Schwimmer JL, Schaaf JA. Clozapine-induced agranulocytosis. *New Engl J Med.* 1993;329:162–167.

75. Zhang M, Owen RR, Pope SK, Smith R. Cost-effectiveness of clozapine monitoring after the first 6 months. *Arch Gen Psychiatry.* 1996;53:954–958.

76. Atkin K, Kenadll F, Gould D, Freeman J, Liberman J, O'Sullivan D. Neutropenia and agranulocytosis in patients receving clozapine in the UK and Ireland. *Br J Psychiatry.* 1996;169:483–488.

77. Freeman DJ, Oyewumi LK. Will routine therapeutic drug monitoring have a place in clozapine therapy? *Clin Pharmacokinet.* 1997;32:93–100.

78. Kleinerman MJ. Controversy grows over monitoring system for new schizophrenia drug. *JAMA.* 1990;264:2488.

79. Casey DE. Clozapine for the treatment-resistant schizophrenic: a double-blind comparison with chlorpromazine. *Arch Gen Psychiatry.* 1988;99:S47–S53.

80. Peacock L, Solgaard T, Lublin H, Gerlach J. Clozapine versus tupical antipsychotics: a retro- and prospective study of extrapyramidal side effects. *Psychopharmacology.* 1996;124:188–196.

81. Casey DE. Side effcet profile of new antipsychotic agents. *J Clin Psychiatry.* 1996;57:40–45.

82. Muller-Spahn F, Group TIRR. Risperidone in the treatment of chronic schizophrenic patients: an international double-blind parallel-group study versus haloperidol. *Clin Neuropharmacol.* 1992;15 (suppl 1):90A–91A.

83. Vanden Bussche G, Heykants J, De Coster R. Pharmacokinetic profgile and neuroendocrine effects of the new antipsychotic risperidone. 16th Congress of the Collegium Internationale Neuro-Psychopharmacologicum, Munich, West Germany, 1988.

84. Huang M, Van Peer A, Woestenborghs R, et al. Pharmacokinetics of the novel antipsychotic agent risperidone and the prolactin response in healthy subjects. *Clin Pharmacol Ther.* 1993;54:257–268.

85. Heykants J. Pharmacokinetics of risperidone. 1st International Risperidone Investigators Meeting, Paris, France, March, 1992.

86. Ames D, Marder SR, Wirshing WC. Risperidone: clinical applications. In A Brieir, ed. *The New Pharmacotherapy of Schizophrenia.* Washington, DC: American Psychiatric Press, Inc;1996:15–40.

87. Van Beijsterveldt L, Geerts RJF, Leysen J, et al. The regional brain distribution of risperidone and its active metabolite 9-hydroxy-risperidone in the rat. *Psychopharmacology* (Berl). 1994;114:53–62.

88. Ereshefsky L. Pharmacokinetics and drug interactions: update for new antipsychotics. *J Clin Psychiatry.* 1996;57(S11):12–25.

89. Fischer W, Vogels B, Maurer G, Tynes R. The antipsychotic clozapine is metabolized by the polymorphic human microsomal and recombinant cytochrome p450 2D6. *J Pharmacol Exp Ther.* 1992;260:1355–1360.

90. Claus A, Bollen J, De Cuyper H, et al. Risperidone versus haloperidol in the treatment of chronic schizophrenic inpatients: a multicentre double-blind comparative study. *Acta Psychiatr Scand.* 1992;85:295–305.

91. Castelao JF, Ferreira L, Gelders YG, Heylen SLE. The efficacy of the D and 5-HT antagonist risperidone (R64 766) in the treatment of chronic psychosis: an open dose-finding study. *Schizophr Res.* 1989;2:411–415.

92. Chouinard G, Jones B, Remington G, et al. A Canadian multicenter placebo-controlled study vs fixed doses of risperidone and haloperidol in the treatment of chronic schizophrenic patients. *J Clin Psychopharmacol.* 1993;13:25–40.

93. Davis JM, Erickson S, Dekirmenjian H. Plasma levels of antipsychotic drugs and clinical response. In Lipton MA, DiMascio A, Killam KF, eds. *Psychopharmacology: A Generation of Progress.* New York: Raven Press; 1978:905–915.

94. Rifkin A, Quitkin F, Klein DF. Akinesia: a poorly recognized drug-induced extrapyramidal behavioral disorder. *Arch Gen Psychiatry.* 1975;32:672–674.

95. Van Putten T, Marder SR. Behavioral toxicity of antipsychotic drugs. *J Clin Psychiatry.* 1987;48:13–19.

96. Gelenberg AJ, Mandel MR. Catatonic reactions to high-potency neuroleptic drugs. *Arch Gen Psychiatry.* 1977;34:947–950.

97. Marder SR, Meibach R. Risperidone in the treatment of schizophrenia. *Am J Psychiatry.* 1994;151:825–835.

98. Lee H, Ryan J, Mullett G, et al. Neuroleptic malignant syndrome associated with the use of risperidone, an atypical antipsychotic agent. *Human Psychopharmacology.* 1994;9:303–305.

99. Najara JE, Enikeev I. Risperidone and neuroleptic malignant syndrome. *J Clin Psychiatry.* 1995;56:534–535.

100. Webster P, Wijeratne C. Risperidone-induced neuroleptic malignant syndrome. *Lancet.* 1994;344:1228–1229.

101. Limited L. Summary of product charactersitics, Serdolect: United Kingdom, 1996.

102. McEvoy J, Borison R, Small J, et al. The efficacy and tolerability of sertindole in schizophrenic patients: a pilot, double-blind, placebo-controlled, dose-ranging study. *Schizophr Res.* 1993;9:244–254.

103. van Kammen DP, McEvoy JP, Targum SD, Kardatzke D, Sebree TB. A randomized, controlled, dose-ranging trial of sertindole in patients with schizophrenia. *Psychopharmacology.* 1996;124:168–75.

104. Zimbroff DL, Kane JM, Tamminga CA, et al. Controlled, dose-response study of sertindole, and haloperidol in the treatment of schizophrenia. *Am J Psychiatry.* 1997;154:782–791.

105. Schultz SC, Bark NM, Zborowski J, Zchmitz P, Sebree T, Wallin B. *Efficacy and safety of sertindole in two double-blind, placebo-controlled trials for schizophrenic patients.* In Institute Proceedings and Syllabus Summary, American Psychiatric Association 47th Institute on Psychiatric Services, Washington, D.C., 1995. American Psychiatric Association.

106. Daniel D, Targum S, Zimbroff D, et al. *Efficacy, safety, and dose response of three doses of sertindole and three doses of haloperidol in schizophrenic patients.* 34th Annual Meeting of the American College of Neuropsychopharmacology, San Juan, Puerto Rico, December 15, 1995.

107. Garson AJ. How to measure the QT interval—what is normal? *Am J Cardiol.* 1993;72:14B–16B.

108. Pilowsky LS, O'Connel P, Davies N, et al. In vivo effects of striatal dopamine D2 receptor binding by the novel atypical antipsychotic drug sertindole—a 123I IBZM single photon emission tomography (SPET) study. *Psychopharmacology.* 1997;130:152–158.

109. Bymaster FP, Calligaro DO, Falcone JF. Radioreceptor binding profile of the atypical antipsychotic olanzapine. *Neuropsychopharmacology.* 1996;14:87–96.

110 Roth BL, Craigo MS, Choudhary MS, et al. Binding of typical and atypical antipsychotic agents to 5-hydroxytryptamine-6 and 5-hydroxytryptamine-7 receptors. *J Pharmacol Exp Ther.* 1994;268:1403–1410.

111 Fulton B, Goa KL. Olanzapine. A review of its pharmacological and therapeutic efficacy in the management of schizophrenia and related psychoses. *Drugs.* 1997;53:281–298.

112. Boyd D, Obermeyer BD, Nyhart EH. The disposition of olanzapine in healthy volunteers. *Pharmacologist.* 1993;35:176.

113. Ring BJ, Binkley SN, Vandenbranden M. Identification of the human cytochrome responsible for the in vitro formation of the major oxidative metabolites of the antipsychotic agent olanzapine. *J Pharmacol Exp Ther.* 1996;276:658–666.

114 Demolle D, Onkelinx C, Muller-Oerlinghausen B. Interaction between olanzapine and lithium in healthy male volunteers. *Therapie.* Abstract # 486. 1995;50(Suppl).

115 Beasley CMJ, Sanger T, Satterlee W, et al. Olanzapine versus placebo: results of a double-blind, fixed-dose olanzapine trial. *Psychopharmacology.* 1996;124:159–67.

116 Beasley CM, Tollefson G, Tran P, et al. Olanzapine versus placebo and haloperidol: acute phase results of the North American double-blind olanzapine trial. *Neuropsychopharmacology.* 1996;14:111–123.

117 Tollefson GD, Sanger TM. Negative symptoms: a path analytic approach to a double blind, placebo and haloperidol controlled clinical trial with olanzapine. *Am J Psychiatry.* 1997;154:466–474.

118 Tollefson GD, Beasley CMJ, Tran PV, et al. Olanzapine versus haloperidol in the treatment of schizophrenia and schizoaffective and schizophreniform disorders: results of an international collaborative trial. *Am J Psychiatry.* 1997;154:457–465.

119 Tran PV, Tollefson G, Hamilton S, Kuntz A. *Olanzapine vs risperidone in the treatment of psychosis: preliminary report.* American College of Neuropsychopharmacology, San Juan, Puerto Rico, December 9–13, 1996. Vol. 35th Annual Meeting.

120. Tran PV, Dellva MA, Tollefson GD, Beasely CM, Potvin JH, Kiesler GM. Extrapyramidal symptoms and tolerability of olaznapine versus haloperidol in the acute treatment of schizophrenia. *J Clin Psychiatry.* 1997;58:205–211.

121. Saller CF, Salama AI. Seroquel: biochemical profile of a potential atypical antipsychotic. *Psychopharmacology*. 1993;112:285–92.

122. Goldstein JM, Arvantitis LA. ICI 204,636 (seroquel): a dibenzothiazepine atypical antipsychotic: review of preclinical pharmacology and highlights of phase II clinical trials. *CNS Drug Reviews*. 1995;1:50–73.

123. Goldstein JM. Pre-clinical pharmacology of new atypical antipsychotics in late stage development. *Expert Opinion on Investigational Drugs*. 1995;4:291–298.

124. Wong YWJ, Ewing BJ, Thyrum PT, Yeh C. The effect of phenytoin and cimetidine on the pharmacokinetics of Seroquel. *Schizophr Res*. 1997;24:200.

125. Potkin SG, Thyrum PT, Bera R, et al. Pharmacokinetics and safety of lithium co-administered with Seroquel (Quetiapine). *Schizophr Res*. 1997;24:199.

126. Meltzer HY, Hirsch SR, Arvanitis LA, Miller BG, Group ISS. *Quetiapine, an atypical antipsychotic: an open-label international multicenter trial of efficacy and safety in patients with acute psychotic symptoms*. Submitted.

127. Link CGG, Smith A, Miller B, Ryan J, Group SS. A multicenter, double-blind controlled comparison of Seroquel and chlorpromazine in the treatment of hospitalized patients with acute exacerbation of subchronic and schronic schizophrenia. *Eur Neuropsychopharmacol*. 1994;4:385.

128. Small JG, Hirsch SR, Arvanitis LA, Miller BG, Link CGG. Quetiapine in patients with schizophrenia: a high- and low-dose, bouble-blind comparison with placebo. *Arch Gen Psychiatry*. 1997;54:549–557.

129. Arvanitis LA. Seroquel (ICI 204,636), a new atypical antipsychotic: overview of clinical development. 34th Annual Meeting of the American College of Neuropsychopharmacology, San Juan, Puerto Rico, December, 1995.

130. Borison RL, Arvanitis LA, Miller BG. ICI 204,636, an atypical antipsychotic: efficacy and safety in a multicenter, placebo-controlled trial in patients with schizophrenia. *J Clinical Psychopharmacol*. 1996;16:158–69.

131. Casey DE. 'Seroquel' (quetiapine): preclinical and clinical findings of a new atypical antipsychotic. *Expert Opinion on Investigational Drugs*. 1996;5:939–957.

132. Fleishhacker WW, Link CGG. A multicenter, double blind randomized comparison of dose and dose regimen of Seroquel in the treatment of patients with schizophrenia. 34th Annual Meeting of the American College of Neuropsychopharmacology, San Juan, Puerto Rico, 1995.

133. Seeger TF, Seymour PA, Schmidt AW, et al. Ziprasidone (CP-88, 059): a new antipsychotic with combined dopamine and serotonin receptor antagonist acivity. *J Pharmacol Exp Ther*. 1995;275:101–113.

134. Reeves K, Harrigan EP. Efficacy and safety of ziprasidone: an update. American College of Neuropsychopharmacology, 1996. Vol. December.

135. Janiszewski JS, Fouda HG, Cole RO. Development and validation of a high-sensitivity assay for an antipsychotic agent, CP-88,059, with solid-phase extraction and narrow-bore high-performance liquid chromatography. *J Chromatogr A*. 1995;668:133–139.

136. Lebel M, Proulx MJ, Allard S, Tremblay J, Miceli J, Wilner K. Influence of a high fat breakfast on the absorption and the pharmacodynamics of CP-88,059, a new antipsychotic. *Clin Invest Med*. Abstract #117. 1993;16:B18

137. Harrigan E, Morrisey M. The efficacy and safety of 28-day treatment with ziprasidone in schizophrenia/schizoaffective disorder. 149th American Psychiatric Association Meeting, New York, 1996. Vol. May.

138. Harrigan EP, Reeves K. The efficacy and safety of two fixed doses of ziprasidone in schizophrenia. *Psychopharmacol Bull.* 1996;32:456.

139. Reeves KR, Harrigan EP. The efficacy and safety of two fixed doses of ziprasidone in schizophrenia and schizoaffective disorder. 149th Annual Meeting of the American Psychiatric Association, New York, 1996. Vol. May.

140. Wilner KD, Anziano RJ, Johnson AC, Miceli JJ, Fricke JR, Titus CK. Anxiolytic effects of ziprasidone compared with diazepam and placebo prior to dental surgery. *European Psychiatry.* 1996;11:380S.

141. Miceli JJ, Hunt T, Cole MJ, Wilner KD. The pharmacokinetics (PK) of CP-88,059 (CP) in healthy male volunteers following oral (PO) and intravenous (IV) administration. *Clin Pharmacol Ther.* 1994;55:142.

142. Muirhead GJ, Holt PR, Oliver S, Harness J, Anziano RJ. The effect of ziprasidone on steady-state pharmacokinetics of a combined oral contraceptive. *European Psychiatry.* 1996;11:4195.

143. Arvanitis LA. Clinical profile of Seroquel (quetiapine): an overview of recent clinical studies. In Holliday SG, Ancill RJ, MacEwan GW, eds. *Schizophrenia: Breaking Down the Barriers.* New York: John Wiley & Sons, Ltd; 1996;209–236.

144. Wirshing WC, Wirshing DA, Green MF, Marshall BD, McGurk SR. Risperidone efficacy beyond conventional symptoms. CINP Conference, 9 May, 1997, United Kindom.

145. Ames D, Wirshing WC, Marder SR, et al. Efficacy of clozapine vs. haloperidol in a long term clinical trial: preliminary result. *Biol Psychiatry.* 1995,37:661

146. Tran PV,Tollefson G, Hamilton S, Kuntz A. Olanzapine vs risperidone in the treatment of psychosis. Preliminary Report Presented at the Annual Meeting of the American College of Neuropsychopharmacology in Puerto Rico, December 1996.

147. Quietapine package insert.

148. Frye MA, Altshuler LL, Bitran JA. Clozapine in rapid cycling bipolar disorder. *J Clin Psychopharmacol.* 1996;16:87–90.

149. Suppes T, Phillips KA, Judd CR. Clozapine treatment of nonpsychiatric rapid cycling bipolar disorder: a report of three cases. *Biol Psychiatry.* 1994;36:338–340.

10 The Psychopharmacology of Negative Symptoms

Rajiv P. Sharma, MD

Dr. Sharma is Associate Professor of Psychiatry, University of Illinois at Chicago.

Supported in part by PHS MH48888 to RPS. The author is grateful to Nijole Grazulis, MS, for editorial comments.

Editor's Note

In this chapter, we are reminded of the distinction between two types of primary negative symptoms in schizophrenia: deficit state symptoms which do not covary with positive symptoms, and nonenduring symptoms which usually improve when positive symptoms abate. Secondary negative symptoms, of course, include post-psychotic depression, post-psychotic regressive states, antipsychotic side effects such as akinesia and extrapyramidal effects, environmental deprivation as a result of institutionalization, and nonspecific depressive syndromes. The author offers us guidelines for the management of each of these situations. For example, managing akinesia would entail reducing dosage, using targeted antipsychotic plasma levels, administering anticholinergics, or using atypical antipsychotics, which have fewer of such side effects. Negative symptoms secondary to environmental deprivation, such as decreased spontaneity, opportunity for "pay" activity, and curiosity and exploration are best handled through social skills training, vocational and cognitive rehabilitation, and case management that links individuals to community resources.

Primary negative symptoms that occur during the active phase of illness respond to treatment with conventional antipsychotics; some improvement in the deficit state can occur as well, except in early-onset patients. A variety of medications that have been used to improve enduring negative symptoms are reviewed in this chapter, including disinhibitory antipsychotics of the benzamide class (e.g., amisulpride) and the diphenylbutylpiperidine class (e.g., pimozide), and atypical antipsychotics (e.g., risperidone, olanzapine, clozapine). All groups seemed to have some beneficial effects on deficit symptoms, although it now appears that clozapine's effect is essentially secondary to its effect on primary symptoms. Glycine has also been shown to have some effect, but the effect of dopamine agonists (e.g., amphetamine) are equivocal, and, in fact, methylphenidate has been shown to induce a worsening of negative symptoms. Agents which increase available serotonin, such as the SSRIs, appear to improve negative symptoms, although it is sometimes hard to distinguish these from signs and symptoms of depression. The usefulness of anticholinergic drugs (e.g., trihexyphenidyl) and neuropeptides, (e.g., neurotensin, β-endorphin, cholecystokinin) appears to be equivocal at best.

Given the efficacy and safety of both olanzapine and risperidone, the author recommends these medications as the first-line treatment of psychotic symptoms. He also recommends the adjunctive use of SSRIs, since there is some evidence of a modest degree of effectiveness against negative symptoms, whether primary or secondary to depression.

Introduction

Efficacy in the treatment of negative symptoms has become the new benchmark for the evaluation of novel therapies in schizophrenia. Research in this area has benefitted greatly from the demonstration that negative symptoms can be reliably assessed and categorized into primary and secondary subtypes, with further subclassifications based on putative pathophysiology. Indeed, numerous operationalized assessments are now available to the interested researcher or clinician. The purpose of this chapter is to review relevant theories and the evidence for the efficacy of several different classes of psychotropic medications in the treatment of the negative symptoms of schizophrenia.

Secondary negative symptoms may be more amenable to therapeutic interventions. Therefore, the initial clinical objective must be to differentiate primary from secondary negative symptoms. Generally, secondary symptoms appear to dominate during the early years of

the illness, when variable levels of demoralization and despair are present in the aftermath of the onset of a devastating illness. They also dominate during psychotic exacerbations requiring acute pharmacologic intervention, when there is a higher likelihood of experiencing side effects. Secondary negative symptoms can be resolved if the appropriate causative sources are identified and treated (e.g., observing and treating extrapyramidal side effects [EPS]).

Primary negative symptoms are presumed to be expressions of the schizophrenic disease process. The *primary nonenduring* type fluctuates with the level of positive symptoms for reasons elaborated on below. The *primary enduring* type does not fluctuate with the level of positive symptoms, and is best observed during the interepisodic remitted state. Thus, it is considered loosely equivalent to the *"deficit state,"* as defined by Carpenter et al.[1] Indeed the deficit state may be that aspect of schizophrenia wherein structural brain pathology is finally encountered as the only reliable pathophysiological explanation.

Treatment of Secondary Negative Symptoms

The entire negative syndrome, as well as individual symptoms, has been described in other clinical conditions. A brief review of the major themes is presented below.

Table 10.1
Classifying Negative Symptoms

Primary Negative Symptoms
a) Primary enduring or deficit state (these do not covary with positive symptoms)
b) Primary nonenduring (these may covary with positive symptoms)

Secondary Negative Symptoms *as a Result of*:
a) Postpsychotic depression
b) Postpsychotic regressive states
c) Antipsychotic side effects (akinesia, extrapyramidal)
d) Environmental deprivation (institutionalization)
e) Nonspecific depressive syndromes

Negative Symptoms Secondary to Antipsychotic Side Effects:

These include (a) extrapyramidal symptoms (EPS) (including mask-like facies) and akinesia (b) cognitive blunting, possibly resulting from anticholinergic effects; and (c) increased apathy, diminished spontaneity, and diminished affective arousal due to diminished frontal cortex dopamine function.

Akinesia is a motor anomaly the expanded definition of which includes a lack of emotional reactivity, social ineptitude, retarded spontaneous speech, sluggishness, diminished spontaneity, diminished social initiative, and decreased physical movement. In addition, patients may manifest the characteristic mask-like facies of EPS, which readily mimic the "unchanging facial expression" component of primary negative symptoms.

Treatment of these symptoms includes reducing the dose of antipsychotics; using targeted antipsychotic plasma levels; administering anticholinergics; and using atypical antipsychotics, which have fewer EPS. We have demonstrated that those patients who respond to haloperidol (Haldol) will do so equally well at haloperidol plasma levels ranging from less than 5 ng/ml to greater than 25 ng/ml. In those patients who do not show an initial response to haloperidol (regardless of plasma level), the best long-term results may be obtained by adjusting the haloperidol dose to achieve a plasma level in the range of 5–15 ng/ml.[2]

Negative Symptoms Secondary to Depression:

Affective disturbances could occur during a psychotic episode because of (a) depression due to the onset of a devastating illness, (b) depressive effect of antipsychotic medications, and (c) depression as a secondary manifestation of impaired stress management.

Descriptions of postpsychotic depression include unchanging facial expression, lack of initiative, poverty of speech, hypersomnia, social withdrawal, anhedonia, lack of interest, fatigue, and neurasthenic complaints. Unfortunately, such effects are included among negative symptoms. Psychotic patients have a difficult time verbalizing their inner experiences, further complicating the psychiatrist's ability to diagnose depression in this population. The presence of the classical depression triad symptoms—guilt, worthlessness, and hopelessness—

may help the physician pinpoint depression, but there is often no clear-cut approach here. Treatment includes the use of antidepressants; use of individual, family, and group therapy; and training in stress management techniques.[3]

Negative Symptoms Secondary to Environmental Deprivation:

Environmental deprivation can result in (a) decreased spontaneity, (b) decreased opportunity for playing activity, and (c) decreased curiosity and exploration. "Institutionalization" is a term that can be applied to behaviors that emerge from impoverished, degrading, or emotionally unresponsive environments. Institutional behaviors are presumably learned in an environment that is easily alarmed by spontaneity and patient-initiated behaviors and that encourages passivity and submissiveness.

Treatment includes social skills training, vocational and cognitive rehabilitation, and case management that links individuals to community resources.

Treatment of Primary Negative Symptoms

The subject of the remainder of this will be pharmacologic interventions aimed at treating primary negative symptoms (both deficit state and nonenduring). Recent antipsychotic trials are attempting to demonstrate separate improvement of the deficit state and the of the primary nonenduring symptoms by the use of statistical techniques through which the variance in negative-symptom response attributed to improvement in positive symptoms is parceled out. Any remaining improvement can be attributed to changes in the deficit state (orthogonality for the deficit state assumes that changes in symptoms attributable to the deficit state are entirely independent of changes in positive symptoms; this will be accepted implicitly for the purposes of this chapter).

Several theories attempt to explain the covariance of positive symptoms and primary nonenduring negative symptoms as a pathological expression of the imbalance between two or more neurotransmitter systems (dopamine versus norepinephrine, acetylcholine, serotonin, or most recently glutamate). **However, there are also several clinical reasons why negative symptoms could occur as *epiphenom-***

ena to positive symptoms, such as disintegration of stress management functions; internal preoccupation with psychotic experiences; demoralization and despair; social withdrawal as a consequence of paranoia; and the need to reduce sensory stimulation because of poor sensory gating. These clinical reasons may be very useful in charting out treatment strategies.

Typical Antipsychotics:
Conventional Antipsychotics

Even though several major neurobiological theories of negative symptoms would predict at best the absence of effect and at worst a detrimental effect on negative symptoms, **there is substantial evidence supporting a significant therapeutic role for conventional antipsychotics.**[4] **Specifically, the negative symptoms that occur during the active phase of illness** (i.e., primary nonenduring) **clearly respond to treatment with conventional antipsychotics.**[4,5] For example, in 82 drug-free inpatients with schizophrenia or schizoaffective disorder treated for 4 weeks with conventional antipsychotics, we found significant improvement in negative symptoms as measured by the Brief Psychiatric Rating Scale negative-symptom factor (R.P. Sharma, MD, unpublished results).

Because the primary nonenduring type of negative symptoms covary with the level of positive symptoms, treatments that improve positive symptoms should provide a secondary relief from these negative symptoms. Thus, although there is substantial evidence that conventional antipsychotics will improve primary nonenduring negative symptoms occurring during an acute episode, these drugs have not been credited with independent effects on the deficit state. **Therefore, it is encouraging to note evidence that some improvement of even the deficit state can occur with conventional antipsychotics.** Meltzer and colleagues[5] found significant improvement in deficit-type negative symptoms in 48 schizophrenic patients treated for 6 weeks, even after adjusting for changes in positive symptoms.

The improvement in negative symptoms due to conventional antipsychotic drugs may also depend on other factors that have neurobiological significance. We have noted a differential response of negative symptoms to conventional antipsychotics in early-onset patients: the early onset patients do not have significant improvements in negative symptoms even when positive symptoms are concurrently improving (R. P. Sharma, unpublished results).

Disinhibitory Antipsychotics

In France, there is a tradition of antipsychotic classification, extending back to the original work of Delay and Deniker,[6] that ascribes disinhibitory or "energizing effects" to low doses of certain classes of antipsychotics.[7] Evidence now exists to suggest that low doses of antipsychotics from the benzamide class (e.g., amisulpride) have a specific therapeutic effect on the primary enduring or deficit type of negative symptoms.

Amisulpride (Solian) is a substituted benzamide with high affinity and preferential selectivity for dopamine D2 and D3 receptors in the limbic system rather than the striatum. It also blocks dopamine autoreceptors at low doses and postsynaptic receptors at higher doses, but has low affinity for receptors of other neurotransmitters.[8] Behaviorally, amisulpride has activating effects at lower doses and appears not to induce catalepsy at higher doses. Clinical studies have found amisulpride to have "activating" properties on the EEG of patients with schizophrenia (i.e., increases in beta and/or alpha activity, and increases in the centroid activity), especially in those who are demonstrating improvement of negative symptoms.

There are three double-blind, placebo-controlled studies examining the effects of amisulpride on patients with schizophrenia with significant negative symptoms. Two of these studies were short-term (six weeks),[9,10] and the third was six months.[8] All three trials include patients with minimal positive symptoms (i.e., relatively pure negative symptoms), and all conclude that low-dose amisulpride is an effective treatment for negative symptoms. **In fact, these studies report improvement of negative symptoms independent of any changes in positive symptoms, which, according to our working definition, is tantamount to an improvement of the deficit state.**

In actual clinical practice, patients with schizophrenia will experience exacerbations of positive symptoms during the course of the illness; it is uncommon to see schizophrenia patients with consistently "pure" negative symptoms.[11] Amisulpride is effective on negative symptoms in the dose range of 50–300 mg but requires doses of up to 300–1200 mg for the treatment of positive symptoms. Therefore, its use in the routine treatment of schizophrenic patients with both positive and negative symptoms may be problematic.

Diphenylbutylpiperidine Antipsychotics

Gould and coworkers reported that antipsychotics of the diphenyl-butylpiperidine class antagonize calcium channels (of the same type antagonized by verapamil [Calan]) and could have therapeutic potential in the treatment of negative symptoms.[12] These drugs include pimozide (Orap), which is available in the United States. Meltzer and colleagues[5] have reviewed the evidence for the efficacy of pimozide in schizophrenia, indicating beneficial effects on "work or recreation," emotional blunting, and social withdrawal. These studies are encouraging but need to be supplemented with prospective trials that use behavioral measurements specifically designed to examine the currently recognized primary type of negative symptoms.

Atypical Antipsychotics:

The advent of the atypical antipsychotics brought with it great expectations, particularly with regard to three types of patients: (a) those with treatment-resistant positive symptoms, (b) those with dominant negative symptoms, and (c) those at risk for tardive dyskinesia. The atypical antipsychotics have been proven effective in the treatment of primary nonenduring negative symptoms (as a secondary response to their better efficacy on positive symptoms); however, their effect on the deficit state (or primary enduring negative symptoms) is increasingly a subject of debate.

Clozapine

Clozapine (Clozaril) is the prototype of this new generation of antipsychotics. It has been proven to have significant efficacy in patients with schizophrenia who were not responsive to other treatments. Clozapine's reputation, however, rests equally on its ability to improve the more challenging (and historically nonresponsive) negative symptoms. Much of the initial excitement came from the belief that clozapine has a unique mode of action, with a symptom-response profile different from that of the earlier, typical antipsychotics. This position is now contested, and new evidence suggests that the nature of the clozapine response is not qualitatively different from that of the conventional antipsychotics. Also, the efficacy of clozapine with regard to negative symptoms is now largely attributed to improvement in the primary nonenduring type, occurring as a consequence of the superior response of positive symptoms.[13,14] For example, Tandon et al. and Miller et al. have observed that the response of negative symptoms to clozapine is significantly correlated with the improvement of positive symptoms.[15,16] Furthermore, findings from other studies highlight the difficulties in differentiating improved response of primary negative symptoms from the reduced occurrence of extrapyramidal side effects known to be characteristic of clozapine. There are two studies that directly examine the efficacy of clozapine on the deficit state. Conley et al., in an open-labeled study with treatment-resistant patients, found no effect on negative symptoms, although there was improvement of positive symptoms.[17] Brier et al., in a double-blind comparison of clozapine and haloperidol in patients with schizophrenia, were not able to demonstrate a beneficial effect on the deficit state.[18]

Risperidone

Risperidone (Risperdal) is another atypical antipsychotic for which sufficient data exist to address efficacy on the two specific types of primary negative symptoms. **A recent review indicates that four of six open-label, single-blind studies and three of four double-blind studies report that risperidone** (Risperdal) **is efficacious for negative symptoms.**[14] **Interestingly, improvement of negative symptoms was observed to diminish with doses higher than 10 mg a day.** There are two multicenter studies, the North American multicenter Study and the European multicenter study, comparing the effects of risperidone versus haloperidol on negative and positive symptoms. In the European study, 1–6 mg of risperidone was not significantly better than 10 mg of haloperidol for negative symptoms.[19] In the North American Study, it appeared that 2–16 mg of risperidone was more efficacious than 20 mg of haloperidol for the treatment of negative symptoms.[20] Considering the two multicenter studies together, risperidone was marginally better than 20 mg of haloperidol but not better than 10 mg of haloperidol. **In summary, the existing literature indicates that lower doses of risperidone** (10 mg or less) **are better for negative symptoms than haloperidol given in doses of 20 mg or more. Both risperidone and haloperidol, however, cause EPS, particularly at higher doses. The question that arises is whether the risperidone advantage results from a lower**

incidence of EPS side effects and thus a lower frequency and intensity of secondary negative symptoms. Möller and coworkers[21] reanalyzed the data from the North American study to look specifically at risperidone's effect on primary negative symptoms. They found through path analysis that the improvement in negative symptoms induced by risperidone is significantly associated with improvement in positive symptoms and a lower incidence of extrapyramidal effects. Above and beyond this secondary effect, however, the authors statistically adjusted for the improvement in the positive symptoms and *also* detected a primary effect of risperidone on deficit-type negative symptoms.

Olanzapine

Olanzapine (Zyprexa), the third atypical antipsychotic in widespread use, has been compared with both haloperidol and placebo in another North American double-blind study. In the context of negative symptoms, Tollefson and Sanger have also performed a path analysis on this data set.[22] By adjusting for changes in positive symptoms and/or extrapyramidal effects, they were able to examine the direct effect of olanzapine on deficit-type negative symptoms. **Besides a significant "indirect" effect on negative symptoms** (secondary to improvement on positive symptoms)**, they report a "direct" and significant effect of olanzapine on negative symptoms compared with both placebo and haloperidol** (doses of 10 to 20 mg). **Olanzapine had a superior effect on the dimensions of "affective flattening" and "avolition-apathy" when compared with haloperidol.**

Glutamate NMDA Receptor Modulators:

The glutamate hypothesis of schizophrenia serves as possibly the most comprehensive neurotransmitter hypothesis to date, having the ability to explain the involvement of dopamine in schizophrenic pathology.

The essence of the glutamate dysfunction theory is that there is an excessive excitation of cortical pyramidal neurons secondary to a hypofunction of N-methyl-D-Aspartate (NMDA) glutamate receptor-mediated neurotransmission on GABA inhibitory interneurons. This excitation of pyramidal neurons ultimately results (after involvement of several other circuits) in excessive release of glutamate from pyramidal efferents onto kainic acid glutamate receptors of neighboring pyramidal neurons.[23] Persistent and excessive excitation of these receptors may lead to the degeneration of these neighboring pyramidal neurons.

Thus, **the NMDA receptor channel has become a new target for therapeutic intervention,** and its relevant components are noted here. The NMDA receptor channel is occluded by magnesium at resting-membrane potential; the magnesium is dislodged only on depolarization. There exists a recognition site for glycine (Paynocil); glutamate can open the channel only in the presence of glycine at its respective site. Other modulatory sites include a binding site within the channel for MK-801 and related drugs such as phencyclidine and ketamine (Ketalar), which are noncompetitive antagonists. **The strongest support for this NMDA receptor hypofunction theory is the observation that NMDA noncompetitive antagonists** (e.g., phencyclidine, ketamine) **induce psychotic symptoms in control volunteers and that this induced psychosis is more similar to the actual positive and negative symptoms experienced by schizophrenic patients than the psychosis induced by dopamine-mimetic drugs, such as amphetamine and methylphenidate.**

The glutamate theory would predict that pharmacologic agents that increase NMDA receptor-mediated glutamatergic activity should be beneficial for schizophrenic symptoms, including negative symptoms. The literature provides modest evidence for two such NMDA coagonists. **Glycine, which has an allosteric modulatory effect on the NMDA receptor by binding to its glycine-specific site, has proven effective in the improvement of negative symptoms.**[24-26] For example, Javitt et al. examined the effects of somewhat higher doses of glycine, administered as adjunctive therapy in 14 male patients with schizophrenia on stable doses of antipsychotics.[26] Glycine was titrated in a double-blind, placebo-controlled paradigm to a maximum dose of 0.4 g/kg body weight (~30g/day) for a period of up to 8 weeks. They found significant effects on negative symptoms, not only on measurements obtained during the double-blind phase, but also in patients who switched from placebo to open-labeled glycine at the end of the controlled phase of the study.

As glycine does not readily cross the blood-brain barrier, current investigations are focusing on agents that do cross the blood-brain barrier. The antitubercular drug D-cycloserine (Seromycin) is a partial agonist at the glycine site, inhibitory at low doses and excitatory at higher doses. **D-cycloserine crosses the blood-brain barrier and has been found to be effective in the treatment of primary negative symptoms of the deficit type.** Goff and colleagues[27] compared D-cycloserine in doses of 5, 15, 50, and 250 mg, administered consecutively for 2 weeks each, with placebo in nine schizophrenic outpatients concurrently on stable doses of antipsychotics.[27] Significant therapeutic effect on negative symptoms was achieved only on the 50 mg dose of D-cycloserine. Other agents that cross the blood-brain barrier such as milacemide, are currently being investigated.

Dopamine Agonists:

Hypodopaminergia in selected brain regions is an appealing pathophysiological explanation for negative symptoms (for review see Rao and Möller).[28] **Besides the many clinical similarities between negative symptoms and parkinsonian symptoms, further support for this concept also comes from the negative symptom-like side effects of dopamine antagonist medications** (i.e., antipsychotics). **If regional hypo-dopaminergia is assumed as one possible cause of negative symptoms, then the treatment objective in schematic terms would be to concomitantly induce—albeit in different regions—both hypodopaminergia to treat the positive symptoms and hyperdopaminergia to treat or prevent the negative symptoms.**

Earlier reports of improvement in negative symptoms with amphetamine are often cited to support the use of nonselective dopamine agonists for treating negative symptoms. **The effects of acute administration of dopamine agonists on negative symptoms, however, are equivocal.** For example, Angrist and colleagues noted modest improvement in negative symptoms in drug-free remitted schizophrenic inpatients after an acute administration of d-amphetamine, as measured by the Brief Psychiatric Rating Scale (BPRS).[29] **Conversely, Sanfilipo and colleagues did not find acute amphetamine administration to improve negative symptoms.[30] Lieberman and colleagues found significant deterioration on scores of negative symptoms in patients given methylphenidate (Ritalin), another amphetamine-like stimulant; deterioration of negative symptoms was significantly correlated with deterioration of positive symptoms, and patients who had no positive symptom activation had no increase in negative symptoms.[31]**

Likewise, our group did not find any improvement in negative symptoms measured in drug-free schizophrenic patients administered intravenous methylphenidate in a double-blind placebo-controlled challenge paradigm.[32]

The long-term administration of dopamine agonists carries the risk of psychotic exacerbation, especially in patients who are acutely ill or are not currently receiving antipsychotics. In one long-term study of amphetamine in patients with schizophrenia, 50 mg of amphetamine were administered in an open-label design. Nine of 17 patients with prominent negative symptoms showed improvement, but another 5 patients deteriorated, particularly those not receiving antipsychotics.[33]

The evidence that levodopa (L-dopa), a dopamine precursor that increases the availability of dopamine in the synapse, improves negative symptoms is considerably more robust (for review see Meltzer et al.[5]). Levodopa has beneficial effects on overall symptom response, with specific improvement in the BPRS item "withdrawal" as noted by one of the studies reviewed. Furthermore, it appears that levodopa does not exacerbate psychotic symptoms with the same intensity and frequency as do amphetamine and methylphenidate.[5]

Bromocriptine, an ergot alkaloid, is another dopamine agonist examined as a possible treatment for negative symptoms; its results were inconsistent. The need to distinguish improvement in extrapyramidal symptoms from improvement in negative symptoms, especially in response to dopamine agonists, is evident retrospectively.

An alternate strategy is the use of dopamine agonists with preferential action on the dopamine autoreceptors. These drugs selectively stimulate dopamine presynaptic receptors and decrease dopamine synthesis and release, thereby causing an upregulation of postsynaptic dopamine receptors. Supersensitive postsynaptic dopamine receptors could increase regional dopamine transmission, either in response to release of endogenous dopamine or as a result of partial agonist postsynaptic effect. This formulation would be consistent with a hypodopaminergic theory of negative symptoms. Roxindole is a selective dopamine-autoreceptor agonist with an affinity for D_2 0receptors in the nanomolar range and with serotonin-uptake inhibitory and 5HT1a-receptor stimulatory effects. Talipexole is another selective autoreceptor agonist with partial agonist effects at the postsynaptic dopamine receptor, and terguride is an ergot dopamine autoreceptor agonist. These agents have been examined for their efficacy on negative symptoms; Wetzel and Benkert have reviewed the extant studies and found these agonists to have (at best) modest effects (20%–30% improvement) on negative symptoms.[34] Because the literature on dopamine autoreceptor agonists is limited to a few small-sample open studies, we consider the results inconclusive.

Antidepressants:

The use of antidepressants for schizophrenic negative symptoms can be supported by numerous theoretical considerations. **Clinically, the similarities between depression and negative symptoms in themselves provide a compelling reason to administer a trial of antidepressants. Pharmacologically, antidepressants have modulating properties on the neurotransmitters that are specifically implicated in negative symptoms, such as norepinephrine, serotonin (5HT), and acetylcholine (Ach). Unfortunately, interpretation of clinical findings is confounded by the clinical similarities between depression and negative symptoms. In terms of the published literature, the general strategy is to add an antidepressant to an otherwise stable regimen of antipsychotic medications.**

Siris and coworkers reported the significant therapeutic effects of a double-blind trial of imipramine (Tofranil) administered adjunctively in adequate doses to schizophrenic patients suffering from *both* negative symptoms and a post-psychotic depression.[35] Other investigations of tricyclic antidepressants administered as adjunctive therapy to patients with primarily negative symptoms have not reported beneficial effects.[36]

The combination of maprotiline (Mylan) with antipsychotic drugs was noted to reduce negative symptoms in schizophrenia.[37] Maprotiline and imipramine both block the reuptake of norepinephrine, suggesting a possible therapeutic mode of action in the therapy of negative symptoms.

The use of monoamine oxidase inhibitors is supported by findings of high-platelet monoamine oxidase activity and decreased catecholamine levels in patients with pronounced negative symptoms.[28] Bucci has observed improvement in 28 of 30 chronically ill patients with schizophrenia treated with tranylcypromine (Parnate) and chlorpromazine (Thorazine) over a period of 4 months.[38]

More recently, the safety and efficacy of the selective serotonin-reuptake inhibitors has encouraged several trials with these agents in patients with treatment-resistant schizophrenia. The rationale for the use of serotonergic potentiating agents in treating negative symptoms seems contradictory to the prevailing theories of serotonergic involvement in the pathophysiology and treatment of schizophrenia (i.e., 5HT2 receptor antagonism). **Besides its expediency, however, the use of selective serotonin-reuptake inhibitors for negative symptoms can also be supported by several new theoretical formulations. Brier has suggested that serotonergic hypofunction may be a possible mechanism for negative symptoms.[18] Using the acute tryptophan-depletion paradigm to lower brain serotonin under double-blind, placebo-controlled, randomized conditions, we have observed a significant worsening of negative symptoms in patients with schizophrenia.[39] We have consequently proposed the involvement of the 5HT1a receptor system and its interactions with the dopamine system as a possible avenue for therapeutic intervention for negative symptoms.[40]**

Goff and coworkers have reported that the addition of fluoxetine (Prozac) to ongoing antipsychotic therapy will improve clinical response in otherwise nonresponsive patients with schizophrenia.[41] Silver and Nassar have examined the effects of adjunctive treatment with fluvoxamine (Luvox) in a double-blind, placebo-controlled trial in schizophrenic patients on stable doses of conventional antipsychotics.[42] **Fluvoxamine was significantly better than placebo on measures of negative symptoms, with minimal effects on other dimensions of psychopathology such as depression, positive symptoms, and global symptomatology. More recently, Thakore and colleagues have reported the significant efficacy of an open trial of sertraline (Zoloft) on negative symptoms.[43] Sertraline was administered in doses of 50 mg/day for 12 weeks in 20 outpatients with schizophrenia on concurrently stable doses of antipsychotics.**

Finally, Alphs et al. have examined fenfluramine (Pondimin), an indirect serotonin agonist with no known antidepressant properties.[44] These investigators administered fenfluramine over a period of 14–16 weeks during a placebo-controlled crossover study that used several dosages in 11 patients with schizophrenia. **Patients were selected for having prominent negative symptoms. Higher dosages of fenflu-**

ramine (up to 100–180 mg/day) **were found to be significantly better than placebo on negative symptoms measured by ratings of the Negative Symptoms Assessment, but not by the BPRS negative symptom factor.** This study complements the studies with selective serotonin-reuptake inhibitors in that it demonstrates a therapeutic benefit to serotonergic potentiation for negative symptoms because fenfluramine is not known to improve symptoms of depression, which is an important confounding source of secondary negative symptoms.

Anticholinergics:

The known functions and interactions of the cholinergic system pose **at least two implications for the treatment of negative symptoms. The first relates to the therapy of primary nonenduring symptoms and focuses on interactions with the dopamine system. The second addresses interactions with the glutamate system, which may provide opportunities for prophylactic treatments directed towards the deficit state.** The use of anticholinergics to resolve secondary negative symptoms resulting from extrapyramidal side effects has already been noted earlier (see introduction).

The observation that patients with schizophrenia have a tendency to "abuse" anticholinergic drugs to feel energized, stimulated, and sociable suggested therapeutic implications for these agents.[45] Tandon and Greden proposed cholinergic hyperactivity as a neurotransmitter basis for the primary nonenduring type of negative symptoms.[4] The proposal suggested that there exists a physiological balance between dopamine (DA) and Ach neurotransmission. **When DA activity increases (resulting in increasing psychotic activity), muscarinic Ach activity increases as a compensatory response to maintain balance by exerting a damping influence on increasing DA activity. A consequence of the increasing Ach activity, however, is an increase in negative symptoms. This formulation would predict a beneficial effect of anticholinergic medications on negative symptoms. Tandon and coworkers initially reported beneficial effects on negative symptoms in schizophrenic patients treated with biperiden (8 mg a day) for 2 days in a single-blind study.**[46] However, Goff et al. examined the effects of trihexyphenidyl (Artane) in unmedicated patients, in a placebo-controlled double-blind random-order crossover trial, and found it to be ineffective on negative symptoms.[47] **Overall, evidence from five trials** of anticholinergic agents only equivocally supports their efficacy for negative symptoms.[48]

Cholinergic neurotransmission may also have therapeutic implications based on interactions with the glutamate excitatory neurotransmitter system. (Olney and Farber detail this interaction as it pertains to schizophrenic symptoms.)[23] In essence, hypofunction of the NMDA glutamate receptor ultimately may cause neurodegeneration.[23] Numerous other neurotransmitters network with the glutamate system, and their modulation can block neurodegeneration. Thus, muscarinic, sigma, and non-NMDA antagonists, as well as α_2-adrenergic agonists, can block this induced neurodegeneration. **Although no prospective clinical studies exist, the observation that early intervention with antipsychotic drugs** (which usually have adjunct anticholinergic properties) **can alter the long-term course of schizophrenia may suggest a protective or prophylactic role for the use of anticholinergic agents in this disorder.**[49]

Neuropeptides:

Several neuropeptides have been examined in schizophrenic populations. These are neurotensin, β-endorphin, and cholecystokinin. Interest in these peptides derives from early observations that they exhibit antipsychotic-like pharmacologic effects. **de Wied originally suggested that endorphins might be endogenous, naturally occurring antipsychotics and that they could be implicated in schizophrenia.**[50] **Two other aspects of neuropeptide neurobiology make them relevant to negative symptoms. The first is the high concentration of receptors for these neuropeptides in areas of the brain that could be involved in negative symptoms, such as the amygdala, the cingulate cortex, and the entorhinal cortex.**[51] **The second is the multiple levels of interaction with the dopamine neuronal system.**[52–54]

The β-endorphin peptide is metabolized into two fragments, α-endorphin and γ-endorphin. **It is the γ-endorphin fragment that has ascribed to it the antipsychotic properties.** γ-endorphin has been administered to schizophrenic patients as an antipsychotic medication, either independently or as an adjunct to conventional antipsychotics. **Although earlier clinical trials of γ-endorphin in patients with schizophrenia supported the notion that it could have antipsychotic properties, more recent evidence is equivocal.**[55]

Cholecystokinin (or its related decapeptide, cerulein) also has been administered to patients with schizophrenia in clinical trials. Nair et al. have reviewed these studies and have found some modest favorable effects in 8 of 11 studies.[56]

Neurotensin (NT) is an endogenous tridecapeptide neurotransmitter heterogeneously distributed in the mammalian CNS with close neuroanatomical and functional associations with the dopamine neurotransmitter system.[53] **The hypothesis that NT functions as an endogenous antipsychotic is based on the preclinical and clinical investigations in which reduced CSF-NT concentrations have been reported in drug-free schizophrenic patients, especially those with negative symptoms** (for review see Sharma et al.).[39] **We have additionally reported a significant association between antipsychotic-induced increases in CSF-NT levels and improvement of negative symptoms.**[39] Neurotensin does not cross the blood-brain barrier, and, to our knowledge, currently no chemical analogues with agonist action at the neurotensin receptor are available for human evaluation.

There is one published report examining the effects of vasopressin on negative and positive symptoms in schizophrenia.[57] The investigators administered desglycinamide-(Arg)[8]-vasopressin to 10 undifferentiated patients with schizophrenia being treated with stable doses of antipsychotics. They observed a significant improvement on the BPRS negative symptom items, in the absence of improvement of positive symptoms.

Future Directions

Serotonergic Antagonists:

Because 5HT2-receptor antagonism is considered an important contributor to the putative action of the atypical antipsychotics, selective 5HT2-antagonist drugs are being evaluated in the treatment of schizophrenia in general. Ritanserin, a selective 5HT2/5HT1c antagonist, has demonstrated modest therapeutic effects on negative symptoms. MDL 100907 is another selective 5HT2 antagonist that is in the initial stages of clinical testing.

D_1 Receptors:

Dopamine D_1-receptor antagonism does not appear to be necessary for antipsychotic activity, but recent studies indicate decreased specific D_1-receptor binding in the prefrontal cortex of patients with schizophrenia, especially those with negative symptoms.[58] D_1-receptors lie on dendritic spines of prefrontal pyramidal neurons, and are possibly part of synaptic triads on these spines, in conjunction with 5HT2a receptors. **Of some significance is the observation that clozapine (Clozaril) is an effective antagonist at both D_1 and 5HT2 receptors. Overall, therefore, it is possible to formulate a role for D_1 -receptor drugs in treating negative symptoms. In this context, it is interesting to note the therapeutic effects of a D_1 antagonist, SCH-39166, on negative symptoms in schizophrenia in the absence of any significant effects on positive symptoms.**[59]

Conclusions

The increased focus on the treatment of schizophrenic negative symptoms is encouraging, especially because these symptoms are a major obstacle to the social and vocational rehabilitation of the patient. Equally evident, however, is the difficulty in identifying the treatment of choice when everything works but nothing works well enough or consistently enough. **Because negative symptoms may be pleomorphic** (i.e., become expressed in different forms and for different reasons)**, specific treatments for negative symptoms may have to vary with the phase of the illness.** Thus, modification of synaptic transmission (e.g., increasing dopamine or serotonin activity, or reducing cholinergic activity) may be sufficient for the primary nonenduring type and all the secondary types of negative symptoms. However, prevention of excitotoxic neuronal cell death, predicted by the glutamate hypothesis, may be required to prevent or curtail the progression of the primary enduring type (or deficit state). Negative symptoms noted during the prepsychotic period of the illness (i.e., in childhood and adolescence), possibly because of neurodevelopmental abnormalities, have not yet been adequately addressed either theoretically or therapeutically.

Prospective trials that demonstrate improvement of the deficit state are possibly the most important next step. Currently, improvement in the deficit state is largely inferred from statistical analysis of data emerging from studies that were not originally designed to address the deficit state.

At the present, use of the atypical antipsychotics seems the most reasonable approach. At all times, however, the vigilant clinician will test and retest the possibility of secondary negative symptoms and will proceed to treat with the appropriate adjunctive strategies. **Given the efficacy and safety of risperidone and olanzapine, the author would recommend these medications as the first-line approach to antipsychotic treatment, primarily for their lesser tendency to cause akinesia and EPS. If conventional antipsychotics are required, titration to achieve the maximum improvement of positive symptoms on the minimum dose is a useful guideline. Because SSRIs are well tolerated and because there is evidence that they induce a modest improvement in negative symptoms, either primary or secondary to a depression, their use as adjuncts to antipsychotics is also recommended.**

References

1. Carpenter WT, Heinrichs DW, Alphs LD. Deficit and nondeficit forms of schizophrenia: the concept. *Am J Psychiat.* 1988;145:578–583.

2. Janicak PG, Javiad JI, Sharma RP, et al. A two phase double blind randomized study of three haloperidol plasma levels for acute psychosis with reassignment of initial non-responders. *Acta Psychiat Scand.* 1997;2:343–350.

3. Janicak PG, Davis JM, Preskorn SH, Ayd FJ Jr. *Principles and Practice of Psychopharmacology.* 2nd ed. Baltimore: Williams & Wilkins;1997;243.

4. Tandon R, Jibson MD, Taylor SF, DeQuardo JR. Conceptual models of the relationship between positive and negative symptoms. In: Shriqui CL, Nasrallah H, eds. *Contemporary Issues In The Treatment of Schizophrenia.* Washington DC: American Psychiatric Press;1997;121.

5. Meltzer HY, Sommers A, Luchins DJ. The effect of neuroleptics and other psychotropic drugs on negative symptoms in schizophrenia. *J Clin Psychopharm.* 1986;6:329–338.

6. Delay J, Denker P. Caracteristiques psychophysioloques des medicaments neuroleptiques. Rapport au symp. Intern. Sur les Medicaments Psychotropes. Milan, May, 9–11, 1957. In: *Psychotropic Drugs.* Amsterdam: Elsevier;1957;485–501.

7. Colonna L. Antideficit properties of neuroleptics. *Acta Psychiat Scand.* 1994;89(suppl 380):77–82.

8. Loo H, Littre MFP, Theron M, Rein W, Fleurot O. Amisulpride versus placebo in the medium-term treatment of the negative symptoms of schizophrenia. *Brit J Psychiat.* 1997;170:18–22.

9. Boyer P, Lecrubier Y, Puech AJ, Dewailly J, Aubin F. Treatment of negative symptoms in schizophrenia with Amisulpride. *Brit J Psychiat.* 1995;166:68–72.

10. Paillere-Martinot M, Lecrubier Y, Martinot J, Aubin F. Improvement of some schizophrenic deficit symptoms with low doses of amisulpride. *Am J Psychiat.* 1995;152(1):130–133.

11. Gerbaldo H, Fickinger PM, Wetzel H, et al. Primary enduring negative symptoms in schizophrenia and major depression. *J Psychiat Res.* 1995;29(4):297–302.

12. Gould RJ, Murphy KMM, Reynolds IJ, Snyder SH. Antischizophrenic drugs of the diphenyl-butylpiperidine type act as calcium channel antagonists. *Proc Natl Acad Sci.* 1983;80:5122–5125.

13. Carpenter WT, Conley RR, Buchanan RW, Breier A, Tamminga CA. Patient response and resource management: another view of clozapine treatment of schizophrenia. *Am J Psychiat.* 1995;152(6):827–832.

14. Buchanan RW, Gold JM. Negative symptoms: diagnosis, treatment and prognosis. *Internat Clin Psychopharm.* 1996;11(suppl 2):3–11.

15. Tandon R, Goldman R, DeQuardo JR, et al. Positive and negative symptoms covary during clozapine treatment in schizophrenia. *J Psychiatr Res.* 1993;27:341–347.

16. Miller DD, Perry PJ, Cadorer RJ, Andeasen NC. Clozapine's effect on negative symptoms in treatment refractory schizophrenics. *Compr Psychaitry.* 1994;35:8–13.

17. Conley R, Gounaris C, Tamminga C. Clozapine response varies in deficit vs. nondeficit schizophrenic subjects. *Biol Psychiatry.* 1994;35:746–747.

18. Brier A. Serotonin, schizophrenia and antipsychotic drug action. *Schiz Res.* 1995;14:187–202.

19. Peuskens J. Risperidone in the treatment of patients with chronic schizophrenia: a multinational, multi-center double blind parallel-group study versus haloperidol. *Brit J Psychiat.* 1995;166:712–726.

20. Chouinard G, Jones B, Remington G, et al. A Canadian multicenter placebo controlled study of fixed doses of risperidone and haloperidol in tht treatment of chronic schizophrenic patients. *Psychopharmacology.* 1993;13:25–40.

21. Möller HJ, Muller H, Borison RL, Schooler NR, Chouinard G. A path analytical approach to differentiate between direct and indirect drug effects on negative symptoms in schizophrenic patients: a revaluation of the North American risperidone study. *Eur Arch Psychiat Clin Neuroscience.* 1995;245:45–49.

22. Tollefson GD, Sanger TM. Negative symptoms: a path analytic approach to a double blind, placebo and haloperidol controlled clinical trial with olanzapine. *Am J Psychiatry.* 1997;154(4):466–474.

23. Olney JW, Farber NB. Glutamate receptor dysfunction and schizophrenia. *Arch Gen Psychiat.* 1995;52:998–1007.

24. Waziri R. Glycine therapy of schizophrenia (letter). *Biol Psychiatry.* 1988;23:210–211.

25. Rosse RB Theut SK, Banay-Schwartz M, et al. Glycine adjuvant therapy to conventional neuroleptic treatment in schizophrenia: an open label pilot study. *Clin Neuropharm.* 1989;12:416–424.

26. Javitt DC, Zylberman I, Zukin SR, Heresco-Levy U, Lindenmeyer J. Amelioration of negative symptoms in schizophrenia by glycine. *Am J Psychiatry.* 1994;151(8):1234–1236.

247

27. Goff D, Tsai G, Manoach DS, Coyle JT. Dose finding trial of D-Cycloserine added to neuroleptics for negative symptoms in schizophrenia. *Am J Psychiat.* 1995;152:1213–1215.

28. Rao ML, Möller HJ. Biochemical findings of negative symptoms in schizophrenia and their putative relevance to pharmacologic treatment. *Pharmacopsychiatry.* 1994;30:160–172.

29. Angrist B, Peselow E, Rubinstein M, Corwin J, Rotrosen J. Partial improvement in negative schizophrenic symptoms after amphetamine. *Psychopharmacology.* 1982;78:128–130.

30. Sanfilipo M, Wolkin A, Angrist B, et al. Amphetamine and negative symptoms of schizophrenia. *Psychopharmacology.* 1996;123:211–214.

31. Lieberman JA, Jody D, Alvir JMJ, et al. Negative symptoms in schizophrenia. In: Marneros A, Andreasen NC, Tsuang MT, eds. *Negative Versus Positive Schizophrenia.* Berlin: Springer-Verlag;1991.

32. Sharma RP, Javaid JI, Pandey GN, Janicak PG, Davis JM. Behavioral and biochemical effects of methylphenidate in schizophrenic and nonschizophrenic patients. *Biol Psychiat.* 1991;5:459–466.

33. Cesarec Z, Nyman AK. Differential response to amphetamine in schizophrenia. *Acta Psychiat Scand.* 1985;71:523–528.

34. Wetzel H, Benkert O. Dopamine autoreceptor agonists in the treatment of schizophrenic disorders. *Prog Neuro-Psychopharmacol & Biol Psychiat.* 1993;17:525–540.

35. Siris SG, Bermanzohn PC, Gonzalez A, et al. The use of antidepressants for negative symptoms in a subset of schizophrenic patients. *Psychopharm Bull.* 1991;27:331–335.

36. Plasky P. Antidepressant usage in schizophrenia. *Schiz Bull.* 1991;17:4:649–657.

37. Yamagami S, Soejima K. Effect of maprotiline combined with conventional neuroleptics aganist negative symptoms of chronic schizophrenia. *Drugs Exp Clin Res.* 1986;15:171–176.

38. Bucci L. The negative symptoms of schizophrenia and the monoamine oxidase inhibitors. *Psychopharmacology.* 1987;91:104–108.

39. Sharma RP, Janicak PG, Bissette G, Nemeroff C. CSF Neurotensin concentrations and antipsychotic treatment in schizophrenia and schizoaffective disorder. *Am J Psychiat.* 1997;154:1019–1021.

40. Sharma RP, Shapiro L. The 5HT1a receptor system: possible implications for schizophrenic negative symptomatology. *Psychiat Annals.* 1996;26(2): 88–92.

41. Goff D, Beotman A, Waiter RN, et al. Trials of fluoxetine added to neuroleptic-resistant schizophrenic patients. *Am J Psychiatry.* 1990;147:492.

42. Silver H, Nassar A. Fluvoxamine improves negative symptoms in treated chronic schizophrenic patients. Proceedings of the ACNP annual meeting. December 6–10, 1992, San Juan, Puerto Rico.

43. Thakore JH, Berti C, Dinan TG. An open trial of adjunctive sertraline in the treatment of chronic schizophrenia. *Acta Psychiat Scand.* 1996;94:194–197.

44. Alphs LD, Lafferman JA, Ross L, Bland W, Levine J. Fenfluramine treatment of negative symptoms of schizophrenia. *Psychopharm Bull.* 1989;25:149–153.

45. Tandon R., Greden JF, Silk KR. Treatment of negative schizophrenic symptoms with trihexyphenidyl. *J Clin Psychopharm.* 1988;8(3):212–215.

46. Tandon R, Dequardo JR, Goodson J, Mann NA, Greden JF. Effect of antipcholinergics on positive and negative symptoms in schizophrenia. *Psychopharm Bull.* 1992;28(3):297–302.

47. Goff DC, Amico E, Dreyfuss D, Ciraulo D. A placebo controlled trial of trihexyphenidyl in unmedicated patients with schizophrenia. *Am J Psychiatry.* 1994;151(3):429–431.

48. Buchanan RW, Brandes M, Breier A. Treating negative symptoms: pharmacological strategies. In: Alan Breier, ed. *The New Pharmacotherapy of Schizophrenia.* Washington DC: American Psychiatric Press;1996.

49. Wyatt RJ. Early intervention with neuroleptics may decrease the long-term morbidity of schizophrenia. *Schiz Res.* 1991;5:201.

50. de Wied D. Psychopathology as a neuropeptide dysfunction. In: van Ree JM, Terenius L, eds. *Characteristics and Function of Opioids.* Amsterdam: Elsevier/North-Holland Biomedical Press;1978;113–122.

51. Ronken E, Tonnaer JADM, de Boer T, et al. Autoradiographic evidence for binding sites for des-enkephalin gamma endorphin in rat forebrain. *Eur J Pharmacol.* 1989;162:189–191.

52. Van Ree JM, Innemee H, Louwerens JW, et al. Non-opiate ß-endorphin fragments and dopamine, I: the neuroleptic like g-endorphin like fragments interfere with behavioral effects elicited by low doses of apomorphine. *Neuropharmacology.* 1982;21:1095–1101.

53. Cohen SL, Knight M, Tamminga CA, et al. Cholecystokinin effects on conditioned avoidance behavior, stereotypy and catalepsy. *Eur J Pharmacol.* 1982;83:213–222.

54. Bissette G, Nemeroff CB. The neurobiology of neurotensin. In: Bloom F, Kupfer D, eds. *Psychopharmacology: The Fourth Generation of Progress.* New York: Raven Press;1995.

52. Elkashef AM, Issa F, Wyatt RJ. The biochemical basis of schizophrenia. In: Shriqui SL, Nasrallah HA, eds. *Contemporary Issues in the Treatment of Schizophrenia.* Washington DC: American Psychiatric Association;1995;3.

53. Nair NPV, Lal S, Bloom DM. Cholecystokinin and schizophrenia. *Prog Brain Res.* 1986;65:237–258.

54. Brambilla F, Boniolotti GP, Maggioni M, et al. Vasopressin (DDAVP) therapy in schonic schizophrenia: effects of negative symptoms and memory. *Neuropsychobiology.* 1988;20:113–119.

55. Okubo Y, Suhara T, Suzuki K, et al. Decreased prefrontal dopamine D1 receptors in schizophrenia revealed by PET. *Nature.* 1997;385:634.

56. Den Boer JA, van Megen H, Fleischhacker W, et al. Differential effects of the D1-DA receptor antagonist SCH39166 on positive and negative symptoms of schizophrenia. *Psychopharmacology.* 1995;121:317–322.

11 Pharmacotherapy During the Perinatal Period

Laura J. Miller, MD

Dr. Miller is Associate Professor, Department of Psychiatry, University of Illinois at Chicago.

Editor's Note

The potential risks related to the use of psychopharmacologic agents in pregnant women include increased likelihood of spontaneous abortion, major or minor structural congenital anomalies, enduring behavioral changes in the child, toxicity to the fetus or newborn, fetal or neonatal withdrawal symptoms due to drug discontinuation, premature labor, and increased side effects of the medication due to pharmacokinetic and other physiological changes. These issues are further complicated by other variables, such as other medications, nutritional status, genetic influences, and effects of the psychiatric illness on self-care.

A major pharmacokinetic change in pregnancy is related to the slowing down of gastrointestinal motility. Gastric fluid becomes less acidic, so that weak acids like valproate are less well absorbed while weak bases like imipramine are better absorbed. For drugs like lithium, increased plasma volume and total body water has a dilutional effect, thereby reducing efficacy.

Tricyclic antidepressants and fluoxetine are not associated with major congenital anomalies, nor are these drugs behavioral teratogens. Anticholinergic side effects have been noted occasionally in fetuses and newborns, and newborns exposed to fluoxetine throughout pregnancy have occasionally been observed to manifest restlessness and agitation.Tricyclic antidepressant serum levels tend to decrease during pregnancy if the dose is held constant. Maprotoline and MAOIs should be avoided when possible.

Lithium, carbamazepine, and valproate have all been associated with adverse effects on the fetus and the newborn. If they must be used during preganacy, very careful monitoring is essential. Electroconvulsive treatments are a viable alternative.

One should avoid the use of low potency phenothiazines such as chlorpromazine and, if necessary, use high potency agents such as haloperidol or trifluoperazine, since a slight increase in relative risk of nonspecific congenital anomalies has been found with the use of the former group. New antipsychotics have not been systematically studied thus far.

Routine prophylaxis against extrapyramidal symptoms is not recommended.

Among the benzodiazepines, agents which do not accumulate in fetal tissue, such as lorazepam, appear to be preferable to those which do, such as diazepam. There may be an association between first trimester benzodiazepine use and oral clefts. Newborns can experience both intoxication and withdrawal symptoms.

Various medications are present in breast milk, and precautions must be taken to minimize complications to the nursing infant.

Introduction

Many psychiatric disorders are more common in women than in men.[1] **Symptoms of such mental illnesses as major depression, bipolar mood disorder, anxiety disorders, and schizophrenia first appear, for most patients, in the childbearing years.** As a result, women of childbearing age are prescribed more psychotropic medication than men of comparable age.[2] **For decades, however, potentially fertile women have been excluded from most clinical trials of pharmacologic agents.** Few systematic data have been available to clinicians trying to determine recommendations for a woman with disabling psychiatric symptoms who wants to give birth and/or breast feed, or becomes pregnant unintentionally.

Although there is still a relative paucity of research, recent efforts have provided more systematic information with which to make decisions about psychopharmacology in women who are pregnant, potentially pregnant, or lactating. As a result, we are now able to inform patients about a range of treatment options and specific prescribing techniques to minimize the risks of some psychotropic agents. This chapter will summarize these advances, and recommend clinical guidelines based on currently available data.

Potential Pregnancy-Related Risks of Pharmacologic Agents

The same chemical properties that allow psychotropic drugs to cross the blood-brain barrier allow them to largely cross the placental barrier. In addition to side effects experienced by non-pregnant patients, the following pregnancy-related effects can potentially occur with exposure to medications:

- *Decreased likelihood of conceiving: This theoretical risk can be weighed against the possibility that some drugs promote conception indirectly by alleviating symptoms of mental illness.*

- *Increased likelihood of spontaneous abortion.*

- *Morphologic teratogenicity: major or minor structural congenital anomalies.*

- *Behavioral teratogenicity: enduring behavioral changes due to effects on neuroanatomic and/or neurochemical development in utero.*

- *Fetal and/or neonatal side effects, including toxic side effects.*

- *Fetal and/or neonatal withdrawal due to sudden discontinuation of medication during pregnancy or at birth.*

- *Premature labor.*

- *Increased side effects for the pregnant woman due to pharmacokinetic and other physiologic changes.*

It is a major methodologic challenge to determine whether any specific medication contributes to any of the above risks. Confounding variables, which are impossible to fully control, include:

- **Other drugs:** *Concomitant use of other prescription and non-prescription drugs, including teratogens like cigarettes and alcoholic beverages, may be independent risk factors or may enhance the teratogenicity of a given medication. For example, in rats, lithium (Eskalith) and ethanol taken together result in significantly more anomalies than either agent does alone.*

- **Nutritional status:** *In addition to being an independent risk factor, nutritional deficiencies sometimes increase the teratogenicity of specific psychotropic drugs.[4]*

- **Genetic influences:** *Babies may inherit vulnerability to physical and/or behavioral abnormalities. In addition, inherited levels of enzymes that metabolize drugs can determine whether a drug is teratogenic in a particular fetus.[5]*

- **Effects of illness:** *Maternal mental illness may markedly influence self care and prenatal care, thus affecting outcome independently of medication.[6a] Concomitant medical illness is a further confounding variable.*

- **Environmental toxins:** *These may occur through work or other exposure, and are often unidentified.*

- **Maternal age:** *The risk of certain abnormalities in offspring increases with either adolescent pregnancy or with increased maternal age.*

- **Time of gestation:** *The effects of medications may differ depending on the gestational age of the fetus at the time of exposure. For example, most major organs are formed within the first eight weeks after conception. Cortical neuroarchitecture is actively forming throughout much of the second trimester of pregnancy. Drug metabolism may significantly change as pregnancy progresses. Further, intermittent exposure and/or varying drug levels over time may have different effects than prolonged* *exposure to a constant dose. For example, the administration of large doses of carbamazapine (Tegretol) during the period of neural tube closure may result in spina bifida,*[6b] *while ongoing use later in pregnancy will not. Regular use of benzodiazepines late in pregnancy can lead to neonatal withdrawal, whereas occasional use will not.*

- **Stress and rearing:** *Environmental stress may influence pregnant women's physiology and behaviors, which may have an impact on pregnancy outcome.*[7] *Early parenting has a major impact on children's behavior,*[8] *which is a significant confounding variable when assessing behavioral teratogenicity.*

To date, there is no single study of any specific drug which has successfully controlled for all of the above variables. Confidence in research findings is increased when a pattern emerges over several studies. It is usually at least several years after a medication is first marketed that there are enough systematic data to feel adequately informed about its risks during pregnancy.

Pharmacokinetic and Pharmacodynamic Changes During Pregnancy

Due to the physiologic changes inherent to pregnancy, the effects of a given dose of medication may be different than in the non-pregnant state, and, therefore, are less predictable.[9] **A physician administering psychotropic medications to a pregnant patient must be prepared to carefully monitor her. Both pharmacokinetics** (processes by which a drug is delivered to, and removed from, its site of action) **and pharmacodynamics** (the drug action itself) **may be affected by pregnancy. One major pharmacokinetic change is related to the slowing down of the gastrointestinal tract during pregnancy. Drugs spend more time in the stomach, which allows gastric enzymes more time to metabolize them before they are absorbed. However, the intestine is also slower, allowing more time for absorption of whatever made it through the stomach. Further, gastric fluid is less acidic during pregnancy, which means that weak acids** (e.g., valproic acid [Depakene] and divalproex sodium [Depakote]) are more ionized and less well absorbed. Weak bases (e.g., imipramine [Tofranil]) remain more in their non-ionized state and are better absorbed.

Once absorbed, the levels of active drug are affected by plasma volume, protein binding, and metabolism. Plasma volume, along with total body water, increases during pregnancy. This means that the same amount of drug is being distributed in a greater volume of fluid. For drugs like lithium, this dilution effect can be significant. Protein binding decreases for many drugs during pregnancy, so that the free (biologically active) drug level may increase if the total drug level is constant. Further, the glomerular filtration rate increases during pregnancy, increasing the renal clearance of some medications.

For any given drug, some of the above factors cancel one another out, and others have additive effects. For each class of medication, there are generalizations about dose changes during pregnancy that usually apply. However, since there are wide individual differences in these pharmacokinetic changes, it is important to consider these as possible factors if a drug is causing problematic side effects, or is failing to deliver the desired therapeutic effects.

Much less is known about pharmacodynamic changes during pregnancy, but some have been demonstrated. For example, propranolol (Inderal) slows the heart rate more during pregnancy than it does in the non-pregnant state.[10]

Antidepressant Medications During Pregnancy

Antidepressant drugs are used to treat major depression, panic disorder, obsessive compulsive disorder, dysthymic disorder, and a number of other medical and psychiatric conditions. Some of those disorders, if untreated, pose major risks during pregnancy. A woman with major depression may have difficulty maintaining prenatal care or the nutritional needs of pregnancy. She may fail to experience an emotional bond with her fetus, risking early attachment problems.[11] She may attempt suicide.[12] Severe panic attacks during pregnancy have been associated with pregnancy complications such as placental abruption.[13] Agoraphobia can preclude visits to a prenatal clinic, or to a hospital during labor.[14]   Obsessions and compulsions about food can interfere with the nutritional requirements of pregnancy.

Symptoms such as these, when unresponsive to non-pharmacologic interventions, raise the need to consider pharmacotherapy. **To date, the antidepressant agents most systematically studied are the tricyclic antidepressants and fluoxetine** (Prozac). Less commonly used drugs like monoamine oxidase inhibitors, and agents newer than fluoxetine, have not yet been adequately studied.

Teratogenicity:

A number of studies and case collections have examined offspring exposed to tricyclic antidepressants in utero.[15-22] Although each study has methodologic flaws, in the aggregate, the results are reassuring in that **none demonstrated an increased likelihood of congenital anomalies after tricyclic exposure. Further, the types of anomalies that did develop after tricyclic exposure were varied, with no unique pattern emerging.**

Studies and case collections examining babies exposed to fluoxetine in utero have similarly shown no increase in major congenital anomalies.[21-24] However, one study[24] showed an increase in multiple minor anomalies in babies exposed to fluoxetine, as compared to a control group. Minor anomalies were defined as structural defects that occur in less than 4% of the general population, but have no cosmetic or functional importance. There was no particular pattern of anomalies noted. It is difficult to interpret this study, since the index and control groups differed significantly on important variables other than fluoxetine use. Index (fluoxetine-exposed) women were significantly older, and presumably had psychiatric disorders. Further, 30% of them were using other psychotropic drugs in addition to fluoxetine. Although complete confidence awaits further data, at this point overall results suggest fluoxetine is unlikely to be a significant human teratogen.

Children up to 7 years old have been followed after in utero tricyclic or fluoxetine exposure.[22] IQ, language, and other neurodevelopmental measures did not differ significantly from those of control (unexposed) children, suggesting that these medications are not behavioral teratogens in humans.

257

Fetal and Neonatal Side Effects:

Tricyclic antidepressants cause anticholinergic side effects in adults; similar side effects are occasionally observed in fetuses and newborns. The most problematic of these include tachycardia (which can lead to tachyarrhythmia) and urinary retention.[25,26] These are rare and transient phenomena; no reports to date describe permanent damage to babies resulting from these side effects.

Fluoxetine can cause weight loss and restless, agitated feelings in adults. One study found similar symptoms in newborns exposed to fluoxetine throughout pregnancy.[24] The mean birth weight and length of full term fluoxetine-exposed infants were significantly less than those of full term nonexposed infants. Behaviorally, fluoxetine-exposed infants showed higher rates of poor neonatal adaptation, the descriptions of which corresponded to the jitteriness reported by many adults on fluoxetine. Since this was the same study that found an increase in multiple minor anomalies, these findings are subject to the methodologic criticisms mentioned above. However, these side effects are plausible, since they correspond closely to common adult side effects.

Fetal and Neonatal Withdrawal:

Just as adults can experience symptoms upon sudden discontinuation of antidepressants, similar symptoms have been observed in fetuses and newborns.[27,28] In most cases, symptoms are mild and not clinically significant. In rare instances, they are more severe. Symptoms can include irritability, tachypnea, tachycardia, peripheral cyanosis, diaphoresis, tremor, increased tone, clonus, spasm, and seizures.

Preterm Labor:

The incidence of prematurity (defined as spontaneous delivery at less than 37 weeks gestation) was found in one study to be significantly greater for women who took fluoxetine throughout their pregnancies than for women who took no fluoxetine.[24] No other studies to date have replicated this finding, for either fluoxetine or other antidepressants. This was the same study described above in which confounding variables make it difficult to interpret the results.

Maternal Side Effects:

Some of the common side effects of tricyclic antidepressants are similar to the physiologic changes of pregnancy, and thus can be more difficult to tolerate while pregnant. These include tachycardia, constipation, and sedation. Further, significant orthostatic hypotension, even if not directly affecting the fetus, can have an indirect effect by decreasing placental perfusion.

Dosing Changes:

Due to pharmacokinetic changes, tricyclic antidepressant serum levels tend to decrease over the course of pregnancy if the dose is held constant.[29] Breakthrough depression can occur if the dose is not adjusted accordingly.

Guidelines for Using Antidepressants During Pregnancy

1   *When possible, use agents that have been systematically studied during pregnancy and that pose the fewest side effects. Currently, that includes desipramine* (Pertofrane), *nortryptiline* (Pamelor), *and fluoxetine.*

2   *When possible, avoid agents that could pose additional problems during pregnancy. These include monoamine oxidase inhibitors, which can cause hypertensive crises, and maprotiline* (Ludiomil), *which can lower the seizure threshold and increase the likelihood of seizures in pre-eclamptic women.*

3   *When using tricyclics, serum levels should be monitored more frequently than usual* (e.g., about once per trimester, or whenever depressive symptoms return).

4   *To minimize the likelihood of neonatal withdrawal, some women prefer to taper down their antidepressant dose gradually if they are asymptomatic, beginning at about three weeks before the expected date of delivery. Since women with prior episodes of depression are especially vulnerable to postpartum recurrence,[30] it is usually best not to completely discontinue the medication, and to resume a full therapeutic dose after delivery. Likewise, if*

*a woman decides to discontinue her antidepressant upon learn-
ing that she is pregnant, a gradual taper will cause less fetal distress than sudden discontinuation.*

5   *We have better knowledge of what constitutes therapeutic serum
    levels with the TCAs (specifically, desipramine and nortrypti-
    line), which is the reason we prefer these agents over the newer
    antidepressants as initial treatment options. With these drugs, we
    can make more accurate dosage adjustment in women who experi-
    ence clinically significant pharmacokinetic changes throughout
    their pregnancies. However, some women may have difficulty tol-
    erating tricyclic side effects, especially during pregnancy. In such
    cases, the SSRIs may be used with caution.*

To minimize the likelihood of neonatal withdrawal, some women
prefer to taper down their antidepressant dose gradually if they are
asymptomatic, beginning at about three weeks before the expected
date of delivery. Since women with prior episodes of depression are
especially vulnerable to postpartum recurrence,[30] it is usually best not
to completely discontinue the medication, and to resume a full therapeutic dose after delivery. Likewise, if a woman decides to discontinue
her antidepressant upon learning that she is pregnant, a gradual taper
will cause less fetal distress than sudden discontinuation.

Mood Stabilizing Medications During Pregnancy

**Untreated mania during pregnancy can pose significant hazards.
Impulsive behavior can include unprotected sexual intercourse,
increasing the risk of HIV infection for both mother and fetus.**[31]
Lack of realistic risk appraisal may lead to refusal of prenatal care and
failure to plan for the baby. **Impaired judgment can increase the likelihood of becoming a perpetrator or victim of violence. However, medications known to be effective mood stabilizing agents** (lithium, carbamazepine, and valproate [Depakote]) **pose significant risks during
pregnancy.** Weighing these risks to develop an optimal treatment plan
involves knowing as much as possible about specific risks and about the
individual patient.

Teratogenicity:

As lithium came into widespread clinical use, a *Registry of Lithium Babies* was established for voluntary reporting by physicians of any lithium use during pregnancy. Initial results were reassuring in that, despite a probable bias toward overreporting abnormalities, the incidence of anomalies in registry babies was not significantly higher than expected in the general population. **However, the ratio of cardiac to other anomalies was significantly higher than expected.[32] In particular, the rare right-sided Ebstein's anomaly showed up significantly more often than would otherwise be expected.[33] This led to the recommendation to avoid lithium during pregnancy.**

Subsequent prospective and case-control studies[34-36] have presented a different picture. Based on those studies, the relative risk of congenital heart disease is either slightly elevated, or not elevated, by lithium exposure in utero. Animal studies provide a clue, although not proof, to explain why lithium might be a weak cardiac teratogen. **In some species, the combination of lithium and ethanol is significantly more teratogenic than either substance alone.[3] Studies to date have not determined whether ethanol and lithium have a similar interaction in humans. Mental and behavioral development have not been found to be adversely affected by in utero lithium exposure.[37]**

Anticonvulsant mood stabilizers, such as carbamazepine and valproate, are also teratogens. Both are associated with an increased likelihood of minor and major malformations, particularly neural tube defects, after first trimester exposure.[38-47] The incidence of malformations is, in most studies, somewhat higher for valproate than for carbamazepine, and higher with the combination of both drugs than with either alone. **With valproate, there is some evidence that risk is dose-dependent, with more neural tube defects among babies whose mothers took higher doses during pregnancy.[48]** Although initial data suggested a higher incidence of developmental delay among babies exposed to either anticonvulsant,[39,48] subsequent prospective studies have found no significant differences in neurodevelopment or IQ related to carbamazepine exposure.[49,50]

Additive risk factors may explain why only a small percentage (1%–2%) of babies exposed to these anticonvulsants in utero develop neural tube defects. **Folate deficiency can increase the risk of neural** tube defects in offspring of pregnant women on anticonvulsants.[51] Maternal obesity, an independent risk factor for fetal neural tube defects,[52] may add to the anticonvulsant risk. Another risk factor may be genetic. Inheriting low levels of epoxide hydrolase, a major enzyme in metabolizing several anticonvulsants, may produce a higher likelihood of developing neural tube defects in the presence of those anticonvulsants.[5]

Fetal and Neonatal Side Effects:

Lithium can produce side effects in newborns that resemble "floppy baby syndrome": flaccidity, lethargy, difficulty sucking, and decreased Moro reflex.[53] (The Moro reflex, present in normal newborns, is a startle reflex elicited by any stimulus which suddenly moves the head in relation to the spine.) Rarely, it has been reported to cause toxic neonatal effects such as abnormal breathing, cyanosis, cardiac arrhythmias, and poor myocardial contractility.[53-55] Other reported side effects are similar to common adult side effects. Transient hypothyroidism has been reported in newborns, with no known permanent sequelae.[56] Nephrogenic diabetes insipidus can cause a fetus to urinate excessively, increasing the volume of amniotic fluid to the point of polyhydramnios.[57-59] No permanent renal damage has been reported to date.

Anticonvulsants can deplete Vitamin K-dependent clotting factors, increasing the risk of neonatal hemorrhage.[60,61] This risk can be eliminated by administering Vitamin K to the pregnant woman and to the newborn. Both carbamazepine and valproate have, in rare instances, been reported to affect neonatal liver function;[62,63] in the case of valproate, this can result in fatal liver toxicity. Another rare, potentially fatal neonatal side effect of valproate is fibrinogen depletion.[64]

Fetal and Neonatal Withdrawal:

Some infants exposed to valproate in utero have developed irritability, jitteriness, abnormal tone, seizures, and/or feeding problems beginning 12–24 hours after birth, consistent with withdrawal manifestations.[48]

Preterm Labor:

Lithium use in late pregnancy has been associated with an increased likelihood of preterm labor.[65]

Maternal Side Effects:

When lithium causes fetal nephrogenic diabetes insipidus, the pregnant woman may experience shortness of breath. This occurs when amniotic fluid volume becomes so great that the woman's lungs do not have adequate room to expand.[57-59]

Dosing Changes:

Lithium serum levels often decline over the course of pregnancy; doses must be increased to maintain a therapeutic level. At the time of delivery, the new mother often loses a great deal of fluid, and could become lithium toxic if the dose were not reduced.

With anticonvulsant mood stabilizers, the most relevant pharmacokinetic change is the degree of plasma protein binding. **Carbamazepine and its major metabolite are more extensively protein bound in maternal plasma than in fetal plasma.**[66] **Further, in some women the amount of protein binding decreases somewhat during pregnancy. At a given carbamazepine dose, this decreases total serum levels while free, biologically active levels remain constant.**[67] When serum levels are needed during pregnancy, obtaining free levels may be more accurate than obtaining total levels, and will avoid unnecessarily increasing fetal exposure.

Unlike carbamazepine, valproate accumulates in fetal blood.[66] **Further, free** (biologically active) **concentrations of valproate may increase by an average of 25% in maternal serum, even when total serum levels decrease.**[67] Using total serum levels to determine dose could lead to increased adverse effects for both the pregnant woman and her fetus.

Guidelines for Using Mood Stabilizing Agents During Pregnancy

1. *Since all mood stabilizing medications with demonstrated efficacy pose significant risks during pregnancy, and since mania can cause hypersexuality and impaired judgment, it is especially important to discuss family planning with patients of reproductive age. As much as possible, plan ahead with patients about what to do in case of a desired or unintended pregnancy. Involving significant others in this planning may enhance its efficacy.*

2.   *For patients who have mild to moderate disease, can recognize prodromal symptoms, and can seek help, it is often possible to discontinue mood stabilizing medication during the first trimester of pregnancy. Although some women prefer to discontinue medication while trying to conceive, this is not likely to be necessary to protect the embryo. Urine pregnancy tests can detect pregnancy early enough so that no significant effect of medication on the embryo has yet occurred.*

3.   *If a woman who has discontinued medication becomes symptomatic during the first trimester, electroconvulsive therapy (ECT) is a low risk, effective alternative for mood stabilization, provided the technique is modified appropriately for pregnancy.*[68]

4.   *Women with brittle and severe disease can opt for either maintenance ECT or maintenance medication.*

5.   *Folate supplementation* (present in standard prenatal vitamins), *particularly for women on anticonvulsants, should begin as soon as a woman plans to become pregnant.*

6.   *For women who have used lithium during the first trimester, ultrasound examination can detect most cardiac anomalies, some of which are surgically treatable.*[69,70] *For women who have used anticonvulsants during the first trimester, the standard screening test for neural tube defects, serum alpha fetoprotein (AFP), is not sufficient, since there will be a high rate of false negatives in this high-risk group.*[71] *Supplementing with amniocentesis and/or ultrasound will detect most neural tube defects.*

7.   *For women who opt to use lithium after the first trimester, monitoring uterine size and amniotic fluid levels will help detect fetal nephrogenic diabetes insipidus. Lithium should be discontinued if polyhydramnios develops. Serum lithium levels should be monitored and kept as low as possible while maintaining efficacy.*

8.   *For women who opt to use anticonvulsants after the first trimester, the risk of neonatal hemorrhage can be reduced by administering Vitamin K, 20 mg po daily, during the last one to two months of pregnancy, followed by 1 mg IM for the newborn at birth.*[72] *Dosing should be based on clinical response. If serum*

levels are needed, free levels are more accurate than total (free plus protein-bound) levels, especially for valproate.

9. *If a woman is taking lithium at the time of labor onset, the dose should be cut in half to avoid postnatal toxicity. Since women with bipolar mood disorder are at high risk for postpartum psychoses, this is usually preferable to discontinuing lithium completely. Serum lithium levels can be checked about a week after delivery, when acute fluid changes have mostly stabilized, and the dose can be adjusted as needed.*

10. *Verapamil (Calan) and other calcium channel blockers may prove to be safer alternatives for some pregnant women,[73] but their efficacy as mood stabilizers is not well established. Newer anticonvulsants which are being investigated for their efficacy as mood stabilizers (e.g., lamotrigine [Lamictal] and gabapentin [Neurontin]) have not yet been adequately studied during pregnancy.*

Antipsychotic Medications During Pregnancy

Active psychosis during pregnancy can pose significant risks for the pregnant woman and her fetus. Psychotic symptoms can compromise nutrition and prenatal care, and can lead to precipitous and/or unassisted deliveries. **In rare but tragic cases, psychosis can contribute to fetal abuse and/or neonaticide.**[74]

Antipsychotic agents have been prescribed for control of nausea and vomiting during pregnancy. Some studies of antipsychotic use during pregnancy have been done with predominantly non-mentally ill subjects who are exposed to lower doses and less continuous use. However, data from mentally ill and non-mentally ill samples seem comparable, and will be summarized below.

Teratogenicity:

A meta-analysis of published outcomes after first trimester phenothiazine exposure revealed a slight increase in relative risk of nonspecific congenital anomalies after exposure to low potency phenothiazines (*chlorpromazine [Thorazine] in most cases*).[75] This increase is on the order of 0.4%; in other words, if the baseline incidence of congenital anomalies is about 2%, the risk for babies exposed to low potency phenothiazines in utero is about 2.4%. **A similar increase has not been found for high potency antipsychotic agents, such as haloperidol** (Haldol) **and trifluoperazine** (Stelazine), **that have been studied.**[76-79] **Newer medications, such as clozapine** (Clozaril), **risperidone (Risperdal), and olanzapine** (Zyprexa), **and quetiapine** (Seroquel) **have not yet been systematically studied.** Clozapine poses theoretical risks because it can accumulate in fetal tissue,[80] can decrease the seizure threshold, and can cause agranulocytosis.

Antipsychotic exposure in utero has no demonstrable effect on IQ and behavior in children. However, exposed children were significantly taller and/or heavier than control children in one study.[81] This raises the possibility that in utero neuroleptic exposure causes enduring changes in dopaminergic neurotransmission which, in turn, affects growth hormone.

Fetal and Neonatal Side Effects:

Rarely, newborns develop withdrawal dyskinesias after neuroleptic exposure throughout pregnancy.[82] Signs can include tremors, hand posturing, increased tone, jerky eye movements, hyperreflexia, arching back, tongue thrusting, irritability, and a shrill cry. These signs develop hours to days after birth, and gradually resolve spontaneously over several months, leaving no enduring sequelae. Newborns can also have side effects related to the anticholinergic properties of neuroleptics, such as functional intestinal obstruction.[83]

Maternal Side Effects:

Neuroleptic side effects like sedation, constipation, tachycardia, and orthostatic hypotension may be more difficult to tolerate during pregnancy, since the physiologic changes of pregnancy may also have these effects.

Dosing Changes:

Pregnancy is not known to affect the dose of antipsychotic agents. **Clinical observation suggests, however, that antipsychotic medications may be more poorly absorbed during pregnancy, so that intramuscular administration may become more effective for some women. Keeping the dose as low as possible without compromising** efficacy will also minimize the likelihood of extrapyramidal side effects (EPS). This is particularly important during pregnancy, since agents commonly used to counteract EPS (benztropine [Cogentin], diphenhydramine [Benadryl], and amantadine [Symmetrel]) have been associated with increased rates of congenital anomalies, pregnancy complications, and neonatal side effects.[84-89] For akathisia, however, β-adrenergic blocking agents such as propranolol and atenolol are effective and pose no major risks during pregnancy, provided they do not excessively lower blood pressure or heart rate.[90]

Guidelines for Using Antipsychotic Agents During Pregnancy

1. *It is best to use relatively well-studied, high potency agents such as haloperidol or trifluoperazine and to avoid, when possible, low potency phenothiazines such as chlorpromazine.*

2. *Routine pharmacologic prophylaxis against EPS is not recommended. Calcium supplementation may protect against EPS in some women.[91]*

Anxiolytic Medications During Pregnancy

Mild anxiety during pregnancy is the norm. Extreme, ongoing anxiety can contribute to pregnancy complications such as hyperemesis gravidarum, preterm labor, and prolonged labor.[92,93] Psychotherapeutic techniques such as relaxation exercises, stress reduction, cognitive-behavioral therapy, and hypnosis are often effective treatments for anxiety. However, there are patients for whom such techniques are ineffective, and clinicians are often left considering whether anxiolytic medication is warranted. Several studies of benzodiazepine use during pregnancy have been done; no systematic data are currently available on non-benzodiazepine agents like buspirone (BuSpar).

Teratogenicity:
Studies of benzodiazepine teratogenicity are plagued with methodologic flaws, and have contradictory results. Some early studies of

diazepam linked first trimester use with an increased likelihood of oral clefts.[94-96] Subsequent studies of diazepam and other benzodiazepines did not find this link.[97-101] Meta-analysis of data from all relevant studies reveals a positive association between first trimester benzodiazepine use and oral clefts.[75] Because there has been no population-wide increase in oral clefts corresponding with widespread use of benzodiazepines among women of reproductive age, most investigators have concluded that benzodiazepines are weakly teratogenic, if at all.

Investigations of behavioral teratogenicity are equally controversial. While one group found evidence of motor immaturity and general developmental delay in toddlers exposed to benzodiazepines in utero,[102,103] others found no significant increase in neurodevelopmental problems.[100,104] The methodologies of these studies are not comparable, and none of the methodologies employed could rule out significant confounding variables.

Fetal and Neonatal Side Effects:

Newborns can experience both intoxication and withdrawal from benzodiazepines. Infants can develop a "floppy baby syndrome," consisting of lethargy, hypotonia, hyporeflexia, difficulty sucking, poor respiratory efforts, and difficulty maintaining body temperature.[105,106] Intoxication can also develop in a fetus if a pregnant woman overdoses on benzodiazepines; this can be detected by decreased beat-to-beat variability on fetal cardiac monitoring.[107] If exposed to long-term benzodiazepine use, withdrawing newborns can develop hypertonia, hyperreflexia, and tremor.[108-110] These intoxication and withdrawal manifestations are transient and self-limited, but may require supportive care. Rarely, neonatal functional intestinal obstruction may also result from benzodiazepine exposure in utero.[111]

Guidelines for Using Anxiolytic Agents During Pregnancy

1. *Agents which do not accumulate in fetal tissue, such as lorazepam (Ativan), have at least a theoretical advantage compared to agents such as diazepam, which can accumulate.*[112]

2. *Fetal or neonatal intoxication can be reversed with the benzodi- azepine antagonist flumazenil* (Mazicon).[113]

3. *If long-term use of benzodiazepines is being discontinued due to pregnancy, it is probably safer to taper them by a maximum of 10% per day, rather than discontinue them suddenly. For women who have taken benzodiazepines throughout pregnancy, such tapering can also be attempted within the last month of pregnancy to avoid sudden neonatal withdrawal.*

Psychotropic Medications During Lactation

Breast feeding has significant benefits for mothers and babies.[114] It is less expensive than formula feeding, and precludes errors in formula prepa- ration. It promotes babies' digestion, absorption, and immune responses. **Breast fed babies have fewer infectious diseases, lower mortality rates, and higher IQ's than bottle-fed babies. Breast feed- ing also provides some natural contraception, and promotes feelings of relaxation, bonding, and maternal competency in many mothers.** For these reasons, it is not a simple matter to advise a woman not to breastfeed if she is taking psychotropic medications.

Several factors, besides the mother's dose, influence the dose a nursing baby will experience when a breastfeeding mother takes medication.[115] These include the drug's solubility, degree of protein binding, pH (with weak acids being less soluble in acidic breast milk), neonatal absorption, and neonatal metabolism. Further, nursing pat- terns vary widely, with some babies taking in nothing but breast milk, and others supplementing their diets with breast milk.

Infant drug metabolism changes rapidly after birth.[116] For about the first two weeks of life, most babies' livers can only metabolize at about 1/3 to 1/5 the rate of an adult liver. After that, oxidative capacity increases; by age two to three months, most babies metabolize at about two to six times adult capacity. Glomerular filtration rate in newborns is about 30%–40% of the adult rate, which makes it more difficult for babies to clear drugs via renal excretion.

To date, there are no large scale systematic outcome studies of chil- dren exposed to psychotropic medication via breast milk. Available data consists of reported cases and clinical experience, and will be sum- marized below.

Antidepressant Medications and Lactation:

Most of the time, antidepressants and their active metabolites are not detectable in nursing babies when their mothers are on therapeutic doses. The few exceptions reported have mostly been in babies who are less than 10 weeks old. Sedation and respiratory depression resulted in one reported case of doxepin (Sinequan) ingestion via breast milk.[116] Fluoxetine ingestion via breast milk has been associated with "colic" (inconsolable crying and disturbed sleep) in one infant.[117] Perhaps due to its long half-life, weight-adjusted relative doses of fluoxetine are greater than those of other selective serotonin reuptake inhibitors (SSRIs) (e.g., about 1.2%–6.2% of the mother's dose for fluoxetine, compared to 0.3%–0.5% for paroxetine [Paxil] or fluvoxamine [Luvox]).[118]

Mood Stabilizing Medications and Lactation:

Lithium concentrations in breast milk are about 20%–60% of maternal serum concentrations.[115] This causes detectable levels of lithium in the sera of nursing infants. In some cases, side effects have been reported, including hypotonia, hypothermia, and cyanosis.[119] Since long-term lithium use can cause hypothyroidism and nephrogenic diabetes insipidus in adults, these are additional potential risks in babies.

By contrast, valproate, as a weak acid, is present in much lower concentrations in breast milk—up to about 10% of the levels in maternal serum.[120] No adverse effects have been reported in nursing infants. Carbamazepine has intermediate concentrations in breast milk, and sometimes produces detectable infant serum levels.[63] Adverse effects in infants whose sole exposure was through breast feeding have not yet been reported, but there are two reports of transient hepatic dysfunction in babies exposed to carbamazepine both in utero and subsequently, through breast milk.[63,121]

Antipsychotic Medications and Lactation:

Antipsychotic medications are present in breast milk in lower concentrations than in maternal serum.[115] An exception is clozapine, which may accumulate in breast milk.[80] Sedation has been noted in one infant exposed to chlorpromazine via breast milk.[122] Adverse effects from higher potency antipsychotic agents have not been noted to date.

Anxiolytic Medications and Lactation:

Some benzodiazepines may accumulate in nursing infants.[123] Acute effects can include sedation and weight loss.[124] Prolonged exposure could lead to withdrawal signs in babies upon weaning. Nevertheless, a number of infants have been reported to have no adverse effects from low doses of benzodiazepines.

Guidelines for Prescribing During Lactation

Prescribing psychopharmacologic agents during lactation involves the following steps:

1. *Compare with patients the risks and benefits of breast feeding with medication, breast feeding without medication (and with untreated symptoms), and weaning in order to take medication.*

2. *Discuss these risks and benefits with the patient and, whenever possible, this discussion should include the father of the baby and the pediatrician. The limitations of our knowledge should be explained.*

3. *Encourage parents to describe their baby's baseline behavior before starting the medication.*

4. *Find the lowest effective dose.*

5. *If the infant's behavior changes, or if the parents or pediatrician are worried for any reason, measure the baby's serum level of the drug and its active metabolites. Because this is not a routine test for many laboratories, contact a laboratory in advance that can perform this test to get specific collection instructions.*

6. *If there are detectable serum levels but no symptoms, the mother may opt to continue breast feeding, but recheck infant serum levels in a week. By then, they may be nondetectable due to elimination of leftover medication from in utero exposure, and due to hepatic maturation.*

7. *If levels are still detectable a week later and/or the baby has adverse effects, weaning is usually advisable.*

Conclusion

Many women who are pregnant, desire to become pregnant, or are nursing are faced with the difficult decision of whether to take medication when they develop symptoms of a psychiatric disorder. They can be helped to make optimal decisions in these ways:

1. *Review the risks of untreated symptoms.*

2. *Consider interventions other than medication that might be effective for the duration of the pregnancy.*

3. *Review all potentially effective medications to find those with fewest risks during pregnancy.*

4. *Use dosing strategies that minimize risks.*

5. *Decrease additive risk factors, such as cigarette smoking and alcohol drinking.*

6. *Add protective supplements when applicable* (e.g., folate and Vitamin K for anticonvulsant mood stabilizers).

Offer extra support, both directly (via increased frequency of visits) and indirectly (by involving significant others in treatment plans and referring to support groups).

References

1. Seeman MV, ed. *Gender and Psychopathology*. Washington, DC: American Psychiatric Press;1995.

2. Jensvold MF, Halbreich U, Hamilton JA, eds. *Psychopharmacology and Women: Sex, Gender, and Hormones*. Washington, DC: American Psychiatric Press;1996.

3. Sharma A, Rawat AK. Teratogenic effects of lithium and ethanol in the developing fetus. *Alcohol*. 1986;3:101–106.

4. Brioni JD, Orsingher OA. Operant behavior and reactivity to the anticonflict effect of diazepam in perinatally undernourished rats. *Physiol & Behav*. 1988;193–198.

5. Finnell RH, Buehler BA, Kerr BM, et al. Clinical and experimental studies linking oxidative metabolism to phenytoin-induced teratogenesis. *Neurology*. 1992;42(suppl 5):25–31.

6a. Miller LJ. Psychiatric disorders during pregnancy. In: Stewart DE, Stotland NL, eds. *Psychological Aspects of Women's Health Care: The Interface Between Psychiatry and Obstetrics and Gynecology*. Washington, DC: American Psychiatric Press; 1993:55–70.

6b. Little BB, Santos-Ramoz R, Newell JF, et al. Megadose carbamazepine during the period of neural tube closure. *Obstet Gynecol.* 1993;82:705–708.

7. Hensleigh PA, Brown EL. Psychosocial stress and pregnancy. In: Gleicher N, ed. *Principles of Medical Therapy in Pregnancy.* New York: Plenum; 1985:885–888.

8. Reder P, Lucey C, eds. *Assessment of Parenting: Psychiatric and Psychological Contributions.* London: Routledge; 1995.

9. Cupit GC, Rotmensch HH. Principles of drug therapy in pregnancy. In: Gleicher N, ed. *Principles of Medical Therapy in Pregnancy.* New York: Plenum; 1985:77–90.

10. Rubin PC, Butters L, McCabe R et al. The influence of pregnancy on drug action: concentration-effect modelling with propranolol. *Clin Sci.* 1987;73:47–52

11. Jacobsen T (in press). The effects of postpartum disorders on parenting and on offspring. In: Miller LJ, ed. *Postpartum Mood Disorders.* Washington, DC: American Psychiatric Press.

12. Lester D, Beck AT. Attempted suicide and pregnancy. *Am J Obstet Gynecol.* 1988;158:1084–1085.

13. Cohen LS, Rosenbaum JF, Heller VL. Panic attack-associated placental abruption: a case report. *J Clin Psychiatry.* 1989;50:266–267.

14. Olsen ME, Toeppen-Sprigg B, Krell MA. Prenatal care and delivery in an agoraphobic woman: a case report. *J Reprod Med.* 1992;37:466–468.

15. Scanlon FJ. Use of antidepressant drugs during the first trimester (letter). *Med J Australia.* 1969;2:1077.

16. Banister P, Dafoe C, Smith ESO, et al. Possible teratogenicity of tricyclic antidepressants (letter). *Lancet.* 1972;1:838–839.

17. Crombie DL, Pinsent RJFH, Fleming D. Imipramine in pregnancy (letter). *Brit Med J.* 1972;1:745.

18. Kuenssberg EV, Knox JDE. Imipramine in pregnancy (letter). *Brit Med J.* 1972;2:292.

19. Rachelefsky GS, Flynt JW, Ebbin AJ, et al. Possible teratogenicity of tricyclic antidepressants (letter). *Lancet.* 1972;1:838.

20. Misri S, Sivertz K. Tricyclic drugs in pregnancy and lactation: a preliminary report. *Int J Psychiatry Med.* 1991;21:157–171.

21. Pastuszak A, Schick-Boschetto B, Zuber C, et al. Pregnancy outcome following first-trimester exposure to fluoxetine (Prozac). *JAMA.* 1993;269:2246–2248.

22. Nulman I, Rovet J, Stewart DE, et al. Neurodevelopment of children exposed in utero to antidepressant drugs. *N Engl J Med.* 1997;336:258–262.

23. Goldstein DJ. Effects of third trimester fluoxetine exposure on the newborn. *J Clin Psychopharmacol.* 1995;15:417–420.

24. Chambers CD, Johnson KA, Dick LM, et al. Birth outcomes in pregnant women taking fluoxetine. *N Engl J Med.* 1996;335:1010–1015.

25. Prentiss A, Brown R. Fetal tachyarrhythmia and maternal antidepressant treatment (letter). *Brit Med J.* 1989;298:190.

26. Elia J, Katz IR, Sinpson GM. Teratogenicity of psychotherapeutic medications. *Psychopharmacol Bull.* 1987;23:531–586.

273

27. Webster PAC. Withdrawal symptoms in neonates associated with maternal antidepressant therapy. *Lancet*. 1973;2:318–319.

28. Eggermont E. Withdrawal symptoms in neonates associated with maternal imipramine therapy (letter). *Lancet*. 1973;2:680.

29. Wisner KL, Perel JM, Wheeler SB. Tricyclic dose requirements across pregnancy. *Am J Psychiatry*. 1993;150:1541–1542.

30. Steiner M, Tam WYK (in press). Postpartum depression in relation to other psychiatric disorders. In: Miller LJ, ed. *Postpartum Mood Disorders*. Washington, DC: American Psychiatric Press.

31. Sacks MH, Silberstein C, Weiler P, et al. HIV-related risk factors in acute psychiatric inpatients. *Hosp Community Psychiatry*. 1990;41:449–451.

32. Weinstein MR, Goldfield MD. Cardiovascular malformations with lithium use during pregnancy. *Am J Psychiatry*. 1975;132:529–531.

33. Nora JJ, Nora AH, Toews WH. Lithium, Ebstein's anomaly, and other congenital heart defects (letter). *Lancet*. 1974;2:594–595.

34. Kallen B, Tandberg A. Lithium and pregnancy: a cohort study on manic-depressive women. *Acta Psychiatr Scand*.1983;68:134–139.

35. Zalzstein E, Koren G, Einarson T, et al. A case-control study on the association between first trimester exposure to lithium and Ebstein's anomaly. *Am J Cardiology*. 1990;65:817–818.

36. Jacobson SJ, Jones K, Johnson K, et al. Prospective multicentre study of pregnancy outcome after lithium exposure during first trimester. *Lancet*. 1992;339:530–533.

37. Schou M. What happened later to the lithium babies? A follow-up study of children born without malformations. *Acta Psychiatr Scand*. 1976;54:193–197.

38. Murasaki O, Yoshitake K, Tachiki H, et al. Reexamination of the teratological effects of antiepileptic drugs. *Japanese J Psychiatry Neurol*. 1988;42:592–593.

39. Jones KL, Lacro RV, Johnson KA, et al. Pattern of malformations in the children of women treated with carbamazepine during pregnancy. *N Engl J Med*. 1989;320:1661–1666.

40. Dravet C, Julian C, Legras C, et al. Epilepsy, antiepileptic drugs, and malformations in children of women with epilepsy: a French prospective cohort study. *Neurology*. 1992;42(Suppl 5):75–82.

41. Gladstone DJ, Bologa M, Maguire C, et al. Course of pregnancy and fetal outcome following maternal exposure to carbamazepine and phenytoin: a prospective study. *Reprod Toxicol*. 1992;6:257–261.

42. Kanecko S, Otani K, Kondo T, et al. Malformation in infants of mothers with epilepsy receiving antiepileptic drugs. *Neurology*. 1992;42(suppl 5):68–74.

43. Koch S, Losche G, Jager-Roman E, et al. Major and minor birth malformations and antiepileptic drugs. *Neurology*. 1992;42(suppl 5):83–88.

44. Yerby MS, Leavitt A, Erickson DM, et al. Antiepileptics and the development of congenital anomalies. *Neurology*. 1992;42(suppl 5):132–140.

45. Kallen AJB. Maternal carbamazepine and infant spina bifida. *Reprod Toxicol*. 1994;8:203–205.

46. Waters CH, Belai Y, Gott PS, et al. Outcomes of pregnancy associated with antiepileptic drugs. *Arch Neurol.* 1994;51:250–253.

47. Nulman I, Scolnik D, Chitayat D, et al. Findings in children exposed in utero to phenytoin and carbamazepine monotherapy: independent effects of epilepsy and medications. *Am J Med Genet.* 1997;68:18–24.

48. Thisted E, Ebbesen F. Malformations, withdrawal manifestations, and hypoglycaemia after exposure to valproate in utero. *Arch Dis Child.* 1993;60:288–291.

49. van der Pol MC, Hadders-Algra M, Huisjes HJ, et al. Antiepileptic medication in pregnancy: late effects on the children's central nervous system development. *Am J Obstet Gynecol.* 1991;164:121–128.50.   Scolnik D, Nulman I, Rovet J, et al. Neurodevelopment of children exposed in utero to phenytoin and carbamazepine monotherapy. *JAMA.* 1994;271:767–770.

51. Dansky LV, Rosenblatt DS, Andermann E. Mechanisms of teratogenesis: folic acid and antiepileptic therapy. *Neurology.* 1992;42(suppl 5):32–42.

52. Shaw GM, Velie EM, Schaffer D. Risk of neural tube defect-affected pregnancies among obese women. *JAMA.* 1996;275:1093–1096.

53. Woody JN, London WL, Wilbanks GD. Lithium toxicity in a newborn. *Pediatrics.* 1971;47:94–96.

54. Nishiwaki T, Tanaka K, Sekiya S. Acute lithium intoxication in pregnancy (letter). *Int J Gynecol Obstet.* 1996;52:191–192.

55. Wilson N, Forfar JC, Godman MJ. Atrial flutter in the newborn resulting from maternal lithium ingestion. *Arch Dis Child.* 1983;58:538-549.

56. Karlsson K, Lindstedt G, Lundberg PA, et al. Transplacental lithium poisoning: reversible inhibition of fetal thyroid (letter). *Lancet.* 1975;1:1295.

57. Ang MS, Thorp JA, Parisi VM. Maternal lithium therapy and polyhydramnios. *Obstet Gynecol.* 1990;76:517–518.

58. Krause S, Ebbesen F, Lange AP. Polyhydramnios with maternal lithium treatment. *Obstet Gynecol.* 1990;75:504–506.

59. Mizrahi EM, Hobbs JF, Goldsmith DI. Nephrogenic diabetes insipidus in transplacental lithium intoxication. *J Pediatrics.* 1979;94:493–495.

60. Morales WJ. Antenatal therapy to minimize neonatal intraventricular hemorrhage. *Clin Obstet Gynecol.* 1991;34:328–335.

61. Moslet U, Hansen ES. A review of vitamin K, epilepsy and pregnancy. *Acta Neurol Scand.* 1992;85:39–43.

62. Legius E, Jaeken J, Eggermont E. Sodium valproate, pregnancy, and infantile fatal liver failure (letter). *Lancet.* 1987;2:1518–1519.

63. Merlob P, Mor N, Litwin A. Transient hepatic dysfunction in an infant of an epileptic mother treated with carbamazepine during pregnancy and breastfeeding. *Ann Pharmacother.* 1992;26:1563–1565.

64. Bavoux F. Neonatal fibrinogen depletion caused by sodium valproate (letter). *Ann Pharmacother.* 1994;28:1307.

65. Troyer WA, Pereira BR, Lannon RA, et al. Association of maternal lithium exposure and premature delivery. *J Perinatol.* 1993;13:123–127.

66. Kuhnz W, Steldinger R, Nau H. Protein binding of carbamazepine and its epoxide in maternal and fetal plasma at delivery: comparison to other anticonvulsants. *Dev Pharmacol.* 1984;7:61–72.

67. Yerby M, Friel PN, McCormick K. Antiepileptic drug disposition during pregnancy. *Neurology.* 1992;42(suppl 5):12–16.

68. Miller LJ. Use of electroconvulsive therapy during pregnancy. *Hosp Community Psychiatry.* 1994;45:444–450.

69. Long WA, Willis PW. Maternal lithium and neonatal Ebstein's anomaly: evaluation with cross-sectional echocardiography. *Am J Perinatol.* 1984;1:182–184.

70. Ferrazzi E, Fesslova V, Bellotti M et al. Prenatal diagnosis and management of congenital heart disease. *J Reprod Med.* 1989;34:207–214.

71. Omtzigt JGC, Los FJ, Hagenaars AM, et al. Prenatal diagnosis of spina bifida aperta after first-trimester valproate exposure. *Prenatal Diagnosis.* 1992;12:893–897.

72. Delgado-Escueta AV, Janz D. Consensus guidelines: preconception counseling, management, and care of the pregnant woman with epilepsy. *Neurology.* 1992;42(suppl 5):149–160.

73. Goodnick PJ. Verapamil prophylaxis in pregnant women with bipolar disorder (letter). *Am J Psychiatry.* 1993;150:1560.

74. Brozovsky M, Falit H: Neonaticide: clinical and psychodynamic considerations. *J Am Acad Child Psychiatry.* 1971;10:673–683.

75. Altshuler LL, Cohen L, Szuba MP, et al. Pharmacologic management of psychiatric illness during pregnancy: dilemmas and guidelines. *Am J Psychiatry.* 1996;153:592–605.

76. Moriarty AJ, Nance MR. Trifluoperazine and pregnancy (letter). *Can Med Assoc J.* 1963;88:375–376.

77. Rawlings WJ, Ferguson R, Maddison TG. Phenmetrazine and trifluoperazine (letter). *Med J Australia.* 1963;1:370.

78. Schrire I. Trifluoperazine and foetal abnormalities (letter). *Lancet.* 1963;1:174.

79. Van Waes A, Van de Velde E. Safety evaluation of haloperidol in the treatment of hyperemesis gravidarum. *J Clin Pharmacol.* 1969;July-Aug:224–227.

80. Barnas C, Bergant A, Hummer M, et al. Clozapine concentrations in maternal and fetal plasma, amniotic fluid, and breast milk (letter). *Am J Psychiatry.* 1994;151:945.

81. Platt JE, Friedhoff AJ, Broman SH, et al. Effects of prenatal exposure to neuroleptic drugs on children's growth. *Neuropsychopharmacology.* 1988;1:205–212.

82. Sexson WR, Barak Y. Withdrawal emergent syndrome in an infant associated with maternal haloperidol therapy. *J Perinatology.* 1989;9:170–172.

83. Falterman CG, Richardson CJ. Small left colon syndrome associated with maternal ingestion of psychotropic drugs. *J Pediatrics.* 1980;97: 308–310.

84. Parkin DE. Probable Benadryl withdrawal manifestations in a newborn infant (letter). *J Pediatrics.* 1974;85:580.

85. Saxen I. Cleft palate and maternal diphenhydramine intake (letter). *Lancet.* 1974;1:407–408.

86. Heinonen OP, Slone D, Shapiro S. *Birth Defects and Drugs in Pregnancy.* Littleton, Mass: Publishing Sciences Group; 1977.

87. Golbe LI. Parkinson's disease and pregnancy. *Neurology*. 1987;37:1245–1249.

88. Rosa F. Amantadine pregnancy experience. *Reprod Toxicol*. 1994;8:531.

89. Brost BC, Scardo JA, Newman RB. Diphenhydramine overdose during pregnancy: lessons from the past. *Obstet Gynecol*. 1996;175:1376–1377.

90. Rubin PC. Beta-blockers in pregnancy. *N Engl J Med*. 1981;305:1323–1326.

91. Kuny S, Binswanger U. Neuroleptic-induced extrapyramidal symptoms and serum calcium levels: results of a pilot study. *Pharmacopsychiatr*. 1989;21:67–70.

92. Hod M, Orvieto R, Kaplan B, et al. Hyperemesis gravidarum: a review. *J Reprod Med*. 1994;39:605–612.

93. Hensleigh PA, Brown EL. Psychosocial stress and pregnancy. In: *Principles of Medical Therapy in Pregnancy*. Gleicher N, ed. New York: Plenum; 1985.

94. Saxen I. Associations between oral clefts and drugs taken during pregnancy. *Int J Epidemiology*. 1975;4:37–44.

95. Aarskog D. Association between maternal intake of diazepam and oral clefts (letter). *Lancet*. 1975;2:921.

96. Safra MJ, Oakley GP. Association between cleft lip with or without cleft palate and prenatal diazepam exposure. *Lancet*. 1975;2:478–480.

97. Rosenberg L, Mitchell AA, Parsells JL, et al. Lack of relation of oral clefts to diazepam use during pregnancy. *New Eng J Med*. 1983;309:1282–1285.

98. Shiono PH, Mills JL. Oral clefts and diazepam use in pregnancy. *New Eng J Med*. 1984;311:919–920.

99. Czeizel A. Lack of evidence of teratogenicity of benzodiazepine drugs in Hungary. *Reprod Toxicol*. 1988;1:183–188.

100. Hartz SC, Heinonen OP, Shapiro S, et al. Antenatal exposure to meprobamate and chlordiazepoxide in relation to malformations, mental development, and childhood mortality. *New Eng J Med*. 1975;292:726–728.

101. St. Clair SM, Schirmer RG. First-trimester exposure to alprazolam. *Obstet Gynecol*. 1992;80:843–846.

102. Laegreid L, Hagberg G, Lundberg A. Neurodevelopment in late infancy after prenatal exposure to benzodiazepines—a prospective study. *Neuropediatrics*. 1992;23:60–67.

103. Viggedal G, Hagberg BS, Laegreid L, et al. Mental development in late infancy after prenatal exposure to benzodiazepines—a prospective study. *J Child Psychol Psychiatry*. 1993;3:295–305.

104. Bergman U, Rosa FW, Baum C, et al. Effects of exposure to benzodiazepine during fetal life. *Lancet*. 1992;340:694–696.

105. Cree JE, Meyer J, Hailey DM. Diazepam in labour: its metabolism and effect on the clinical condition and thermogenesis of the newborn. *Brit Med J*. 1973;4:251–255.

106. Gillberg C. "Floppy infant syndrome" and maternal diazepam. *Lancet*. 1977;2:244.

107. Yeh SY, Paul RH, Cordero L, et al. A study of diazepam during labor. *Obstet Gynecol*. 1974;43:363–373.

108. Athinarayanan P, Perog SH, Nigam SK, et al. Chlordiazepoxide withdrawal in the neonate. *Am J Obstet Gynecol*. 1976;124:212–213.

109. Mazzi E. Possible neonatal diazepam withdrawal: a case report. *Am J Obstet Gynecol.* 129:586–587.

110. Sanchis A, Rosique D, Catala J. Adverse effects of maternal lorazepam on neonates. *DICP, Ann Pharmacother.* 1991;25:1137–1138.

111. Haeusler MCH, Hoellwarth ME, Holzer P. Paralytic ileus in a fetus-neonate after maternal intake of benzodiazepine. *Prenatal Diagnosis.* 1995;15:1165–1167.

112. Whitelaw AGL, Cummings AJ, McFadyen IR. Effect of maternal lorazepam on the neonate. *Brit Med J.* 1981;282:1106–1108.

113. Stahl MMS, Saldeen P. Reversal of fetal benzodiazepine intoxication using flumazenil. *Brit J Obstet Gynaecol.* 1993;100:185–188.

114. Freed GL. Breastfeeding: time to teach what we preach. *JAMA.* 1993;269:243–245.

115. Buist A, Norman TR, Dennerstein L. Breastfeeding and the use of psychotropic medication: a review. *J Affective Disorders.* 1990;19:197–206.

116. Matheson I, Pande H, Alertsen AR. Respiratory depression caused by N-desmethyldoxepin in breast milk. *Lancet.* 1985;2:1124.

117. Lester BM, Cucca J, Andreozzi L, et al. Possible association between fluoxetine hydrochloride and colic in an infant. *J Am Acad Child Adolesc Psychiatry.* 1993;32:1253–1255.

118. Spigset O, Carleborg L, Norstrom A, et al. Paroxetine level in breast milk (letter). *J Clin Psychiatry.* 1996;57:39.

119. Tunnesen WW, Hertz CG. Toxic effects of lithium in newborn infants: a commentary. *J Pediatr.* 1972;81:804–807.

120. Nau H, Kuhnz W, Egger HJ, et al. Anticonvulsants during pregnancy and lactation: transplacental, maternal and neonatal pharmacokinetics. *Clin Pharmacokinetics.* 1982;7:508–543.

121. Frey B, Schubiger G, Musy JP. Transient cholestatic hepatitis in a neonate associated with carbamazepine exposure during pregnancy and breast feeding. *Eur J Pediatr.* 1990;150:136–138.

122. Wiles DH, Orr MW, Kolakowska T. Chlorpromazine levels in plasma and milk of nursing mothers. *Br J Clin Pharmacol.* 5:272–273.

123. Kanto JH. Use of benzodiazepines during pregnancy, labour and lactation, with particular reference to pharmacokinetic considerations. *Drugs.* 1982;23:354–380.

124. Patrick MJ, Tilstone WJ, Reavy P. Diazepam and breast feeding. *Lancet.* 1972;1:542–543

12   Psychoactive Drug–Drug Interactions in Children, Adolescents, and Adults

C. Lindsay DeVane, PharmD, Eve G. Spratt, MD, and Floyd R. Sallee, MD, PhD

Dr. DeVane is Professor of Psychiatry and Behavioral Sciences and Professor of Pharmaceutical Sciences; Dr. Spratt is Assistant Professor of Psychiatry and Behavioral Sciences and Assistant Professor of Pediatrics; and Dr. Sallee is Associate Professor of Psychiatry and Behavioral Sciences and Associate Professor of Pharmacology,Department of Psychiatry and Behavioral Sciences, Medical University of South Carolina, Charleston, SC.

Editor's Note

In the management of patients receiving psychoactive medications, the objective is to obtain a maximum improvement in symptoms while at the same time keeping unpleasant or disabling side effects to a minimum. When two or more drugs are combined, as is often the case, there is frequently a risk of either losing efficacy or intensifying side effects. One important, known reason for this is the competition between and among drugs for metabolism via the cytochrome P450 enzymes in the liver.

For instance, when methylphenidate is combined with an anticonvulsant or a tricyclic antidepressant, the plasma levels of these two drugs rise. It should not be combined with clonipine because there may be serious cardiovascular complications, and several deaths in children have been attributed to this combination.

When clomipramine is combined with fluoxetine, the plasma level of clomipramine rises and there is a risk of seizures. Combining tricyclics with low-potency antipsychotics, benztropine, various antihistamines, or meperidine carries the risk of additive anticholinergic toxicity; when they are combined with SSRIs, the plasma concentration of the TCA rises. SSRIs present a special risk of cardiac arrythmias when combined with nonsedating antihistamines, such as terfenidine; when an antihistamine is required in a patient receiving an SSRI, carboxy-terfenadine, loratadin, or citirizine are preferred. MAOI inhibitors should not be given in conjunction with TCAs or SSRIs because of the danger of overstimulation of catecholamines and cardiovascular toxicity.

The plasma levels of clozapine are reduced by cigarette smoking; they are increased when clozapine is combined with fluvoxamine or ciprofoxacin. Adding fluvoxamine increases the plasma concentration of olanzepine; cigarette smoking reduces benzodiazepines, TCAs, or antipsychotics.

Research in animals and adults has elaborated upon most of the pharmacodynamics of these drugs and their interactions. They are, nonetheless, widely used in children and adolescents as well, where special considerations must be kept in mind.

General Principles of Drug Interactions

Ideally, we would like to treat each mental disorder with a single drug. **However, the effects of psychoactive drugs are often nonspecific; drugs have their major effects on reduction of symptoms, but they more often produce their effects regardless of the patient's diagnosis. Many disorders have symptoms that overlap other disorders. Frequently a single drug will not be sufficient to treat all of the symptoms of a specific disorder.** Thus, drugs are frequently coadministered to achieve therapeutic effects from the combined actions at effect (receptor) sites or to treat the adverse effects caused by one drug with another.[1] **The concurrent administration of multiple drugs to a patient increases the possibility that they may interact in a negative or undesired way.** As additional medications are prescribed in a treatment regimen, the probability increases that both pharmacodynamic and pharmacokinetic interactions will occur.

Drug interactions are graded phenomena. **The degree of interaction depends upon the interacting drugs' pharmacology, the doses administered, the resulting drug concentrations, and the times of administration. Drug interactions are most likely to be meaningful when therapy with an interacting drug is initiated or discontinued.** The clinical significance will depend upon the particular drugs involved, the physiologic state of the patient, the presence of concurrent illness, and other patient factors. **Drugs with a narrow concentration range** for producing their therapeutic effects without incurring toxicity are more likely to be involved in clinically significant drug interactions. This group includes the antipsychotics, anticonvulsants and mood stabilizers, and most drugs with a primary effect on the cardiovascular system. Drugs with a broad range of doses and plasma concentrations that are well tolerated include the selective serotonin-reuptake inhibitors (SSRIs) and the benzodiazepines.

Mechanisms of Drug Interactions

Drug interactions occur through either pharmacokinetic and/or pharmacodynamic mechanisms; a classification is given in Table 12.2 The former are more easily detected and quantified. Analytic methods are available to measure drug concentrations for most drugs in therapeutic use. A pharmacokinetic interaction occurs when one drug alters the absorption, distribution, steady-state concentration, or elimination characteristics of another drug. *Pharmacodynamic interactions occur when coadministered drugs have an affinity for the same receptor sites* and produce additive or synergistic effects, or their actions oppose one another through antagonistic effects at receptor sites. This latter mechanism is the basis for development of naloxone (Narcan) and propranolol (Inderal), two drugs that oppose the actions of opiates and catecholamines at their respective receptor sites.

The most common mechanisms of pharmacokinetic drug interactions involve an alteration of drug metabolism of one drug by another through either induction or inhibition of hepatic cytochrome P450 enzymes. Major differences exist in the pharmacokinetic consequences of these interactions. These situations are shown in Figure 12.1.

An *inducer* is defined as a drug that, upon chronic administration, causes an increase in hepatic enzymes that metabolize either the administered drug itself—a phenomenon known as autoinduction— or other drugs. When an enzyme inducer is initiated, the effects on the steady-state concentration of preceding chronic therapy do not occur immediately. An observable effect may be delayed for several days as additional hepatic enzyme is synthesized. For example, the drug given as Regimen B in Figure 12.1 may remain at a steady-state for several days after the introduction of an inducer. Eventually, an increase occurs in the drug's metabolic clearance secondary to the increased enzyme available for drug metabolism. **This results in a decreased drug plasma concentration to a new steady-state.** The degree to which drug clearance is increased will depend upon the relative importance of the induced enzyme(s) in the overall elimination of the drug. The dose of the enzyme inducer is also important. **Cigarette smoking, anticonvulsant treatment** (with either phenytoin [Dilantin], phenobarbital [Donnatal], or carbamazepine [Tegretol]), **and rifampin** (Rifadin) **are common hepatic enzyme inducers. Examples where induction has been clinically significant include a loss of antipsychotic effect of** haloperidol (Haldol) **and diminished contraceptive effects of estrogens from coadministration of carbamazepine with either drug, and loss of antipsychotic efficacy of clozapine** (Clozaril) **from cigarette smoking. In children receiving anticonvulsants** (phenobarbital, phenytoin)**, hepatic enzymes may be induced before the initiation of psychoactive drug therapy. This situation may result in larger-than-expected drug doses required to achieve desired clinical effects.**

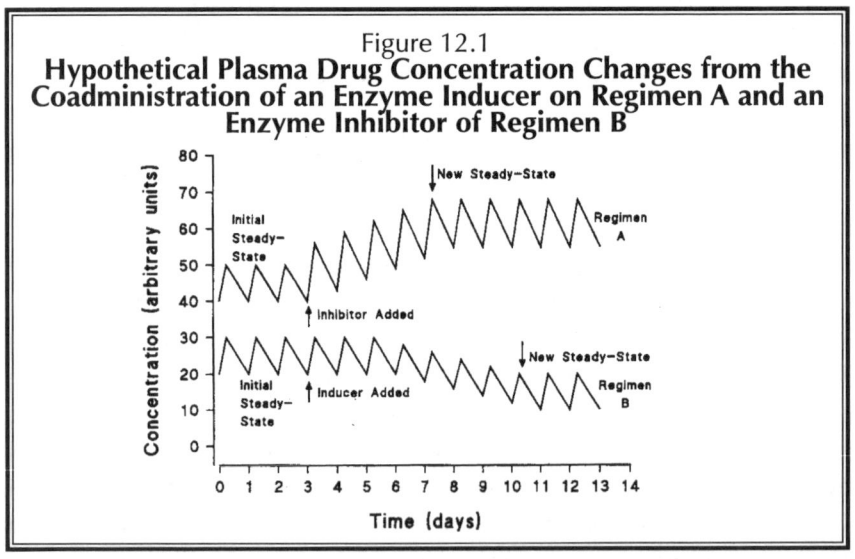

Figure 12.1
Hypothetical Plasma Drug Concentration Changes from the Coadministration of an Enzyme Inducer on Regimen A and an Enzyme Inhibitor of Regimen B

In contrast to the effects of an enzyme inducer, the effect of the addition of an enzyme inhibitor to an existing drug regimen is to cause an immediate increase in the plasma concentration of the previous therapy. This occurs as a result of an enzyme inhibitor possess-

Table 12.1
Mechanism of Drug-Drug Interactions

Pharmacokinetic
    Altered absorption
    Altered metabolic clearance of one or more drugs
        Hepatic enzyme imnduction
        Hapatic enzyme inhibition
    Protein binding displacement
    Altered renal clearance
        Increased or decreased glomerular filtrarion, renal tubular
        secretion or reabsorption

Pharmacodynamic
    Increased response: additive receptor occupancy
    Decreased response: receptor antagonism

ing potent affinity for the same enzyme that metabolizes the drug of interest. The interaction that occurs is one of competitive inhibition as both drugs are essentially competing for the same enzyme for their elimination. The degree of inhibition will depend upon the affinity of both the inhibitor and the inhibitee for the metabolizing enzyme, the concentration of the two drugs at the enzyme sites in the liver, and the doses and times of drug administration. In Figure 12.1, the addition of an enzyme inhibitor causes an immediate increase in the concentration of the drug in Regimen A. A higher steady-state concentration in the body is eventually achieved consistent with a decrease in drug clearance. **As an example of this effect, an asthmatic patient** (many of whom are children) **receiving theophylline is at a risk for theophylline toxicity if fluvoxamine** (Luvox) **therapy is begun without first decreasing the dose of the bronchodilator.** The basis of this interaction, as explained below, is an interference with the hepatic cytochrome enzyme that metabolizes theophylline.

The Cytochrome P450 System

Hepatic drug metabolism is important because it is the mechanism by which the action of most drugs is terminated. **The cytochrome P450 enzymes are involved in the oxidative metabolism of a large number of drugs.**[3,4] **They play additional roles in the metabolism of some endogenous substrates, including prostaglandins and steroids.** At least 30 related enzymes are divided into different families according to their amino acid homology. The majority of psychoactive drugs are metabolized by one or more of these isozymes. It is clear that knowledge of the substrates and inhibitors of the major cytochrome P450 enzymes allows prediction of clinically significant drug interactions. **Table 12.2 lists some commonly used drugs that are substrates for the cytochrome P450 enzymes important in psychiatry; a substrate is a drug or another molecule that combines with an enzyme and results in a chemical reaction forming a new molecule.** Many of the newer antidepressants are inhibitors of one or more different isozymes[5,6] They are shown in Table 12.2 according to their ability to interfere with the metabolism of substrates for each specific cytochrome enzyme. **For example, adding an SSRI to the therapy of a patient taking desipramine** (Norpramin) **will likely increase the tricyclic concentration by an interference with the hydroxylation pathway of this drug's elimination.**[7] Most drugs have reasonable therapeutic indices so that minor alterations in clearance, steady-state plasma concentration, or half-life—all of which may be statistically significant—may be clinically unimportant.

Cytochrome P450 1A2:

CYP1A2 is the major enzyme responsible for metabolizing theophylline, caffeine, and phenacetin. The tertiary amine tricyclic antidepressants undergo demethylation to their secondary amine active metabolites by this enzyme. Clozapine is partially metabolized by CYP1A2.[8] **Fluvoxamine and** ciprofloxacin (Cipro) **are potent inhibitors of CYP1A2, and interactions have been described with theophylline and clozapine.**[9-11] **CYP1A2 is induced by cigarette smoke, charcoal-broiled foods, and some cruciferous vegetables.**[12]

Cytochrome P450 2C9/19:

The cytochrome P450 2C subfamily consists of several closely related enzymes. Major substrates of CYP2C9 and CYP2C19 include diazepam (Valium), clomipramine (Anafranil), amitriptyline (Elavil), and imipramine (Tofranil) (Table 12.2). A genetic polymorphism exists with CYP2C19, with approximately 18% of Japanese and African Americans reported as poor metabolizers of CYP2C19 substrates.[13] Only about 3%–5% of Caucasians inherit this deficiency. Affected persons are easily identifiable by phenotyping with a laboratory test not yet widely available. Poor metabolizers have higher-than-normal plasma concentrations of the CYP2C[19] substrates from usual doses. Some SSRIs (fluvoxamine and fluoxetine [Prozac]) have been implicated in interactions likely involving the inhibition of 2C enzymes.[5,14,15]

Table 12.2
Substrates and Inhibitors of Some Cytochorome P450 Isozymes Important in Pediatric Psychopharmacology

	CYP1A2	CYP2C9/19	CYP2D6	CYP3A4
Substrates	acetominophen	barbituates	chlorpheniramine	alprazolam
	clozapine	diazepam	codeine	diazepam
	haloperidol	mepheynytoin	dextromethorphan	carbamazepine
	phenacetin	propranolol	haloperidol	cisapride
	phenothiazines	tertiary-aimine TCAs[2]	hydrocodone	cyclosporine
	theophylline	buprofen	propranolol	macrolide antibiotics
	tertiary-amine [2]	naproxen	risperidone	erfenadine[3]
	olanzapine	omeprazole	paroxetine	astemizole[3]
		phenytoin	fluoxetine	nefazodone
			secondary-amine TCAs[2]	
Inhibitors				
Potent	fluvoxamine		paroxetine	fluvoxamine
	ciprofloxacin		fluoxetine	nefazodone
				fluoxetine
Moderate		fluoxatine	desiparamine	
		fluvoxamine		
Mild		sertraline	sertraline	sertraline

[1] Many drugs have more than one enzymatic pathway involved in elimination.

[2] Tertiary-amine TCA (imitrptyline, cloramine) undergo demethylation as a primary metabolic step; secondary-amine TCAs (desipramine, nortriptyline) undergo hydroxylation as a primary metabolic step.

[3] Terfenadine and astemizole are contraindicates with CYP3A inhibitors; loratadine and carboxyterfenadine are not.

Cytochrome P450 2D6:

This is the most extensively studied of all cytochrome P450 enzymes. A well-characterized genetic polymorphism exists with 7%–10% of Caucasians inheriting an autosomal recessively transmitted defective allele.[16] Affected persons lack a sufficiently functional enzyme to metabolize normally the CYP2D6 substrates listed in Table 12.2. They will have higher plasma drug concentrations and prolonged elimination half-lives of these drugs. The significance of this metabolic defect is that an exaggerated pharmacologic response is possible following standard doses of drugs which are CYP2D6 substrates.

Several antidepressants are inhibitors of CYP2D6.[5,7] These include fluoxetine, paroxetine, and sertraline, but the potency of inhibition varies widely among these drugs. The degree of inhibition and the clinical consequences will depend upon the substrate inhibited, the dose of both substrate and inhibitor, and other patient factors such as severity of illness. Enzyme induction of CYP2D6 is not a laboratory-reproducible phenomena. Cigarette smoking and chronic administration of barbiturates will reduce the plasma concentration of several CYP2D6 substrates, but this effect probably involves other enzyme pathways or changes in hepatic blood flow.

Cytochrome P450 3A4:

This enzyme metabolizes the largest number of drugs.[17] It is present in the largest amount of all the cytochrome enzymes in the liver and also exerts a substantial effect on the bioavailability of many drugs through its presence in gut mucosa.[18,19] A broad range of compounds—including alprazolam (Xanax), diazepam, the nonsedating antihistamines, calcium channel blockers, and cyclosporine—are metabolized by CYP3A4.[17] There is no convincing evidence of a genetic polymorphism. Everyone possesses the CYP3A4 hepatic enzyme, although the intersubject variability in expressed activity is great. A study of the metabolism of carbamazepine suggested that CYP3A4 activity may peak in children and show a gradual decline to adult levels of activity.[20] This would partly explain why older children and adolescents require larger doses of some drugs than adults. Enzyme induction of CYP3A4 can occur with administration of steroids and rifampin. Inhibition of CYP3A4 substrates occurs potently with administration of nefazodone (Serzone), fluvoxamine, and, to a lessor degree, with fluoxetine.[21,22]

The most potent inhibitors of CYP3A4 are the azole antifungal drugs (e.g., ketoconazole [Nizoral]) and the macrolide antibiotics. A recent report of a sudden death of a child receiving pimozide (Orap) who was treated with clarithromycin (Biaxin) is a case of suspected CYP3A4 inhibition by this antibiotic.[23]

Interactions of Specific Drug Classes

Antidepressants:

Use of tricyclic antidepressants (TCAs) has been declining because of the introduction of the SSRIs and other, newer antidepressants. These newer drugs are far safer in overdosage situations as compared with the TCAs and have a broader spectrum of activity, especially for anxiety disorders.[24] The most convincing evidence for their efficacy in adolescents exists for the treatment of depression and obsessive-compulsive disorder (OCD).[25] **Clomipramine, which is labeled for treatment of OCD, may be combined in occasional recalcitrant cases of OCD with an SSRI. The choice of specific SSRI and dose may result in increased clomipramine plasma concentration.**[5] **In our clinical experience, seizures have been observed at the higher range of approved doses of clomipramine and with the combination of clomipramine and fluoxetine.**

The TCAs have significant anticholinergic effects. **When given in conjunction with traditional low-potency antipsychotics, benztropine (Cogentin), antihistamines, or meperidine (Demerol), the TCAs can produce significant additive atropine-like effects. The general symptoms of anticholinergic toxicity include disorientation; memory impairment; tachycardia; mydriasis** (pupil dilation); **elevated body temperature; hot, dry skin; decreased gastrointestinal motility; and urinary retention. Seizures and arrhythmias may occur in severe cases.**

The use of traditional TCAs within 2 weeks of receiving a monoamine oxidase inhibitor is a risk for precipitating an overstimulation of catecholamines. In severe cases, cardiovascular toxicity is possible. Reports of enhanced clinical effects from drug combinations of TCAs and either phenelzine (Nardil) or methylphenidate also have been published.[26,27] The availability of newer antidepressants makes such combinations unlikely, unless by accident.

The introduction of the SSRIs has emphasized the critical importance for considering these medications' potential to cause drug interactions.[5,6] **The SSRI antidepressants have been shown in vitro and in vivo to be potent inhibitors of some cytochrome P450 enzymes.** The most thoroughly studied reaction is the competitive inhibition of CYP2D6. The combined data from pharma-cokinetic studies in healthy adults, case reports, and in vitro data provide a rank ordering of the cytochrome inhibitory potential of the newer antidepressants. This is shown is Table 12.2.

Depending upon the specific drug and dose, the SSRIs can elevate plasma concentrations of the tricyclics, cardiovascular medications, and other drugs. In the younger population, the most probable combinations appear to be an SSRI and a traditional antipsychotic or a nonsedating antihistamine (e.g., terfenadine [Seldane], astemizole [Hismanal]); **these latter combinations have been contraindicated because of the possibility of precipitating cardiac arrhythmias. Recent studies of terfenadine combined with paroxetine, sertraline (Zoloft) and venlafaxine (Effexor) showed minimal inhibitory effects. Inhibition of terfenadine metabolism by ketoconazole, itraconazole (Sporanox), erythromycin (E-Mycin), or clarithromycin poses a risk of cardiotoxicity.**[28] The noncardioactive metabolite of terfenadine, fexofenadine (Allegra), was recently marketed as a nonsedating antihistamine; either this agent or loratadine (Claritin) are strongly preferred if an antidepressant must be prescribed together with an antihistamine. Cetirizine (Zyrtec) is a recently marketed H1-antihistamine available for treatment of allergic disorders. It is not metabolized by the cytochrome P450 system and is mostly excreted renally as an unchanged drug. It should be relatively free of metabolic drug interactions.

Antipsychotics:

The newer atypical antipsychotic medications (clozapine, risperidone [Risperdal], olanzapine [Zyprexa]) have a significant advantage over the traditional drugs because they tend not to cause extrapyramidal side effects. The cytochrome P450 system has been shown to be important in the metabolism of these drugs and provides a basis for predicting drug interactions.[29–31] **Clozapine is metabolized partly by CYP1A2, and this provides a basis for the observations that cigarette smoking decreases its plasma concentration while the CYP1A2 inhibitors, fluvoxamine and ciprofloxacin, increase its concentration.**[10,11] The role of CYP2D6 is less well understood in the metabolism of clozapine. Evidence exists for inhibition of clozapine by SSRIs

Table 12.3
Drug Interactions Involving Newer Antipsychotics

Agent	Interaction Drug/ Condition	Effects	Possible Mechanism	Suggested Action
Clozapine	Benzodizepines (lorazepam, clonzepam, diazepam)	Delirium, sedation ataxia, rare respiratory arrest	Unknown pharmacodynamic interaction	Avoid when possible
Risperidone	CYP2D6 inhibitors	Altered concentrartion of parent drug and its metabolite	Adverse Effects not described	Cautious use
Olanzapine	CYP1A2 inhibitors (fluvoxamine)	Increased concentration of olanzapine	Theoretical—not yet described	Adjust antipsychotic dosage downward
Pimozide	Clarithromycin	Increased pimozide effects; one case of sudden death suspected	Inhibition of CYP3A4	Avoid known CYP3A4 inhibitors in combination; possible

inhibiting CYP2D6, but a study comparing its concentrations in plasma in slow versus rapid metabolizers of the CYP2D6 substrate debrisoquine found no between-group differences.[32] A summary of clinically important potential interactions is given in Table 12.3.[29–31]

Risperidone is a CYP2D6 substrate, and as such, concurrent therapy with inhibitors of this enzyme would be expected to increase its plasma concentration (Table 12.4). **However, as risperidone is metabolized to an active metabolite, 9-hydroxyrisperidone, the overall effect on patient outcome may be marginal.** Risperidone is a promising agent for the treatment of children and adolescents suffering from schizophrenia, and favorable results have been reported in the treatment of schizophrenia and autistic disorder.[33–35]

Olanzapine is partially metabolized by CYP1A2, and interactions can be predicted to occur with fluvoxamine (enzyme inhibition) **and cigarette smoking** (enzyme induction). Studies of the efficacy of olanzapine have not yet been reported in children and adolescents, but its atypical profile make it a promising agent for this age group.

Miscellaneous Pharmacotherapy:

Clonidine (Catapres), **an α2-adrenergic receptor agonist labeled for the treatment of high blood pressure, reduces peripheral sympathetic activity. It has received considerable use for treatment of tics, Tourette's syndrome, and attention-deficit / hyperactivity disorder.**[36,37] **Three unpublished cases of the combination of clonidine and methylphenidate recently were associated with unexplained sudden death in children 7–9 years old.**[38] Although the circumstances in these three deaths cannot be unequivocally related to the combination of clonidine and methylphenidate, cardiovascular monitoring should be emphasized for future use. Previous cases of abnormal electrocardiogram findings in patients including children taking low doses of clonidine have been described.[39] **General guidelines would suggest blood pressure and pulse monitoring of all children receiving clonidine. A history of a pre-existing cardiac condition is an indication to have an electrocardiogram before and during treatment. Children and adolescents with pre-existing cardiac disease should not be given clonidine for behavioral reasons. Abrupt discontinuation of clonidine should be avoided to minimize any tendency for rebound increases in blood pressure.**

Guanfacine (Tenex) **has received recent interest in the treatment of Tourette's disorder and also for attention-deficit / hyperactivity disorder.**[40,41] It is an α2-adrenoceptor agonist with pharmacologic properties similar to clonidine. Like other centrally acting antihypertensive agents, guanfacine may cause sedation or drowsiness, especially when drug therapy is initiated. A purported advantage in children and adolescents is a decreased propensity to cause sedation, as compared with that of clonidine. **Pharmacodynamic interactions can be predicted, such as additive sedation if guanfacine is combined with benzodiazepines, TCAs, or antipsychotics.**

Fenfluramine (Pondimin) is a serotonergic drug that has been used in the treatment of autism, a disorder associated with elevated blood concentration of serotonin. Its active stereoisomer, dexfenfluramine (Redux), was recently approved for the long-term treatment of obesity. A risk of inducing a serotonin syndrome exists if either of these drugs is combined with any of several other serotonergic drugs.[42] **These would include the monoamine oxidase inhibitors, the SSRIs** (fluoxetine, sertraline, paroxetine [Paxil], fluvoxamine, and citalopram); **some newer antidepressants** (venlafaxine and nefazodone), **trazodone (Desyrel), buspirone (BuSpar), and lithium salts. Although dexfenfluramine has been prescribed in Europe for over 10 years without reported cases of the serotonin syndrome, symptoms suggestive of an emerging syndrome should result in prompt discontinuation of the drug. These would include mental status and behavioral changes** (i.e., disorientation, confusion, restlessness, agitation), **motor system changes** (i.e., myoclonus, tremor, rigidity, hyperreflexia, incoordination), **and autonomic nervous system instability** (i.e., fever, diaphoresis, shivering, tachycardia, tachypnea, mydriasis, diarrhea).

Evidence in the form of case reports exists that fenfluramine may be a hepatic enzyme inhibitor that can cause an elevation of TCA plasma concentration; however, the results from formal studies are not available. Thus, caution should be exercised when adding this appetite suppressant to any pre-existing drug therapy.

Psychostimulants:

Psychostimulants are the most frequently prescribed class of psychoactive drugs in children and adolescents. Their interactions are summarized in Table 12.4. The most widely prescribed,

Table 12.4
Drug Interactions Involving Psychostimulants

Agent	Interaction Drug/ Condition	Effects	Possible Mechanism	Suggested Action
Methylphenidate	Meals	No effect	Absorption unaffected	Keep administration constant for most consistent effects; less appetite suppresion after meals
	Imipramine	Increased TCA	Inhibition of CYP2D6	Avoid; lower imipramine dosage monitor imipramine Cp
	MAOI, pseudoephedrine phenlypropranolamine, sympathomimetic amines	Possible ↑ blood pressure	Combined sympathomimetic effect	MAOI and psychostimulants are avoid other sympahtomimetics as potentially dangerous
	Phenytoin	Phenytoin toxicity	Impaired anticonvulsant metabolism	Monitor phenytoin Cp closely; toxicity reported in isolated cases; little systematic study of PS and anticonvulsants
	Coumarin anticoagulants	Increased effect	Impaired metabolism	Decrease anticoagulant dosage monitor anticoagulation indices closely
Dextroamphetamine, amphetamine salts	MAOI, symphatomimetic amines	Possible ↑ blood pressure	Combined effects	Avoid as potentially dangerous
Pemoline	MAOI, sympathomimetic amines	Possible ↑ blood pressure	Combined effects	Avoid as potentially dangerous

Cp = plasma concentration; PS = psychostiumulants.

methylphenidate (Ritalin), is approved by the Food and Drug Administration for treatment of attention-deficit / hyperactivity disorder, but it also has been used in autism and mental retardation. It is a mild central nervous system stimulant. **In this regard, it may lower the seizure threshold in patients with a prior history of seizures; therefore, its use in children with a known seizure history is unadvisable. Furthermore, the safe use of methylphenidate with anticonvulsants has not been clearly established.** Reports are available of its combination with phenytoin, resulting in anticonvulsant toxicity and also of having no effect upon plasma concentration of phenytoin, phenobarbital, or primidone (Mysoline).[43,44] **If methylphenidate is to be combined with an anticonvulsant, then the anticonvulsant plasma concentrations should be monitored closely. The more crucial times for interactions to occur are after initiating therapy with a psychostimulant and after dosage changes.**

Methylphenidate has long been known to increase the plasma concentration of tricyclic antidepressants, thereby supporting its status as a mild hepatic enzyme inhibitor; however, the specific enzymes involved have not been identified.[45] In this regard, it can inhibit the metabolism of a variety of drugs, including anticoagulants, anticonvulsants, and tricyclics. The dosages of these drugs may need to be titrated downward if methylphenidate is added to therapy.

Special Considerations in Children and Adolescents

Children and adolescents are increasingly being treated with potent psychoactive drugs.[25,33,46] These drugs are often used in combination to enhance response, to decrease side effects, to treat psychiatric comorbidity or concomitant medical illness.[1] The science of pediatric psychopharmacology is progressing rapidly, and clinical drug trials are in progress for a number of different indications. However, drug use in the pediatric population for treatment of mental disorders and behavioral disturbances is accompanied by several problems. **Most of the drugs used in pediatric psychopharmacology were first tested and proven useful in adults. Although this gives us a database from which to extrapolate experience, drug effects in the younger population may not conform to expectations. For example, the efficacy of tricyclic antidepressants in the treatment of adult mood disorders has been**

293

difficult to establish in adolescents.[47] A frequent problem is the need to treat a medically ill child or adolescent for an emotional or behavioral problem. These include asthma, epilepsy, and a host of infections. Children who have cancer or who have been infected by the human immunodeficiency virus (commonly known as HIV) are especially neglected from the perspective of psychoactive drug treatment studies.

The psychiatric conditions in children and adolescents for which pharmacotherapy may be indicated are listed in Table 12.5. Almost all classes of psychoactive drugs have been used in treating this population. The extent of use is marginal for some disorders, and sparse documentation pertaining to drug efficacy exists for some conditions. Nevertheless, the successful practice of pediatric psychopharmacology demands a broad appreciation for the potentially important drug interactions that may occur across the spectrum of psychoactive drug use. This is a near-impossible task, so reliance upon general principles must be emphasized to bring an orderliness to recognition and management of drug interactions.

Differences in the quantity and activity of the hepatic drug-metabolizing enzymes have not been very well characterized in children and adolescents according to age or to the influence of various factors, such as gestational age or other developmental parameters.[48] (Our understanding of various P450 enzymes comes mostly from animal data and studies in adults.[49]) Functional P450 activity traditionally is viewed as being limited in newborn infants, rapidly increasing in the first year of life. Children and adolescents are frequently dosed with higher mg/kg dosages of various drugs than adults and demonstrate shorter elimination half-lives. Part of the explanation for this apparent enhanced metabolic ability is a greater liver mass-to-body weight ratio in younger patients as compared with adults. However, it is likely that the ability to metabolize drugs by various P450 pathways matures at different rates. For example, theophylline metabolism in children generally exceeds adult capacity.[50] Although age significantly contributes to variability in drug metabolism, considerable intersubject variability exists across all age groups with respect to the capacity to eliminate drugs. This source of variability will directly contribute to the prevalence and degree of drug interactions that occur in the younger population and to the clinical significance of interactions.

Table 12.5
Psychiatric Disorder in Children and Adolescents For Which Pharmacotherapy Has Been Used[1]

DSM-IV Classification	Medications
Mental Retardation	conventional antipsychotics, lithium, naltrexone
Pervasive development disorders: Autistic disorder	buspirone, conventional antipsychotics, methylphenidate, novel antipsychotics, selective serotonin-reuptake inhibitors, fenfluramine, clomipramine
Attention deficit and disruptive behavior disorders	amphetamine, bupropion, clonidine, pemoline, tricyclic antidepressants
Tic disorders: Tourette's disorder	pimozide; clonidine
Elimination disorders: Enuresis	imipramine
Other disorders of infancy, childhood or adolescence: Separation anxiety	alprazolam, buspirone, tricyclic antidepressants
Schizophrenia	conventional antipsychotics, novel antipsychotics
Mood disorders: Major depressive disorder	bupropion, nefazodone, selective serotonin-reuptake inhibitors, tricyclic antidepressants, venlafaxine
Bipolar disorder	carbamazepine, divalproex sodium, lithium

Anxiety disorders:
  Obsessive-compulsive disorder
  Posttraumatic stress disorder
  (acute)
	selective serotonin-reuptake inhibitors, clomipramine
	benzodizepines
	Eating disorders:

Eating disorders:
  Anorexia nervosa
  Bulimia nervosa
	cyproheptadine
	selective serotonin-reuptake inhibitors

Primary sleep disorders	benzodiazepines, imipramine

[1] Efficacy has not been established for many indications and literature documenttaion may be sparse.

Clinical Implications

Some general recommendations can be given to minimize drug interactions. **Polypharmacy should occur only when there is a definite indication. Drugs with a narrow therapeutic index** (e.g., anticonvulsants) **can withstand less alterations in their disposition before producing adverse effects. With predictable clinical interactions, a dose reduction of one or both drugs may be required or may be useful to avoid adverse effects.**

Knowledge of the effects of various drugs on the cytochrome P450 system can help to predict and avoid drug interactions. **Patients who are at higher risk for the consequences of drug interactions would be those on multiple medications and those suffering from concurrent illnesses. When previous therapy includes drugs for which a therapeutic plasma concentration range exits, then monitoring concentration when starting new therapy can help to minimize potentially elevated concentrations associated with toxicity.**

Initiating new therapy slowly with gradual titration of doses helps to identify those patients who may be unable to tolerate standard drug doses. A few patients will be at increased risk for impaired drug metabolism because of their status as poor metabolizers of substrates for CYP2C19 or 2D6. These patients are unidentifiable without specific testing for genetic polymorphism in these enzymes.

The clinician will inevitably be faced with the need to combine drugs without knowledge of whether a drug interaction will occur. Careful clinical monitoring may be the best assurance of avoiding adverse effects and their consequences in this situation. Pulse and blood pressure should be determined at the outset of therapy and with any dosage increases. **Cardiovascular effects may be enhanced through interactions with TCAs, antipsychotics, clonidine, and the psychostimulants. The presence of any abnormal movements may signal enhanced effects from antipsychotics, SSRIs, or psychostimulants. An unexpected change in behavior of any kind should alert the clinician to the possibility of a drug interaction as a precipitating cause.** Increased sedation, confusion, agitation, nervousness, or anxiety may suggest behavioral toxicity as a result of a pharmacokinetic or pharmacodynamic interaction.

References

1. Wilens TE, Spencer T, Biederman J, Wozniak J, Connor D. Combined pharmacotherapy: an emerging trend in pediatric psychopharmacology. *J Am Acad Child Adolesc Psychiatry.* 1995;34:110–112.

2. Aarons L. Kinetics of drug–drug interactions. *Pharmacol Ther.* 1981;14:321–344.

3. Guengerich FP. Human cytochrome P450 enzymes. *Life Sci.* 1992;50:1471–1478.

4. Wrighton SA, Stevens JC. The human hepatic cytochromes P450 involved in drug metabolism. *Crit Rev Toxicol.* 1992;22:1–21.

5. Nemeroff CB, DeVane CL, Pollock BG: Newer antidepressants and the cytochrome P450 system. *Am J Psychiatry.* 1996;153:311–320.

6. Brosen K. Are pharmacokinetic drug interactions with the SSRIs an issue? *Int Clin Psychopharmacol.* 1996;(suppl 1):23–27.

7. von Moltke LL, Greenblatt DJ, Court MH, et al. Inhibition of alprazolam and desipramine hydroxylation in vitro by paroxetine and fluvoxamine: comparison with other selective serotonin reuptake inhibitor antidepressants. *J Clin Psychopharmacol.* 1995;15:125-131

8. Jerling M, Lindstrom L, Bondesson U, Bertilsson L. Fluvoxamine inhibition and carbamazepine induction of the metabolism of clozapine: evidence from a therapeutic drug monitoring service. *Ther Drug Monitor.* 1994;16:368–374.

9. Brøsen K, Skjelbo E, Rasmussen BB, Poulsen HE, Loft S. Fluvoxamine is a potent inhibitor of cytochrome P450IA2. *Biochem Pharmacol.* 1993;45:1211–1214.

10. Markowitz JS, Gill HS, Labia M, Brewerton TD, and DeVane CL. Fluvoxamine-clozapine dose dependent interaction. *Can J Psychiatry.* 1996;41:670–671.

11. Markowitz JS, Gill HS, DeVane CL, Mintzer JE. Fluoroquinolone-mediated inhibition of clozapine metabolism. *Am J Psychiatry.* 1997;in press.

12. Pollock BG. Recent development in drug metabolism of relevance to psychiatrists. *Harvard Rev Psychiatry.* 1994;2:204–213.

13. Wilkinson GR, Guengerich FP, Branch RA. Genetic polymorphism of S-mephenytoin hydroxylation. Pharmacol Ther. 1989;43:53–76.

14. Shader RI, Greenblatt DJ, von Moltke LL. Fluoxetine inhibition of phenytoin metabolism. *J Clin Psychopharmacol.* 1994;14:375–376.

15. Perucca E, Gatti G, Cipolla G, et al. Inhibition of diazepam metabolism by fluvoxamine: a pharmacokinetic study in normal volunteers. *Clin Pharmacol Ther.* 1994; 56:471–476.

16. Eichelbaum M, Gross AS. The genetic polymorphism of debrisoquine/sparteine metabolism: clinical aspects. *Pharmacol Ther.* 1990;46:377–394.

17. Ketter TA, Flockhart DA, Post RM, et al. The emerging role of cytochrome P450 IIIA in psychopharmacology. *J Clin Psychopharmacol.* 1995;15:387–398.

18. Shimada T, Yamazaki H, Mimura M, et al. Interindividual variations in human liver cytochrome P450 enzymes involved in the oxidation of drugs, carcinogens, and toxic chemicals: studies with liver microsomes of 30 Japanese and 30 Caucasians. *J Pharmacol Exp Ther.* 1994;270:414–423.

19. Paine MF, Shen DD, Kunze KL, et al. First-pass metabolism of midazolam by the human intestine. *Clin Pharmacol Ther.* 1996;60:14–24.

20. Korinthenberg R, Haug C, Hannak D. The metabolization of carbamazepine to CBZ-10,11-epoxide in children from the newborn age to adolescence. *Neuropediatrics.* 1994;25:214–216.

21. Barbhaiya RH, Shukla UA, Kroboth PD, Greene DS. Coadministration of nefazodone and benzodiazepines, II: a pharmacokinetic interaction study with triazolam. *J Clin Psychopharmacol.* 1995;15:320–326.

22. DeVane CL, Gill HS, Markowitz JS, Carson WH. Pharmacokinetic interaction between sertraline and amiodarone. *Ther Drug Monitor.* 1997;in press.

23. Flockhart DA, Richard E, Woosley RL, Pearle PL Drici M-D. A metabolic interaction between clarithromycin and pimozide may result in cardiac toxicity [abstract]. *Clin Pharmacol Ther.* 1996;59:189.

24. DeVane CL. The place of selective serotonin reuptake inhibitors in the treatment of panic disorder. *Pharmacotherapy.* 1997;in press.

25. DeVane CL, Sallee FR. Serotonin selective reuptake inhibitors in child and adolescent psychopharmacology: a review of published experience. *J Clin Psychiatry.* 1996; 57:55–66.

26. Feighner JP, Herbstein J, Damlouji N. Combined MAO, TCA, and direct stimulant therapy of treatment-resistant depression. *J Clin Psychiatry.* 1985;46:206–209.

27. Gwirtsman HE, Szuba MP, Toren L, Feist M. The antidepressant response to tricyclics in major depressives is accelerated with adjunctive use of methylphenidate. *Psychopharmacol Bull.* 1994;30:157–165.

28. Kivistö KT, Neuvonen PJ, Klotz U. Inhibition of terfenadine metabolism: pharmacokinetic and pharmacodynamic consequences. *Clin Pharmacokinet.* 1994;27:1–5.

29. Byerly MJ, DeVane CL. Pharmacokinetics of clozapine and risperidone: a review of recent literature. *J Clin Psychopharmacol.* 1996;16:177–187.

30. Ereshefsky L. Pharmacokinetics and drug interactions: update for new antipsychotics. *J Clin Psychiatry.* 1996;57(suppl 11):12–25.

31. Edge SC, Markowitz JS, DeVane CL. Clozapine drug–drug interactions: a review of the literature. *Hum Psychopharmacol.* 1997;12:5–20.

32. Dahl M-L, Llerena A, Bondesson U, Lindstrom L, Bertilsson L. Disposition of clozapine in man: lack of association with debrisoquine and S-mephenytoin hydroxylation polymorphisms. *Br J Clin Pharmacol.* 1994;37:71–74.

33. Findling RL, Grcevich S J, Lopez I, Schulz SC. Antipsychotic medications in children and adolescents. *J Clin Psychiatry.* 1996;57(suppl 9):19–23.

34. Quintana H, Keshavan M. Case study: risperidone in children and adolescents with schizophrenia. *J Am Acad Child Adolesc Psychiatry.* 1995;34:1292–1296.

35. Peterson BS, McDougle CJ, Leckman JF. Risperidone treatment of children and adolescents with chronic tic disorders: a preliminary report. *J Am Acad Child Adolesc Psychiatry.* 1995;34:1147–1152.

36. Schvehla TJ, Mandoki MW, Sumner GS. Clonidine therapy for comorbid attention-deficit / hyperactivity disorder and conduct disorder. *Soc Med J.* 1994;87:692–695.

37. Hunt RD, Minderaa RB, Cohen DJ. Clonidine benefits children with attention deficit disorder: report of a double-blind, placebo-crossover therapeutic trial. *J Am Acad Child Adolesc Psychiatry.* 1985;24:617–629.

38. Maloney MJ, Schwam JS. Clonidine and sudden death. *Pediatrics.* 1995;96:1176–1177.

39. Chandran KSK. ECG and clonidine. *J Am Acad Child Adolesc Psychiatry.* 1994; 33:1351.

40. Hunt RD, Arnsten AFT, Asbell MD. An open trial of guanfacine in the treatment of attention-deficit / hyperactivity disorder. *J Am Acad Child Adolesc Psychiatry.* 1995; 34:50–54.

41. Chappell PB, Riddle MA, Scahill L, et al. Guanfacine treatment of comorbid attention-deficit / hyperactivity disorder and Tourette's syndrome: preliminary clinical experience. *J Am Acad Child Adolesc Psychiatry.* 1995;34:1140–1146.

42. Schenck CH, Mahowald MW. Potential hazard of serotonin syndrome associated with dexfenfluramine hydrochloride (Redux). *JAMA* 1996;276:1220–1221.

43. Kupferberg HJ, Jeffery W, Hunninghake DB. Effect of methylphenidate on plasma anticonvulsant levels. *Clin Pharmacol Ther.* 1972;13:201–204.

44. Mirkin BL. Drug interactions: effect of methylphenidate on the disposition of diphenylhydantoin in man. *Neurology.* 1971;21:1123–1128.

45. Perel JM. Inhibition of imipramine metabolism by methylphenidate. *Fed Proc.* 1969; 28:418.

46. Alessi N, Naylor MW, Ghaziuddin M, Zubieta JK. Update on lithium carbonate therapy in children and adolescents. *J Am Acad Child Adolesc Psychiatry.* 1994;33:291–304.

47. Ryan ND. Heterocyclic antidepressants in children and adolescents. *J Child Adolesc Psychopharmacol.* 1990;1:21–31.

48. Leeder JS. Developmental aspects of drug metabolism in children. *Drug Info J.* 1996;30:1135–1143.

49. Hakkola J, Pasanen M, Purkunen R, et al. Expression of xenobiotic-metabolizing cytochrome P450 forms in human adult and fetal liver. *Biochem Pharmacol.* 1994; 48:59–64.

50. Kraus DM, Fischer JH, Reitz SJ, et al. Alterations in theophylline metabolism during the first year of life. *Clin Pharmacol Ther.* 1993;54:351–359

13 Pharmacotherapy of Dysthymia

Michael E. Thase, MD, Robert H. Howland, MD,
and Edward S. Friedman, MD

*Dr. Thase is Professor of Psychiatry, Dr. Howland is Assistant
Professor of Psychiatry.*

*Dr. Friedman is Assistant Professor of Psychiatry, at the University
of Pittsburgh School of Medicine, Pittsburgh, PA.*

Editor's Note

I am very glad that the old concept of neurotic depression has been
replaced with that of dysthymia, because this new term more appropriately conveys the biopsychosocial nature of this disorder. Somehow,
the term neurotic implied that the condition could best be understood
in the context of psychoanalytic theory. Now, in my own practice, I
approach every such patient with an open mind to the physiological,
interpersonal, and intrapsychic factors which contribute to his or her
distress and dysfunction. And I do so optimistically, because the vast
majority of such patients whom I see do very well in treatment.

It is also reassuring to have a presentation, such as Dr. Thase's, which
systematically reviews the evidence for the effectiveness of various psychopharmacologic agents in dysthymia. He notes that the condition
usually begins in childhood or adolescence, punctuated by periods of
exacerbation that reach the syndromal threshold for a major depressive
disorder, often referred to as "double depression." Nearly half of these
patients have comorbidity with such conditions as social phobia, generalized anxiety disorder, substance abuse and dependence, and
bulimia. Chronic depression is also associated with personality disorders, including avoidant, dependent, and obsessive-compulsive ones.
Symptomatically they may experience classical melancholic symptoms,

such as early morning awakening or diurnal mood variation, or atypical symptoms such as hypersomnia and increased appetite and weight gain. Their work lives and interpersonal relationships are most commonly affected.

In this chapter, the author reviews research into various antidepressants, concluding that because of their relatively benign side-effect profile and ease of administration the SSRIs are the best place to start in dysthymic patients who have never before taken an antidepressant. He offers a number of valuable clues to effective management, such as the observation that patients who experience a partial response to initial treatment are most likely to benefit from an increase in dosage, whereas as absolute nonresponders often warrant a switch to a different antidepressant either in the same or in a different category. He provides valuable guidelines including to be sure to prescribe full dosage; to aim for complete remission; to identify and treat comorbid conditions; and to evaluate the need for psychotherapy and proceed accordingly. Patient education about the nature of his or her depression and about the treatments employed is a key factor in management.

Introduction

Dysthymic disorder, or dysthymia, is a common variant of nonbipolar depression. It is characterized by the combination of chronicity and milder affective and neurovegetative symptomatology when contrasted to major depressive episodes. **The DSM-IV[1] defines dysthymic disorder in adults as a persistently depressed mood presenting with at least two characteristic symptoms for 2 years or longer. During those 2 years, there can be no more than a two-month period of remission and symptoms must be present more days than not. Moreover, there can be no periods of syndromal major depression until the duration criterion has been met.**

Dysthymia is the nosological descendent of neurotic depression, but without inferences regarding unresolved psychodynamic conflicts or introjected anger.[2] Despite such diagnostic categorization, **many people with dysthymia have manifold and long-standing psychosocial problems. Resultingly, both patients and clinicians often view psychotherapy as the most rational initial treatment approach.**[3] This common perception, perhaps supported by the policy design of the

United States Food and Drug Administration not to require psychopharmacologic efficacy trials specifically focusing on dysthymia, has led to a paucity of empirical data on the utility of antidepressant pharmacotherapy for dysthymic disorder.

This chapter will focus on the clinical course of dysthymia, its phenomenology, and the results of recent randomized controlled trials (RCTs) for various psychopharmacologic agents used in its treatment. Evidence pertaining to the efficacy and tolerability of the selective serotonin reuptake inhibitors (SSRIs), as compared to placebo, tricyclic antidepressants (TCAs), and monoamine oxidase inhibitors (MAOIs), will receive the greatest emphasis.

Dysthymia

Clinical Course:

Dysthymia often begins in childhood or adolescence, and it often may smolder for years (see Figure 13.1a). **Most commonly, the course of dysthymia is punctuated by periods of symptomatic exacerbation that reach the syndromal threshold for a major depressive episode.**[4] **This presentation is often referred to as double depression** (see Figure 13.1b). According to DSM-IV, both the chronic and acute depressive diagnoses are coded simultaneously. However, *a protracted residual symptomatic state subsequent to a major depressive episode is not diagnosed as dysthymia in DSM-IV*; this presentation is classified as a major depressive episode with partial remission (see Figure 13.1c). Similarly, *the dysthymia diagnosis is not used if a more severe episode of 2 years duration or longer has persisted at the full syndromal level.* This condition is diagnosed as a chronic major depressive episode (see Figure 13.1d).

The natural histories of these chronic depressive disorders tend to vary as a function of the patient's age of onset, extent of comorbidity, medical status, and treatment utilization. **People with chronic depressions typically have greater psychiatric and general medical comorbidity, and they are high utilizers of health care services.**[4] Paradoxically, despite frequent visits to the doctor, most have never received even a single adequate trial of antidepressant medication.[5,6] Although many treatment resistant patients ultimately become chronically depressed, **a large majority of people with chronic depression are not treatment resistant.**

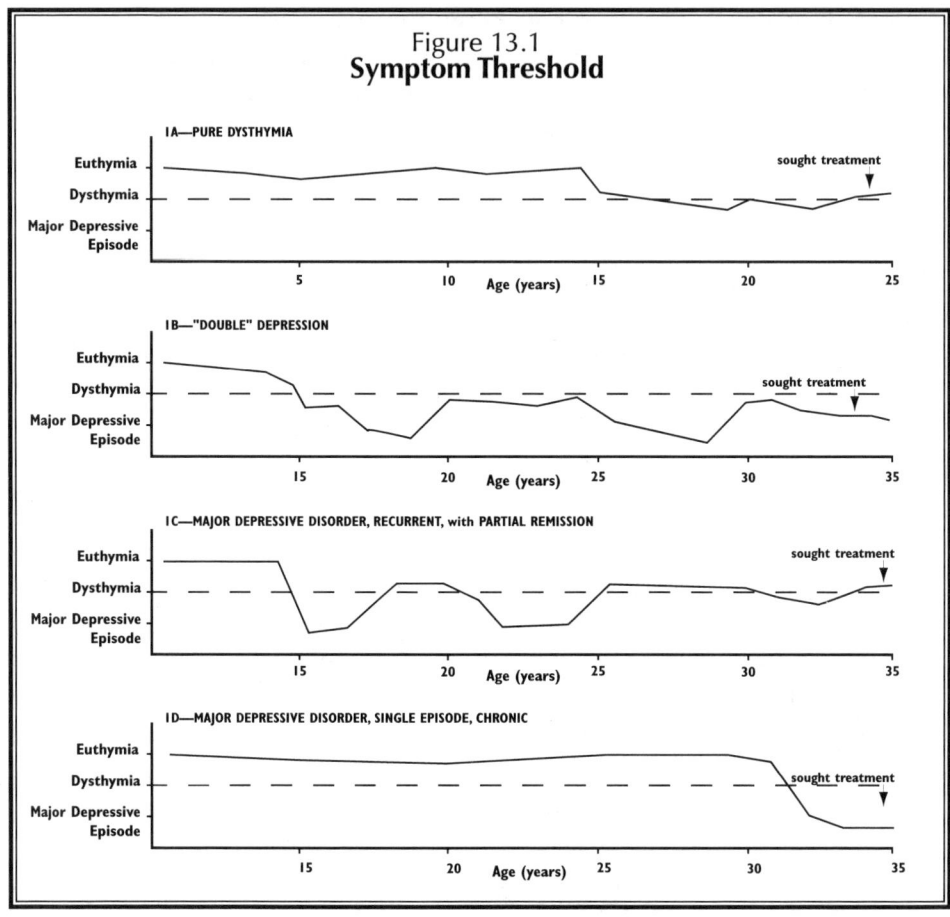

Figure 13.1
Symptom Threshold

Childhood-onset dysthymias often progress to a course of recurrent major depressive episodes or bipolar disorder.[7] Even after 5 or more years of pure dysthymia, young adults remain at high risk for subsequent development of a double depressive disorder,[4] and treatment-emergent hypomanic episodes are not uncommon.[2,4] Spontaneous remission of the underlying dysthymia is rarely observed,[8] although the superimposed episodes of double depression may wax and wane without specific treatment.[4] Whether conceptualized as dysthymia or incomplete remission of a major depressive episode, the presence of persistent residual symptoms represents an important risk factor for relapse or recurrence of major episodes without preventative treatment.[9]

Comorbidity:

At least one-half of people seeking treatment for dysthymia have one or more comorbid conditions.[4] **The more common Axis I nonaffective psychiatric disorders that coaggregate with dysthymia include: social phobia, generalized anxiety disorder, substance abuse and dependence, and bulimia.** Such high comorbidity calls attention to the limitations of our nomenclature, and illustrates the likelihood of more general vulnerability factors with pleomorphic manifestations.[10]

People who develop chronic depressions are also likely to meet criteria for one or more personality disorders.[11,12] **Again, the validity of these comorbid classifications may be questioned because long-standing dysthymic symptoms** (e.g., dysphoria, pessimism, interpersonal sensitivity, self-denigration, or irritability) **undoubtedly have deleterious effects on personality development.**[2,11] **The more common Axis II traits and diagnoses associated with dysthymia are within the Cluster C grouping, which includes avoidant, dependent, and obsessive-compulsive personality disorders.**[11] Some investigators have also reported higher rates of the more unstable, Cluster B personality disorders, including borderline, histrionic, narcissistic, and antisocial personality disorders.[12] Others view these more tempestuous, labile, and impulsive traits to be part of a subaffective or temperamental diathesis to bipolar disorder.[2]

Symptomatology:

Dysthymia, at least in pure form, is a nonmelancholic form of depression. Specifically, the DSM-IV diagnostic criteria for dysthymia essentially excludes the possibility that a patient will meet criteria for melancholia. *This, of course, is an arbitrary convention.* **Many patients with dysthymia have isolated melancholic symptoms, including early morning awakening, psychomotor retardation, pervasive anhedonia, or diurnal mood variation.**[2] **Those with an early age of onset more often present with hypersomnia, increased appetite, or weight gain.**[2] Such reversed neurovegetative symptoms, perhaps coupled with a high prevalence of comorbid anxiety, account for the high incidence of dysthymia or double depression in studies of atypical depression.[13] Cognitive symptoms such as pessimism, complaining, focusing on the negative, and low self-esteem are commonplace.

Akiskal[2] proposed that early onset dysthymia may be characterized as either subaffective or characterologic disorders based on the presence or absence of a number of correlates of affective illness. In this classification, the subaffective subtype was believed to be a subsyndromal variant, or forme fruste, of the major mood disorders, perhaps sharing a common underlying biological or genetic diathesis. By contrast, the characterologic subtype was presumed to be a neurotic personality disorder, unrelated biologically or genetically to the formal mood disorders. He suggested that hypersomnolence, a favorable or hypomanic response to antidepressants, a multigenerational family history of mood disorders, and alterations of sleep neurophysiology were more commonly found in the subaffective form of dysthymia, whereas these factors were unlikely to be found in the characterologic subtype. Although these prototypes are conceptually useful, many patients present with an admixture of both subaffective and characterological features.

Antidepressant Treatment of Dysthymia

Most psychiatrists now use the SSRIs as the treatment of first choice for virtually all depressive disorders.[14] There are several reasons for this practice: the SSRIs have a 5%–10% lower drop-out rate than the TCAs during acute phase therapy, and a substantially lower incidence of annoying anticholinergic and antihistaminic side effects.[14,15] Other advantages include the convenience of single daily dosing, a relatively limited need for dosage titration, and a low risk of cardiovascular complications following overdose. **The SSRIs also may better match for the pathophysiology of early onset, chronic, mild depressions than the more noradrenergically active TCAs. This is because "pure" dysthymia is not typically characterized by the more state-dependent and severity-linked neurobiologic correlates of depression, such as hypercortisolism, elevated peripheral catecholamine metabolites, or marked EEG sleep disturbances.[16]** Moreover, many younger patients, particularly those with weight gain or hypersomnia, have problems tolerating the more sedating TCAs.[13,14]

Data From Clinical Trials:

Early Studies

Howland[17] and Harrison and Stewart[10] have published detailed reviews of the results of open studies and earlier controlled clinical trials. They concluded that, despite the lack of well-controlled trials, it was virtually certain that the TCAs, SSRIs, and MAOIs were effective treatments for chronic depressive disorders. Comparisons across diagnostic groups suggested that chronically depressed patients may be less treatment responsive than those with more acute disorders,[17] a conclusion also reached by reviewers of predictors of antidepressant response.[19,20] This difference is probably explained by a lower likelihood of response to placebo or spontaneous remission among more chronic depressions.[21] If true, the relative drug-placebo differences in acute and chronic depressions actually may be comparable (see Figure 13.2).

One factor that confounds interpretation of the earlier studies is that

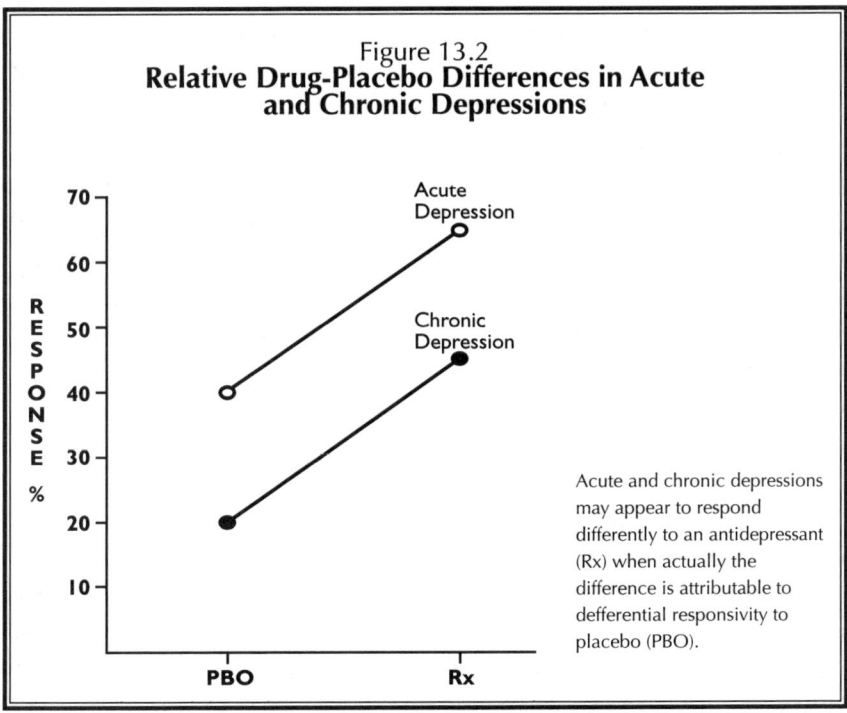

Figure 13.2
Relative Drug-Placebo Differences in Acute and Chronic Depressions

Acute and chronic depressions may appear to respond differently to an antidepressant (Rx) when actually the difference is attributable to defferential responsivity to placebo (PBO).

patients with pure dysthymia, double depression, and chronic major depressive disorder have often been grouped together.[17] This ultimately may not prove to be much of a problem (due to the arbitrary nature of such distinctions), but given the continued debate over the utility of psychologic and pharmacologic treatments, it is important to answer the more specific question: *can pure dysthymia be treated effectively with antidepressants?*

Another problem that continues to plague investigators is the definition of an acceptable response to antidepressant treatment of dysthymia. On the one hand, rating scales that are commonly used in controlled trials of antidepressants, such as the Hamilton[22] and the Montgomery-Asberg[23] rating scales, were developed for use in studies of more severely depressed patients, particularly inpatients. As a result, **these scales are weighted heavily by the presence of melancholic symptoms.** Moreover, unless specifically modified, neither scale addresses the reversed neurovegetative features that characterize many cases of early onset chronic depression. Thus, one cannot assume that threshold scores or change ratios standardized in studies of more severely depressed inpatients will prove to be accurate indicators of a significant response in dysthymia. On the other hand, the self-report Beck Depression Inventory[24] might be too cognitively loaded to detect changes in neurovegetative symptoms. Interviewer and self-report forms of the Cornell Dysthymia Rating Scale[25] have been developed to help deal with these problems, although the incremental validity of this measure (over the earlier scales) has not yet been demonstrated.

Recent Studies of Acute Phase Therapy of Dysthymia:

A summary of the more recent studies of antidepressant treatments of dysthymia is outlined in Table 13.1.

Selective Serotonin Reuptake Inhibitors

One of the first prospective studies of pure dysthymia was conducted by Hellerstein and colleagues.[26] This small (n=32), placebo-controlled study found that **fluoxetine (Prozac) (20–60 mg/day) was an effective and well-tolerated treatment. Approximately 60% of completers responded to treatment with the SSRI, compared to a 19% placebo response rate.**

Nobler and colleagues[27] treated 23 elderly dysthymic patients with 11 weeks of open label fluoxetine (20–60 mg/day). Sixty percent of the completers responded. **This favorable finding contrasts to the rela-**

tively poor showing of fluoxetine in several studies of severe late-life major depression.[28,29] Again, it appears to be at least plausable that the SSRIs are much better treatments for dysthymia and milder major depression than they are for melancholia.

Thase and colleagues[30] conducted the largest controlled clinical trial

---

Table 13.1
Summary of Controlled Trials of Pharmacotherapy of Chronic Depression

Antidperessant Classes

Tricyclic Antidepressants
Imipramine
Bakish et al, Lecrubier et al., Versiani et al.[40]

Desipramine
Kocsis et al.[43]

Monoamine Oxidase Inhibitors
Phenelzine
Stewart et al.[13], Stewart et al.[45]

Moclobemide
Versiani et al.[40]

Selective Serotonin Reuptake Inhibitors
Fluoxetine
Hellerstein et al.[26], Dunneret al.[33], Vanelle et al.[35], Biondi et al.[39]

Sertraline
Thase et al.[30], Ravindran al.[34], Thase et al.[41], Thase et al.[48]

Other
Ritanserin (postsynaptic $5HT_2$ antagonist)
Bakish et al.[36]

Amisulpride (selective limbic D_2 & D_3 agonist)
Lecrubier et al.[38], Biondi et all.[39]

* *Full report not yet published.*

** *Maintenance phase study*

---

of pure dysthymia published to date. Four hundred ten patients were randomly assigned to receive 12 weeks of double-blind treatment with *imipramine* (Tofranil) (mean dose: 190 mg/day), *sertraline* (Zoloft) (mean dose: 154 mg/day), or placebo. **Both active drugs were significantly more effective than placebo, although there were significant** differences in side effects and attrition due to adverse events that favored the SSRI over the TCA (see Figure 13.3). A subsequent report from this study also documented that the benefits of active drug treatment generalized to a variety of quality of life and functional measures.[31] The results of additonal analyses suggest that **there also may be an interesting interaction between gender** (or, perhaps more accurately, sex) **and antidepressant class in this data set.**[32] **Specifically, women responded significantly better to sertraline than to imipramine, whereas the response of men did not differ significantly according to compound. The tolerability advantage for sertraline observed in the main trial appeared to be accounted for entirely by the experience of the younger women patients.** It will be worthwhile to go back to earlier data sets to determine if similar sex/drug type interactions have, heretofore, gone undetected.

Dunner and colleagues[33] randomly assigned 31 dysthymic patients to

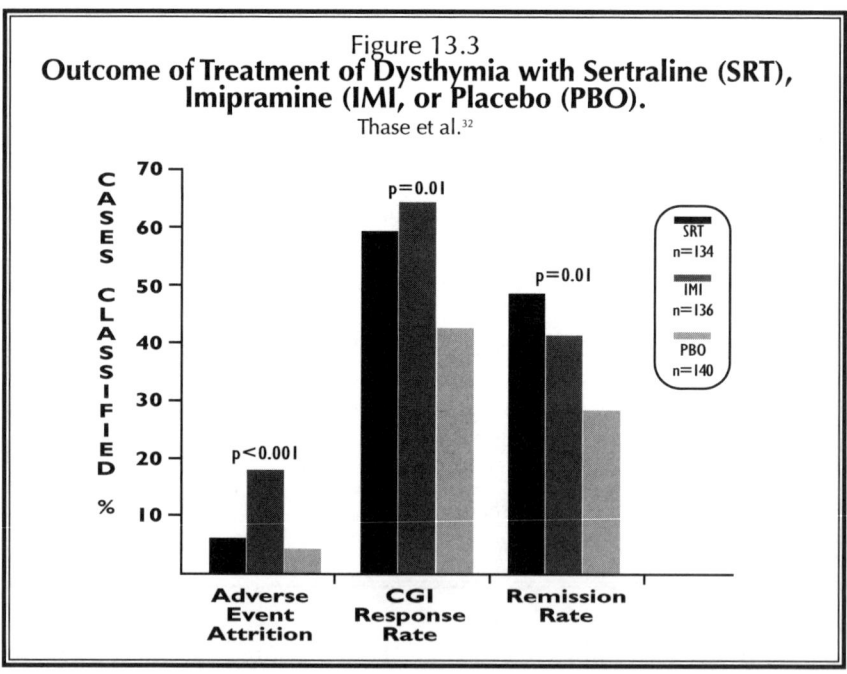

Figure 13.3
Outcome of Treatment of Dysthymia with Sertraline (SRT), Imipramine (IMI, or Placebo (PBO).
Thase et al.[32]

16 weeks of treatment with either *fluoxetine* (20–40 mg/day) or *cognitive therapy*. Although attrition was greater in the fluoxetine group, a consistent pattern of differences suggested that pharmacotherapy

had somewhat better outcomes. However, due to the small size of the study, most of these differences were not statistically significant.

Ravindran and colleagues[34] recently presented preliminary results of a placebo-controlled study comparing sertraline and group cognitive therapy, alone and in combination, among 97 patients with dysthymia. There were 23–25 patients per treatment condition. **The SSRI was significantly more effective than placebo, whereas group therapy was not. The combined treatment condition produced significantly greater improvements on several psychosocial outcome measures. The remission rate was also 18% higher in the combined group as compared to the sertraline alone group, making the latter the second most effective treatment.** However, this potentially clinically meaningful difference was not statistically significant in a study of this size.

Vanelle and colleagues[35] conducted a 3 stage, 6-month placebo-controlled study of *fluoxetine* in 140 patients with pure dysthymia. The results are summarized in Figure 13.4. **During the first 3-month acute phase, 66% of 91 fluoxetine** (20 mg/day) **patients, and only 31% of 49 placebo patients, responded to double-blind treatment. In the second stage of the study, consenting acute phase responders** (fluoxetine, n=42; placebo, n=13) **entered a 3-month continuation phase. Although a few patients relapsed, the proportion of cases achieving full remission by the end of the continuation phase trial was significantly greater in the fluoxetine group. A total of 31 of the nonresponders entered the third phase, during which patients who had received placebo were treated with active fluoxetine** (20 mg/day) **and those who had not responded to fluoxetine had their dosage doubled** (i.e., 40 mg/day). **Response rates of 69%** (switched to active medication) **and 53%** (dosage increase) **and further documented the efficacy of fluoxetine in the treatment of dysthymia.**

Other Agents

Bakish and colleagues[36] compared *imipramine* and *ritanserin* in a placebo-controlled study of 50 patients with dysthymia. Ritanserin, a $5\text{-}HT^2$ receptor antagonist, has a relatively favorable side-effect profile (similar to an SSRI), as well as the added potential advantage of promoting deeper, slow wave sleep. This could be advantageous because decreased slow wave sleep is a trait-like, or state-independent, correlate of depressive disorders that usually is *not* enhanced by standard antidepressants.[37] Bakish and colleagues found that **both active compounds were significantly more effective than placebo. Moreover, ritanserin and imipramine had comparable efficacy.** Despite such apparent promise, it is our understanding that ritanserin is not being developed actively as an antidepressant at this time.

Amisulpride, an atypical antipsychotic unavailable in the United

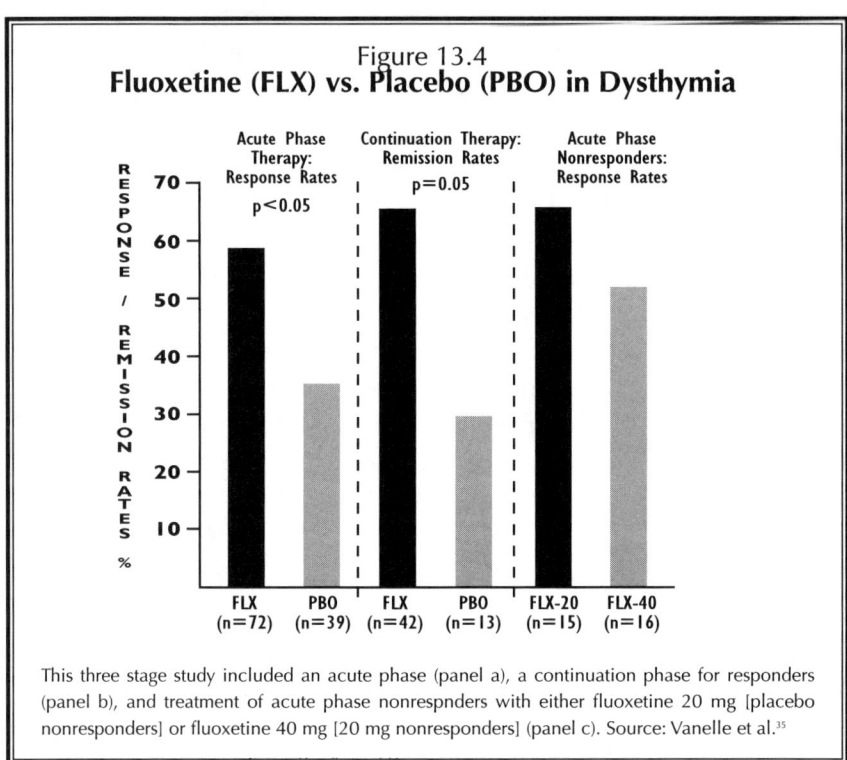

Figure 13.4
Fluoxetine (FLX) vs. Placebo (PBO) in Dysthymia

This three stage study included an acute phase (panel a), a continuation phase for responders (panel b), and treatment of acute phase nonrespnders with either fluoxetine 20 mg [placebo nonresponders] or fluoxetine 40 mg [20 mg nonresponders] (panel c). Source: Vanelle et al.[35]

States, is a relatively selective D_2 and D_3 autoreceptor antagonist at low doses. Because of this property, it enhances dopamine transmission in the limbic system, and has been shown to have antidepressant effects. Two recent European studies have investigated its use in chronic depression. Treatment with amisulpride (50 mg/day) **was as effective as treatment with imipramine** (100 mg/day) **during a 6-month study of a mixed group of patients with dysthymia, double depression, or chronic major depression.**[38] **Both active treatments were more effective than placebo. In addition, amisulpride was better tolerated than imipramine. However, 17% of the women treated with amisulpride** experienced one or more endocrine or gynecological symptoms suggestive of hyperprolactinemia. As amisulpride *blocks* post-synaptic D_2 receptors at higher doses (hence, disinhibiting prolactin release), the optimal dose might even be lower than 50 mg/day for some women. Future studies should include the option for more sensitive patients to reduce the dose to 25 mg/day.

In an as-yet unpublished study, Biondi and colleagues (described by Pages and Dunner[39]) compared *amisulpride* (50 mg/day) and *fluoxetine* (20 mg/day) in a double-blind trial of 268 patients with dysthymia. **Both medications were reported to be well-tolerated and response rates were similar** (amisulpride, 74%; fluoxetine, 67%). Amisulpride appears to be a very promising compound that warrants further study in the treatment of dysthymia. Because of the pronounced interactions of serotonin and dopamine neuronal tracts in the limbic and system prefrontal cortex, it will be interesting to study the use of amisulpride, alone and in combination, to treat patients who do not respond to SSRIs.

Versiani and colleagues[40] studied the MAOI *moclobemide* (Aurorix; not sold in the U.S.) and *imipramine* in an 8-week placebo-controlled trial of 315 patients. **Moclobemide is a reversible inhibitor of MAO type A. Although not available in the United States, it is available throughout much of the world and it does not require the dietary restrictions necessary for use with the older MAOIs. The study showed that both active compounds were significantly more effective than placebo and not significantly different from each other in terms of efficacy. Moclobemide** (mean dose: 675 mg/day) **was generally better tolerated than imipramine** (mean dose: 225 mg/day), **although insomnia was more common in the group receiving the MAOI.**

No placebo-controlled studies of the remaining "newer" antidepressants (i.e., venlafaxine [Effexor], mirtazapine [Remeron], bupropion [Wellbutrin], or nefazodone [Serzone]) **for treatment of dysthymia have been identified. These compounds may be ranked from nonsedating** (bupropion) **to mildly sedating** (venlafaxine and nefazodone) **to very sedating** (mirtazapine); **such sedative effects promise a greater range of treatment options. Moreover, bupropion, nefazodone, and, probably, mirtazapine can be distinguished from the SSRIs by a low incidence of sexual side effects.**[14] **Bupropion can be further differentiated by its weak, but relatively selective, effects on**

dopamine and norepinephrine reuptake. Of these four, bupropion has the least direct effect on 5HT neurotransmission, as well as the smallest track record for treatment of comorbid anxiety. Although probably an SSRI at a low dose, venlafaxine is distinguished from the remainder by potent reuptake inhibition of both serotonin and norepinephrine at dosages above 150 mg/day.

In the absence of data from controlled studies, it is difficult to make recommendations for first-line use of these newer non-SSRI compounds for dysthymia. However, clinical experience and simple logic would suggest that each of these agents will prove to be effective in placebo-controlled studies of dysthymia. It is important to remember that pricing, product loyalty, and other nonpharmacologic factors also influence which agents are used for first-line treatment and which are held in reserve for the more treatment-resistant cases.

Chronic Major Depression and Double Depression:

A large multicenter research program has been conducting a randomized controlled trial comparing sertraline and imipramine in the acute, crossover, continuation, and maintenance treatment of approximately 654 patients with chronic major and double depression. Unpublished data have been analyzed and are being reviewed for publication (see references 6, 30, 32, and 41 for the list of research centers and investigators).

While this project excluded patients with "pure" dysthymia, results are nonetheless relevant to this review. Preliminary analyses revealed that imipramine and sertraline are equally effective as acute phase treatments for both diagnostic subtypes.[6] There was, again, some evidence that the SSRI was better tolerated and more effective than the TCA for the younger female patients.[32]

Thase and colleagues[41] recently presented the results of the crossover treatment phase of a study that included patients who had failed to respond to 12 weeks of double-blind treatment with either imipramine (n=51) or sertraline (n=117). The disparity in cell sizes reflects that, by design, twice as many patients initially received the sertraline. Also, the attrition rate due to side effects during the initial acute phase trial was significantly higher in the imipramine-treated group. **Patients crossed over from imipramine to sertraline were significantly more likely to respond than those switched from sertraline to imipramine**

(60% vs. 44%; see Figure 13.5). **Again, sertraline was better tolerated and had significantly fewer drop-outs due to its side effect profile. Although less than half of the imipramine-treated patients responded to crossover therapy, even this level of response is noteworthy among patients who had not benefitted from 12 weeks of sertraline therapy at maximally tolerated doses (mean=168 mg/day). Thus, one should not assume that failure to respond to one class of antidepressant should preclude trials of alternate classes of medication.**

The combined preliminary results of the acute and crossover phases

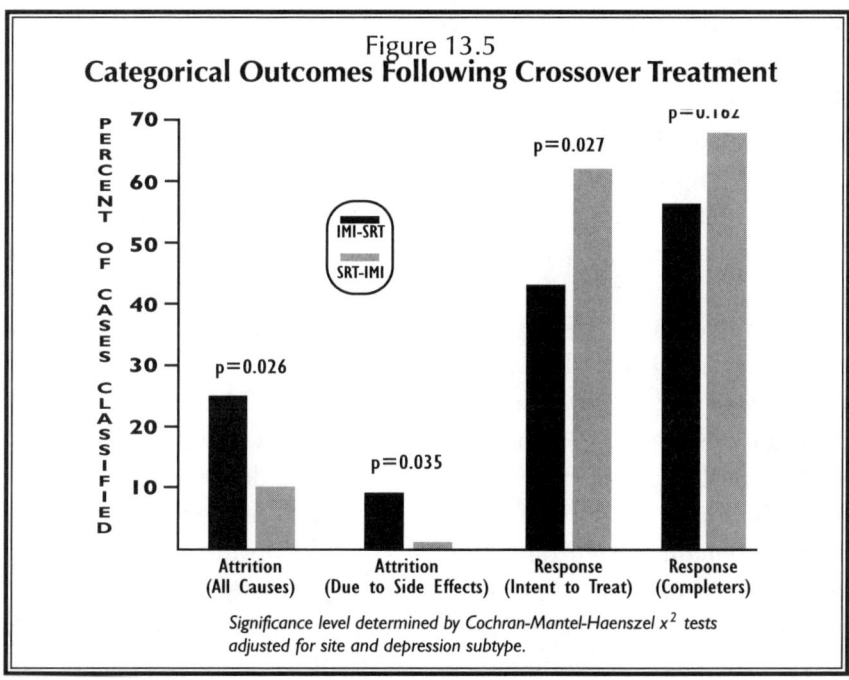

Figure 13.5
Categorical Outcomes Following Crossover Treatment

Significance level determined by Cochran-Mantel-Haenszel x^2 tests adjusted for site and depression subtype.

of this study found that patients who completed a sequence of two drugs (i.e, sertraline followed, if necessary, by imipramine or vice versa) had more than an 80% cumulative response rate.[6,41] Availability of alternate medications with different chemical structures and side effect profiles, as well as numerous augmentation strategies, would suggest that the **conscientious, sequential application of a series of appropriate, empirically verified treatments should yield ambulatory response rates above 90%, even among people with a history of many years of** illness and disability.[42] Moreover, even after failure of multiple medication trials, patients with double or chronic major depression also have at least a 50% chance of responding to a course of bilateral or high energy unilateral ECT.[43] No combination studies have been performed as of yet.

Maintenance Phase Pharmacotherapy:

A 4–6 month period of continuation pharmacotherapy is now recommended for virtually all antidepressant responders to help consolidate response and prevent relapse. Thereafter, an indefinite course of preventative pharmacotherapy may be recommended to lower an ongoing high risk of recurrence. Most specialists have assumed that the chronic depressive disorders, including dysthymia, warrant such maintenance pharmacotherapy. However, until recently there was no empirical data available to validate this practice. Three reports now directly address longer-term treatment in "mixed" samples of chronically depressed patients, although there are still no controlled studies of prophylactic treatment of a sample with pure dysthymia.

Kocsis and colleagues[44] studied the maintenance phase therapy of a group of chronically depressed outpatients treated with *desipramine* (mean dose: 232 mg/day; range: 75–350 mg/day). **The diagnostic composition of the group consisted of about 50% double depression, 40% pure dysthymia, and 10% chronic major depression.** A total of 51 of the initial group of 110 patients (46%) responded to acute phase therapy, remained well throughout a 16-week continuation phase, and consented to random assignment for up to 24 months of maintenance treatment with either active medication or placebo. The results clearly support the value of maintenance pharmacotherapy for depression. For example, **52% of the patients in the placebo condition relapsed as compared to only 15% of the patients taking active desipramine.**

Stewart and colleagues[45] conducted a maintenance phase study of 60 patients with chronic atypical depression who had responded to acute phase therapy with either imipramine (n=32) or phenelzine (Nardil) (n=28). Prior to randomization, patients had remained well throughout a 4-month continuation phase. **The study group was about evenly divided among patients with dysthymia (36%), double depression (28%), and chronic major depression (35%).** Following randomization patients to either continued active pharmacotherapy or double-blind placebo, Stewart and colleagues[45] found that phenelzine had significant prophylactic efficacy, whereas imipramine did not. Interestingly, the phenelzine responders switched to placebo were at greater risk of relapse than either of the groups that had responded to acute phase therapy with imipramine. It is important to note that prior research by this group demonstrated that phenelzine had a much stronger therapeutic effect than imipramine in outpatients with atypical depression (e.g., 65% for the MAOI, 45% for the TCA, and 30% for the placebo).[13] *This suggests that rapid discontinuation of an effective antidepressant (in this case, phenelzine) actually may accelerate the risk of recurrence when compared to the natural history of the disorder.* Research on discontinuation of lithium and neuroleptics has similarly documented an apparent acceleration of relapse risk.[46,47] In practice, such a risk can be lessened by providing a slower medication taper, in addition to patient education, careful and vigilant follow-up, and ongoing psychotherapeutic support.

The final results of the third study are still being analyzed, although several findings have been published in abstract form. Thase and colleagues[48] presented the results of the 18-month maintenance phase of the multi-center clinical trial of double and chronic major depression described previously. Patients who responded to acute phase therapy with sertraline and who remained well during a 16-week continuation phase were randomly assigned to 18 months of treatment with either placebo or active medication. Results demonstrated the superior efficacy of longer-term sertraline therapy as compared to placebo; in fact, the relapse prevention rate was virtually identical to that reported by Kocsis and colleagues.[44] Sertraline was of comparable effectiveness for prophylaxis against recurrence in both double and chronic major depression.

Clinical Issues

Proper acute phase therapy of dysthymia and related chronic depressive disorders should be guided by several principles. Clinicians need to:

1. *Prescribe full dosages of antidepressants;*

2. *Aim for a complete remission if possible;*

3. *Identify and treat comorbid disorders;*

4. *Evaluate, and periodically re-evaluate, the need for psychotherapy; and*

5. *Continue to modify and revise the treatment plan in a timely manner until a remission is achieved.*

When effective, an acute phase therapy can segue naturally into continuation and, as appropriate, maintenance phases of treatment. Generally, this allows a decrease in the frequency of outpatient visits for pharmacologic management (i.e., from twice monthly to monthly to every other month), *but entails* no reduction *of antidepressant dosage.*

It is not yet certain that dysthymic patients or those with chronic major depression who have both achieved a complete remission and have been able to maintain it for longer than six months *require* longer-term therapy. **For those with double depression or chronic major depression, the more conservative strategy is to recommend maintenance phase treatment routinely. Patients with persistent residual symptoms, particularly those associated with significant Axis I comorbidity or personality difficulties, probably have the greatest need for longer-term pharmacotherapy.** Such patients also may be excellent candidates for treatment with a combination of psychotherapy and pharmacotherapy.

Two recently completed studies by Fava and colleagues[49,50] illustrate the value of the sequential use of pharmacotherapy and psychotherapy. The first study[49] randomly assigned 40 patients who had responded to acute phase antidepressant treatment to receive continued pharmacotherapy, either alone or in combination with 12 individual sessions of cognitive-behavioral therapy. Therapy focused on management of residual symptoms, including generalized and specific anxiety. The first study showed that CBT resulted in a significant reduction in residual symptoms.[49] This was subsequently associated with significantly lower risks of relapse and recurrence, according to the second study.[50] One additional study assessed the value of interpersonal psychotherapy for 21 dysthymic patients, who had shown a positive response to antidepressant medication.[51] Psychotherapy resulted in significant improvements in interpersonal and psychosocial functioning. Studies suggest that adding psychotherapy for patients who have responded to pharmacotherapy, but have residual symptoms or psychosocial deficits, may result in an overall superior treatment outcome.

Choosing a Medication:

The typical chronically depressed patient has never before taken an antidepressant; accordingly, the SSRIs are usually a logical place to start. The SSRIs are particularly well-suited for use by primary care physicians working within HMO or point-of-service plans; these physicians have an increasingly greater responsibility for identifying and treating dysthymic patients. Unlike fluoxetine and sertraline, controlled studies of paroxetine (Paxil), fluvoxamine (Luvox), or citalopram (Nitralapram; not available in the U.S.) in dysthymia or related chronic depressions are yet to appear in the literature. Therefore, fluoxetine and sertraline should be used on the basis of demonstrated efficacy in controlled trials. On clinical grounds, the authors can relate no strong reason for favoring a specific choice between fluoxetine and sertraline; each is an excellent choice, each has selective (and debatable) advantages, and neither is perfect. Cost will be an increasingly important consideration in prescribing during the next decade, as the FDA-approved SSRIs begin to go "off patent" (fluoxetine will be the first to do so in the United States, in 2002).

All available evidence suggests that the doses of antidepressants needed to treat dysthymia are comparable to those used to treat major depressive disorder. Thus, no SSRI trial should be considered a failure unless the maximally approved dosage has been tried for at least 2 weeks. Although not proven, many experts believe that chronic depressions may respond more slowly to treatment; therefore, patients may require longer courses of acute phase therapy (i.e., 8–12 weeks instead of the prototypical 4–6 week trial). **In some cases, clinicians** increase the dosage of an SSRI more rapidly than necessary, which may result in greater cost or an increased likelihood of side effects. This can **be most problematic with fluoxetine, because its active metabolite** (norfluoxetine) does not reach steady state until after the fourth week of therapy. Consistent with this notion, studies by Schweizer and colleagues[52] and Nierenberg and colleagues[53] suggest that fluoxetine dosing normally should not be increased above 20 mg/day before the fourth week of therapy. Comparable data are not yet available for sertraline and paroxetine. Until corroborating data become available, **the authors recommend that, at the very least, a 2–3 week trial of sertraline** (50 mg/day) **or paroxetine** (20 mg/day) **should be considered before increasing the dosage above the minimally effective dose.**

In the authors' experience, a trend towards improvement informs the selection of the next treatment option. For example, patients who are experiencing a partial response on a given medication (e.g., 25%–45% improvement in symptoms) **are the most likely to benefit from a dosage increase, whereas absolute nonresponders** (< 20% change) **often warrant a switch to a different antidepressant.** This understanding is consistent with a third study by Fava and colleagues[54] of fluoxetine treatment of patients with recurrent depression. This study found that partial responders to 20 mg of fluoxetine for eight weeks responded significantly better to higher dose fluoxetine than to lithium or desipramine augmentation. Similarly, in a double-blind placebo-controlled study of 20 mg of fluoxetine in patients with dysthymia, Vanelle and colleagues[35] found that 50% of the non-responders (after three months of initial treatment) subsequently responded after three additional months of treatment with 40 mg of fluoxetine.

Common SSRI side effects include nausea, diarrhea, headaches, tremor, insomnia, nervousness, and sexual dysfunction. There are subtle differences between various SSRIs, as well as across individuals, and patients intolerant to one SSRI often can tolerate another SSRI quite nicely.[55,56] Thus, many practitioners should try at least two SSRIs before switching to a different class of medication. It is less certain that for patients who fail to respond to a trial of one SSRI at maximum dosages, they should be switched to a dissimilar type of antidepressant or receive at least one more trial with another SSRI. **However, some data suggest that patients treated maximally with one SSRI may still have about a 40%–50% chance of responding to another SSRI.**[56,57] In our experience, it is clinically reasonable to use a second SSRI in patients who have failed or cannot tolerate an initial SSRI, but a subsequent failure should clearly be an indication for switching to an antidepressant from another class.

Alternate antidepressant choices for SSRI nonresponders include: TCAs, MAOIs, venlafaxine, and the other newer medications. After several SSRI failures, many experts consider the TCAs to be the sine

qua non of efficacy, particularly for treatment of more severe double or chronic major depressions characterized by endogenomorphic features. However, venlafaxine, nefazodone, and mirtazapine also may provide good coverage for many patients with these more severe states.[14] The nonselective MAOIs play a comparable role for treatment of patients with reversed neurovegetative features.[58] Bupropion and moclobemide (outside of the U.S.) provide safe and well-tolerated alternatives to the older MAOIs for the patient with atypical depression. Several of the newer non-SSRI medications have a special utility among patients with sexual dysfunction (e.g., nefazodone, bupropion, and mirtazapine), insomnia (e.g., nefazodone and mirtazapine), or prominent anxiety (e.g., venlafaxine, nefazodone, and mirtazapine).[14] Recently introduced sustained release formulations of venlafaxine[59] and bupropion also should simplify dosing and dosage titration.

When a chronic depressive syndrome responds to antidepressant medications, longer-term preventative pharmacotherapy can significantly improve the subsequent clinical course. Moreover, substantial improvements in vocational and interpersonal functioning typically accompany sustained clinical responses. People with chronic depression have a 50%–60% risk of relapse within the first 6 months of medication withdrawal. Thereafter, a cumulative risk of recurrence of about 10% per year must be faced.[4] When medication must be withdrawn, it makes sense to taper down the medication dosage slowly, over 2–3 months. Focused, problem-oriented psychotherapies may also help reduce the risk of recurrence. For many people with chronic depression, the risks of relapse greatly outweigh the costs associated with an indefinite maintenance treatment. Patient education is a cornerstone of longer-term treatment. It should address the risks and early warning signs of a depressive relapse, the relative effectiveness and safety of long-term antidepressant use, strategies for managing antidepressant side effects, and understanding and coping with life stressors. This should include periodic discussions with patients about the course and outcome of stressors and changes. Such education will greatly enhance adherence to treatment, which will contribute to a better overall long-term outcome.

Conclusion

Research studies and clinical experience during the past 15 years have clearly shown that pharmacotherapy can be an effective treatment modality for many patients with dysthymia. For most such patients, an initial trial of an SSRI antidepressant is appropriate. Patients who fail or cannot tolerate one SSRI can generally be treated with a second SSRI, although especially noxious serotonergic side effects may suggest switching to a dissimilar antidepressant. If an adequate trial of a second SSRI is ineffective or intolerable, switching to a drug from a different class is most appropriate.[60] The choice of an alternative is best dictated by trying to match the side effect profile of a drug to the patient's particular clinical symptoms (e.g., anxiety, sleep disorders) or side effect concerns (e.g., sexual dysfunction, weight gain). Finally, the potential role of psychotherapy in the treatment of dysthymia should not be overlooked or minimized.[61] Practical, behaviorally-oriented, problem-solving psychotherapies, such as cognitive therapy, interpersonal psychotherapy, and social skills training, can be effective alternative treatments for patients who do not respond to or cannot tolerate medication. Moreover, psychotherapy can qualitatively enhance the overall response of some patients by further treating residual symptoms and improving psychosocial deficits.

References

1. American Psychiatric Association. *Diagnostic and Statistical Manual of Mental Disorders*. 4ᵗʰ edition. Washington, DC: Author; 1994.

2. Akiskal HS. Dysthymic disorder: psychopathology of proposed chronic depressive subtypes. *Am J Psychiatry*. 1983;140:11–20.

3. Markowitz JC. Psychotherapy of dysthymia. *Am J Psychiatry*. 1994;151:1114–1121.

4. Keller MB, Hanks DL. Course and natural history of chronic depression. In: Kossis JH, Klein DN, eds. *Diagnosis and Treatment of Chronic Depression*. New York: Guilford Press; 1995:59–72.

5. Shelton RC, Davidson J, Yonkers KA, et al. The undertreatment of dysthymia. *J Clin Psychiatry*. 1997;58:59–65.

6. Keller MB, Harrison W, Fawcett J, et al. Treatment of chronic depression with sertraline or imipramine: preliminary blinded response rates and high rates of undertreatment in the community. *Psychopharmacol Bull*. 1995;31:205–212.

7. Kovacs M, Akiskal HS, Gatsonis C, Parrone PL. Childhood-onset dysthymic disorder: clinical features and prospective naturalistic outcome. *Arch Gen Psychiatry*. 1994;51:365–374.

8. McCullough JP, McCune KJ, Kaye AL, et al. One-year prospective replication study of an untreated sample of community dysthymia subjects. *J Nerv Ment Disord*. 1994;182:396–401.

9. Mueller TI, Keller MB, Leon AC, et al. Recovery after 5 years of unremitting major depressive disorder. *Arch Gen Psychiatry*. 1996;53:794–799.

10. Tyrer P, Seivewright N, Ferguson B, et al. The Nottingham study of neurotic disorder: relationship between personality status and symptoms. *Psychol Med*. 1990;20:423–431.

11. Hirschfeld RMA. Major depression, dysthymia and depressive personality disorder. *Br J Psychiatry*. 1994;165:23–30.

12. Riso LP, Klein DN, Ferro T, et al. Understanding the comorbidity between early-onset dysthymia and cluster B personality disorders: a family study. *Am J Psychiatry*. 1996;153:900–906.

13. Stewart JW, McGrath PJ, Quitkin FM. Relevance of DSM-III depressive subtype and chronicity to antidepressant efficacy in atypical depression. *Arch Gen Psychiatry*. 1989;46:1080–1087.

14. Thase ME, Kupfer DJ. Recent developments in the pharmacotherapy of mood disorders. *J Consult Clin Psychol*. 1996;64:1–14.

15. Martin RM, Hilton SR, Kerry SM, Richards NM. General practitioners' perceptions of the tolerability of antidepressant drugs: a comparison of selective serotonin reuptake inhibitors and tricyclic antidepressants. *Br Med J*. 1997;314:646–651.

16. Howland RH, Thase ME. Biological studies of dysthymia. *Biol Psychiatry*. 1991;30:283–304.

17. Howland RH. Pharmacotherapy of dysthymia: a review. *J Clin Psychopharmacol*. 1991;11:83–92.

18. Harrison WM, Stewart JW. Pharmacotherapy of dysthymic disorder. In: Kocsis JH, Klein DN, eds. *Diagnosis and Treatment of Chronic Depression*. New York: Guilford Press; 1995:124–145.

19. Bielski RJ, Friedel RO. Prediction of tricyclic antidepressant response: a critical review. *Arch Gen Psychiatry*. 1976;33:1479–1489.

20. Joyce PR, Paykel ES. Predictors of drug response in depression. *Arch Gen Psychiatry*. 1989;46:89–99.

21. Thase ME, Howland R. Refractory depression: relevance of psychosocial factors and therapies. *Psychiatric Ann*. 1994;24:232–240.

22. Hamilton M. A rating scale for depression. *J Neurol Neurosurg Psychiatry*. 1960;23:56–62.

23. Montgomery SA, Åsberg M. A new depression scale designed to be sensitive to change. *Br J Psychiatry*. 1979;134:382–389.

24. Beck AT, Ward CH, Mendelson M, Mack J, Erbaugh J. An inventory for measuring depression. *Arch Gen Psychiatry*. 1961;4:561–571.

25. Mason BJ, Kocsis JH, Leon AC, et al. Measurement of severity and treatment response in dysthymia. *Psychiatr Ann*. 1993;23:625–631.

26. Hellerstein DJ, Yanowitch P, Rosenthal J, et al. A randomized double-blind study of fluoxetine versus placebo in the treatment of dysthymia. *Am J Psychiatry*. 1993;150:1169–1175.

27. Nobler MS, Devanand DP, Kim MK, et al. Fluoxetine treatment of dysthymia in the elderly. *J Clin Psychiatry*. 1996;57:254–256.

28. Roose SP, Glassman AH, Attia E, Woodring S. Comparative efficacy of selective serotonin reuptake inhibitors and tricyclics in the treatment of melancholia. *Am J Psychiatry.* 1994;151:1735–1739.

29. Schneider LS, Small GW, Hamilton SH, et al. Fluoxetine Collaborative Study Group. Estrogen replacement and response to fluoxetine in a multicenter geriatric depression trial. *Am J Geriatr Psychiatry.* 1997;5:97–106.

30. Thase ME, Fava M, Halbreich U, et al. A placebo-controlled, randomized clinical trial comparing sertraline and imipramine for the treatment of dysthymia. *Arch Gen Psychiatry.* 1996;53:777–784.

31. Kocsis JH, Zisook S, Davidson J, et al. Double-blind comparison of sertraline, imipramine, and placebo in the treatment of dysthymia: psychosocial outcomes. *Am J Psychiatry.* 1997;154:390–395.

32. Thase ME, Frank E, Kornstein S, Yonkers KA. Sex-related differences in response to treatments of depression. In: Frank E, ed. *Sex, Society, and Madness: Gender and Psychopathology.* Washington, DC: American Psychiatric Press; In press.

33. Dunner DL, Schmaling KB, Hendrickson H, et al. Cognitive therapy versus fluoxetine in the treatment of dysthymic disorder. *Depression.* 1997;4:34–41.

34. Ravindran AV, Telner J, Bialik R, et al. The combined efficacy of cognitive therapy and pharmacotherapy in primary dysthymia. *Biol Psychiatry.* 1997;42:255S.

35. Vanelle JM, Attar-Levy D, Poirier MF, et al. Controlled efficacy study of fluoxetine in dysthymia. *Br J Psychiatry.* 1997;171:345–350.

36. Bakish D, Lapierre YD, Weinstein R, et al. Ritanserin, imipramine and placebo in the treatment of dysthymic disorder. *J Clin Psychopharmacol.* 1993;13:409–414.

37. Thase ME. Depression, sleep, and antidepressants. *J Clin Psychiatry.* 1998;59(Suppl 4):55–56.

38. Lecrubier Y, Boyer P, Turjanski S, Rein W, Amisulpride Study Group. Amisulpride versus imipramine and placebo in dysthymia and major depression. *J Affect Disord.* 1997;43:95–103.

39. Pages KP, Dunner DL. Focus on dysthymic disorder and chronic depression. *Psychiatric Clin N Am Ann Drug Therapy.* 1997;4:91–109.

40. Versiani M, Amrein R, Stabl M. Moclobemide and imipramine in chronic depression (dysthymia): an international double-blind, placebo-controlled trial. *Int Clin Psychopharmacol.* 1997;12:183–193.

41. Thase ME, Keller MB, Gelenberg A, Hirschfeld R, Schatzberg A. Double-blind crossover antidepressant study: sertraline vs. imipramine. *Biol Psychiatry.* 1997;42:230S.

42. Thase ME, Rush AJ. When at first you don't succeed...sequential strategies for antidepressant nonresponders. *J Clin Psychiatry.* 1997;58(Suppl 13):23–29.

43. Prudic J, Haskett RF, Mulsant B, et al. Resistance to antidepressant medications and short-term clinical response to ECT. *Am J Psychiatry.* 1996;153:985–992.

44. Kocsis JH, Friedman A, Markowitz JC, et al. Maintenance therapy for chronic depression. *Arch Gen Psychiatry.* 1996;53:769–774.

45. Stewart JW, Tricamo E, McGrath PJ, Quitkin FM. Prophylactic efficacy of phenelzine and imipramine in chronic atypical depression: likelihood of recurrence on discontinuation after 6 months' remission. *Am J Psychiatry.* 1997;154:31–36.

46. Faedda GL, Tondo L, Baldessarini RJ, Suppes T, Tohen M. Outcome after rapid vs gradual discontinuation of lithium treatment in bipolar disorders. *Arch Gen Psychiatry.* 1993;50:448–455.

47. Viguera AC, Baldessarini RJ, Hegarty JD, van Kammen DP, Tohen M. Clinical risk following abrupt and gradual withdrawal of maintenance neuroleptic treatment. *Arch Gen Psychiatry.* 1997;54:49–55.

48. Thase ME, Keller MB, Gelenberg AJ, et al. Sertraline maintenance therapy in chronic depression. *Psychopharmacol Bull.* 1997;33:482.

49. Fava GA, Grandi S, Zielezny M, Canestrari R, Morphy MA. Cognitive behavioral treatment of residual symptoms in primary major depressive disorder. *Am J Psychiatry.* 1994;151:1295–1299.

50. Fava GA, Grandi S, Zielezny M, Rafanelli C, Canestrari R. Four-year otucome for cognitive behavioral treatment of residual symptoms in major depression. *Am J Psychiatry.* 1996;153:945–947.

51. Markowitz JC. Psychotherapy of the postdysthymic patient. *Journal of Psychotherapy Practice and Research.* 1993;2:157–163.

52. Schweizer E, Rickels K, Amsterdam JD, et al. What constitutes an adequate antidepressant trial for fluoxetine? *J Clin Psychiatry.* 1990;51:8–11.

53. Nierenberg AA, McLean NE, Alpert JE, et al. Early nonresponse to fluoxetine as a predictor of poor 8-week outcome. *Am J Psychiatry.* 1995;152:1500–1503.

54. Fava M, Rosenbaum JF, McGrath PJ, et al. Lithium and tricyclic augmentation of fluoxetine treatment for resistant major depression: a double-blind, controlled study. *Am J Psychiatry.* 1994;151:1372–1374.

55. Brown WA, Harrison W. Are patients who are intolerant to one serotonin selective reuptake inhibitor intolerant to another? *J Clin Psychiatry.* 1995;56:30–34.

56. Thase ME, Blomgren SL, Birkett MA, Apter JT, Tepner RG. Fluoxetine treatment in patients with major depressive disorder who failed initial treatment with sertraline. *J Clin Psychiatry.* 1997;52:16–21.

57. Joffe RT, Levitt AJ, Sokolov STH, Young LT. Response to an open trial of a second SSRI in major depression. *J Clin Psychiatry.* 1996;53:114–115.

58. Thase ME, Trivedi MH, Rush AJ. MAOIs in the contemporary treatment of depression. *Neuropsychopharmacology.* 1995;12:185–219.

59. Thase ME. Efficacy and tolerability of once-daily venlafaxine extended release (XR) in out-patients with major depression. *J Clin Psychiatry.* 1997;58:393–398.

60. Howland RH, Thase ME. Switching strategies for the treatment of unipolar major depression. *Mod Probl Pharmacopsychiatry.* 1997;25:56–65.

61. Howland RH. Psychosocial therapies for dysthymia. In: Flach FF, ed. *The Hatherleigh Guide to Managing Depression.* New York: Hatherleigh Press; 225–241.

14 A Cross-Cultural Perspective on Psychopharmacology

Edmond H. Pi, MD and Gregory E. Gray, MD, PhD

Dr. Pi is Professor of Clinical Psychiatry and Director of Transcultural Psychiatry, University of Southern California School of Medicine, Los Angeles, CA.

Dr. Gray is Professor and Chairman, Department of Psychiatry and Human Behavior, Charles R. Drew University of Medicine and Science, and Director, Augustus F. Hawkins Community Mental Health Center, Martin Luther King, Jr./Drew Medical Center, Los Angeles, CA.

Editor's Note

Doctors Pi and Gray provide us with a most detailed and scholarly analysis of cross-cultural factors in psychopharmacology. The fascination of this topic stems from the range of topics addressed from ethnic differences in cytochrome P450 enzymes to subtle attitudinal differences in psychotropic drug acceptance and use. It is important to emphasize the multiplicity of ethnic and cultural groups throughout the world, of whom relatively few have been studied in any detail. The practical implication is that clinicians must be aware of these factors in their approach to their ethnically disparate patients and in their subsequent use of psychopharmacological agents.

Introduction

As a result of the increasing geographic mobility of populations (including immigration), societies are becoming much more ethnically and culturally diverse. In the United States today, nearly three out of every ten persons is a member of an ethnic minority group, and nearly 20 million Americans are foreign-born.[1]

Because of this increase in ethnic diversity, there has been growing interest in the impact of culture and ethnicity on the diagnosis and treatment of mental disorders. These interests include:

- The incidence, prevalence, and natural history of disorders in various ethnic groups.

- The ways in which members of different ethnic groups seek help from medical and mental health professionals, as well as traditional or folk healers.

- Differences in the way symptoms are expressed in different cultures.

- The impact of cultural differences between patient and professional on the diagnostic and treatment process.

- Differences in response to medications and other therapies.

The understanding of cross-cultural perspectives in psychopharmacology is no longer optional, but has instead become essential for clinicians who are treating an increasing number of psychiatric patients from ethnic and sociocultural backgrounds different from their own. As recent comprehensive reviews[2,3] provide an overview of the impact of culture and ethnicity on psychiatric practice, this article will present a cross-cultural perspective in psychopharmacology which addresses the impact of ethnicity on the pharmacologic therapy of psychiatric illness.

Ethnicity and Culture

Although there is considerable anecdotal evidence that members of different ethnic groups respond differently to psychotropic medications, a number of problems that arise in conducting studies of this phenomena make it difficult to reach definitive conclusions. **The most obvious difficulty concerns the concept of ethnicity itself.** An ethnic group is a subset within the larger society, having a common ancestry and shared social norms, including language and/or religious traditions.[4,5] Although we refer to African American, Asian American, Caucasian, and Hispanic/Latino ethnic groups, it should be clear that considerable variation exists within each group in terms of country of origin of an individual's ancestors, as well as adherence to customs unique to that ethnic group. Within the Latino group, for example, there exists considerable variation between immigrants from Mexico, Central America, Puerto Rico, and other parts of Latin America, especially in terms of their various cultural and health-oriented beliefs.[6]

A related issue is that of genetic diversity within a given ethnic group. For example, African Americans and Latinos may have European, Native American, and African ancestors.[6,7] In recent decades, there has also been a growing number of mixed-race populations with varied backgrounds. Within a given continent, genetic drift[8] may give rise to obvious differences in the physical characteristics of individuals living in different geographic areas;[9] it is therefore likely that some of these differences may affect response to various medications.

There are problems which can influence the results of studies and are related to the diagnostic and prescribing practices of clinicians. For example, clinicians may mistake folk beliefs about witchcraft or spirit possession for delusions.[10,11] Similarly, **it has been noted that African Americans more commonly receive a diagnosis of schizophrenia**[12,13] **and higher doses of antipsychotic medications when in psychiatric emergency rooms than Caucasian patients.**[14] **Incorrect diagnoses and higher dosages of medications can lead to mistaken beliefs about the sensitivity of particular ethnic groups to particular medications. In addition, preconceived notions about the sensitivity of patients of a particular ethnic group may lead the clinician to observe responses that otherwise might not have been noticed, either because of observer bias,**[15] **placebo effects,**[16–18] **or the "Pygmalion effect."**[19]

Pharmacokinetics and Pharmacogenetics

Before focusing on ethnic differences in the response to psychotropic medications, it is helpful to understand the absorption, distribution, metabolism, and elimination of these medications, i.e. pharmacokinetics. **Just as there are inter-individual differences in these processes, so too can there be differences between ethnic groups.**

The first step after administration of a medication is that of absorption. Differences in absorption of a drug can occur because of differences in gastrointestinal motility, the presence of food, and "first-pass" metabolism in the intestinal wall or liver.[20] Dietary factors can alter gastrointestinal motility, absorption, and first pass metabolism;[21] thus, inter-ethnic dietary differences can be responsible for some variation in response to medications.[22–24]

Next, the drug is distributed throughout the body. Most psychotropic medications are transported in the circulation bound to proteins such as albumin.[25] As only the free (unbound) fraction of a medication crosses the blood-brain barrier and interacts with the target receptor, protein-binding plays an important role in determining inter-individual as well as inter-ethnic differences in drug response. **Although ethnic differences in plasma proteins have been noted,[26,27] the significance of these findings has received little study.[28] Plasma concentration of a1-acid glycoprotein, a plasma protein that provides binding sites for psychotropic drugs in the blood, are significantly lower in Asians than in Caucasians and African Americans,[29,30] although levels of albumin are comparable.[30]** Most psychotropic medications are also lipophilic, so they concentrate in adipose tissue.[25] Ethnic differences in the prevalence of obesity[31] could therefore have an impact on drug distribution.

The last two pharmacokinetic processes are drug metabolism and elimination. **Most psychotropic medications are oxidized in the liver, conjugated, and then eliminated in the urine.[20,25]** Most of the research on ethnic differences in pharmacokinetics has focused on differences in the rate of drug metabolism.[32]

There are well-defined pharmacogenetic differences leading to inter-individual, as well as inter-ethnic, differences in rates of drug metabolism.[33] Alcohol metabolism is a well-studied example of a genetically-determined ethnic difference in drug metabolism.[34] Approximately 50% of East Asians lack the active form of the enzyme aldehyde dehydrogenase (ALDH) because of a single amino acid substitution. This enzyme deficiency results in the accumulation of acetaldehyde and the "flushing" response (facial flushing and palpitations). Also, 85%–90% of Chinese and other East Asians possess an "atypical" alcohol dehydrogenase isozyme (ADH) that possesses greater capacity to convert alcohol into acetaldehyde. Another well-studied, genetically-determined ethnic difference in drug response is the deficiency of glucose-6-phosphate dehydrogenase in African Americans, which results in severe hemolytic anemia when taking primaquine, an antimalarial agent.[35]

Acetylation of drugs also demonstrates genetically-determined inter-individual and inter-ethnic differences. Differences in isoniazid toxicity between Asians and Caucasians are due to acetylation enzyme polymorphism. The majority of Chinese and East Asians (78%–93%) are fast acetylators, while only 50% of Caucasians and African Americans are.[36] This is clinically important, as many of the medications used in the treatment of cardiac disorders (e.g., procainamide) and psychiatric conditions (e.g., caffeine, clonazepam [Klonopin], nitrazepam, and phenelzine are metabolized via acetylation.[32]

The activities of the conjugating enzymes (transferases) are genetically determined, but they also can be induced by various environmental factors (e.g., alcohol, coffee, oral contraceptives, diet, tobacco).[37] An example of inter-ethnic differences in conjugation can be seen in the clearance of acetaminophen (85%–90% excreted after glucuronide or sulfate conjugation), which is 20% slower in Asians than in Europeans.

Cytochrome P-450 Enzymes:

A group of enzymes known as the cytochrome P-450 (CYP) system, found mainly in the liver, is involved in the metabolism of a variety of compounds, both endogenous substances and drugs (including most psychotropic medications other than lithium). These enzymes are under genetic control, but certain isozymes can be induced by specific substrates such as phenobarbital, ethanol, and steroids. They can also be inhibited by certain medications which are potent competitive inhibitors of the enzymes, e.g., cimetidine and ketoconazole. In recent years, considerable information about this group of enzymes and its genetic variation has become available.[32,38]

The CYP enzymes show genetic polymorphism, resulting in individuals being classified as either extensive metabolizers (EMs) or poor metabolizers (PMs) depending on whether they carry genetic mutations which alter the amino acid structure and activity of the enzymes.[39–41] Several pharmacologic probes (e.g., antipyrine, debrisoquin, mephenytoin, and sparteine) have been used to study CYP enzyme polymorphism. The two most studied CYP enzymes are 2D6 (debrisoquin hydroxylase) and 2C19 (mephenytoin hydroxylase-CYPmp).[42]

CYP2D6 is involved in the metabolism of a large number of psychotropic medications including beta-blockers (see Table 14.1).[38] A small proportion of the population are PMs who have little or no activity of this enzyme. The proportion who are PMs differs in different ethnic groups (see Table 14.2). In Caucasians, 5%–10% are

PMs, while the proportion of African Americans and Asians who are PMs is 1%–6%.[28,32,38,42] Among the majority of the total population that have adequate CYP2D6 activity (EMs), there also exists considerable variation in the degree of activity due to genetic polymorphism.[38] There are at least nine mutant forms of the enzyme,[43] and 33%–50% of Asian and African EMs appear to have forms of the enzyme that are significantly less active than the form typically found in Caucasians.[32,44] Such individuals are sometimes referred to as "slow metabolizers," in contrast to "poor metabolizers." In addition to genetic differences between various ethnic groups, some of the inter-ethnic differences in enzyme activity may be due to a variety of environmental factors, such as diet, herbal medicines, and other lifestyle differences.[32,44]

Table 14.1
Psychotropic Medications Metabolized by Cytochrome P-450 2D6

Antipsychotics	Chlorpromazine
	Haloperidol
	Perphenazine
	Risperidone
	Thioridazine
Tricyclic antidepressants	Amitriptyline
	Clomipramine
	Desipramine
	Imipramine
	Maprotiline
	Nortriptyline
SSRI antidepressants	Citalopram
	Fluoxetine
	Fluvoxamine
	Paroxetine
	Sertraline
Others	Amphetamine
	Propranolol
	Venlafaxine

Adapted from data compiled by Sjorqvist et al.,[32] Richelson,[38] and Edeki[42]

CYP2C19 (mephenytoin hydroxylase) also shows marked inter-ethnic differences. This enzyme metabolizes diazepam and several antidepressants (see Table 14.3). **Between 2 and 10 percent of**

Table 14.2
Proportion of Population with Little or no Activity
of Cytochrome P-450 2D6

Ethnic group	Country	No. of studies	No. of subjects	% poor metabolizers
Caucasians	U.S.	6	1848	7.5%
	Canada	5	297	7.4%
	Denmark	2	659	8.3%
	France	4	1061	5.5%
	Spain	3	650	8.3%
	Sweden	3	1973	6.5%
	U.K.	2	352	7.4%
Latinos	U.S.	1	22	4.5%
African-Americans	U.S.	1	106	1.9%
Africans	Ghana	3	248	6.0%
	Nigeria	3	426	2.8%
Middle-Easterners	Jordan	3	475	5.1%
Asians	China	4	648	2.0%
	Japan	3	239	1.3%

Adapted from data compiled by Lin et al.[28] and Edeki[42]

Caucasians have little or no activity of this enzyme, while 15%–25% of Asians and African Americans may be PMs (see Table 14.4).[45-48] In addition, there is also evidence of polymorphism among EMs, with some Asian EMs having a form of the enzyme with less activity than the form commonly found in Caucasian EMs.[32]

The third member of the **CYP enzyme displaying inter-ethnic variation in activity is 3A4** (nifedipine oxidase). This enzyme is involved in the metabolism of many psychotropic medications (see Table 14.5). **It appears that Asians have lower CYP3A4 activity than Caucasians, and it is likely that these differences are due to diet or other environmental factors.**[32] This enzyme does not display polymorphism,[38,49] but it is readily inducible (e.g., by carbamazepine [Tegretol] and steroids) as well as inhibited by dietary compounds (e.g., naringin, which is found in grapefruit juice). It is likely that the inter-ethnic differences in CYP3A4 activity are due to dietary differences or other environmental factors.

A fourth member of interest of the CYP enzyme is 1A2 (phenacetin O-deethylase). This enzyme is responsible for the metabolism of clozapine (Clozaril) and several other psychotropic medications

Table 14.3
**Psychotropic Medications Metabolized by
Cytochrome P-450 2C19**

Benzodiazepines	Diazepam
Tricyclic antidepressants	Clomipramine
	Imipramine
SSRI antidepressants	Citalopram
Other	Propranolol

Adapted from Sjoqvist et al.[32]

Table 14.4
**Proportion of Population with Little or No Activity of
Cytochrome P-450 2C19**

Ethnic group	Country	No. of studies	Subjects	No. of % poor metabolizers
Caucasians	U.S.	4	492	3.2%
	Canada	2	201	3.5%
	Denmark	1	358	2.5%
	France	1	132	6.1%
	Sweden	1	253	2.8%
Latinos	U.S.	1	22	4.8%
African-Americans	U.S.	1	27	18.5%
East Indians	India	1	48	20.8%
Asians	China	1	98	17.4%
	Japan	2	300	21.0%

Adapted from data compiled by Lin et al.[28]

(see Table 14.6). Although **there is considerable polymorphism, there are no consistent inter-ethnic differences, with 12%–13% of Caucasians, Asians, and Africans reportedly having little or no activity of this enzyme.**[38] The enzyme is highly inducible (e.g., by charcoal-broiled beef, constituents of tobacco, industrial toxins, and cruciferous vegetables), so inter-ethnic differences are certainly conceivable.

Pharmacodynamics

Whereas pharmacokinetics is concerned with how the body handles drugs, pharmacodynamics is concerned with the effect of a drug on the body. While pharmacokinetic differences between ethnic groups have received the most study, pharmacodynamic differences have also been considered.

Table 14.5
Psychotropic medications metabolized by cytochrome P-450 3A4

Antidepressants	Nefazodone
	Sertraline
	Venlafaxine
Sedative-hypnotics	Alprazolam
	Clonazepam
	Diazepam
	Midazolam
	Triazolam
	Zolpidem
Other	Carbamazepine
	Codeine

Adapted from Sjoqvist et al.[32] and Richelson[38]

Table 14.6
Psychotropic Medications metabolized by Cytochrome P-450 1A2

Antipsychotics	Clozapine
Tricyclic Antidepressants	Amitriptyline
	Imipramine
	Maprotiline
Other	Caffeine
	Propranolol
	Tacrine

Adapted from Sjoqvist et al.[32] and Richelson[38]

One of the best studied examples involves the beta-blocker propranolol (Inderal), which is known to be less effective in treating African Americans with hypertension than Caucasians with the condition. In contrast, Asians not only require substantially lower doses of propranolol, but also experience greater effects on blood pressure and heart rate. These differences are explained by pharmacodynamic factors such as the beta2-adrenoreceptor sensitivity, and not by pharmacokinetic factors.[50]

Some ethnic differences in therapeutic doses and side effects of various psychotropic medications, including neuroleptics, lithium, and tricyclic antidepressants, have also been explained by pharmacodynamic factors, such as tissue/receptor sensitivity.[51–53]

African Americans

There are a number of factors that influence the prescribing of psychotropic medications to African American patients. One of these factors is the care-seeking behavior of the patients themselves. **Compared to Caucasian Americans, African Americans tend to utilize mental health services less frequently.**[54,55] **Instead, they tend to rely more on informal social supports, prayer, folk remedies, non-mental health professionals, or no treatment at all.**[54,56] Some of the underutilization of professional help may come from folk beliefs.[57] In addition, **there is considerable stigmatization associated with mental illness in the African American community.**[56] Patients fear treatment, believing that it will lead to hospitalization.[58] Differences in the ethnicity of the patient and the mental health professional may hinder care seeking (along with having an impact on the therapeutic process itself).[56–59] Lastly, it is important to recognize the "antipsychiatry" movement has targeted the African American community with propaganda that psychiatry and the use of psychotropic medications are part of a genocidal plot.[60]

Antipsychotics:

There is considerable evidence that antipsychotic medications are overprescribed to African-American patients.[58] **African American patients presenting with mania,**[13,61] **depression,**[62] **and alcohol-related symptoms**[63] **are apt to be misdiagnosed as having schizophrenia and prescribed antipsychotic medications. When antipsychotic medications are prescribed, the dosages tend to be higher than in Caucasian patients;**[14,64,65] **also, African American patients are more apt to be prescribed long-acting depot forms.**[66]

Although the dosages prescribed may be higher, **there is a growing suspicion that African Americans may actually be more sensitive to the effects of antipsychotic medications than Caucasians.**[12,58,67] In addition, it has been suggested that African Americans may respond more quickly to antipsychotic agents than Caucasians.[67] Unfortunately, there has been surprisingly little research done on the topic.

Although the studies of CYP2D6 activity suggest that a significant proportion of African Americans may metabolize antipsychotic medications less efficiently than Caucasians,[33] there have been relatively few studies of the pharmacokinetics of these agents in this population. Studies of the pharmacokinetics of trifluoperazine (Stelazine) and fluphenazine (Prolixin) found no differences in clearance between the two ethnic groups.[68,69]

In a study comparing African American patients with Asian, Latino, and Caucasian patients, Jann et al.[70] found no differences between African American and Caucasian patients in the relationship between plasma haloperidol (Haldol) concentration and daily dose. However, the African American patients did have higher concentrations of reduced haloperidol and a higher ratio of reduced haloperidol to haloperidol than the Caucasian patients. Although the ratio may be a marker of CYP2D6 activity, it shows no clear-cut relationship to clinical effect.[71]

A topic that has received more attention is the relationship between ethnicity and risk of tardive dyskinesia. Although Sramek et al.[72] found no difference in the prevalence of tardive dyskinesia among Caucasians, **African Americans, and Latinos in a study of chronic psychiatric inpatients, other more recent studies have found such differences. Glazer et al. found that African American patients were 1.8 times more likely to develop tardive dyskinesia in a 4 year follow-up period than Caucasians.**[73,74] Similarly, Jeste et al., in a study of patients over age 45, found African Americans to have twice the annual incidence of tardive dyskinesia as Caucasians.[75] Whether these differences are due to genetics or environmental factors is unclear. However, they do point to **the need for greater caution in the use of antipsychotic medications for African Americans.**

Finally, it should be noted that there may be inter-ethnic differences in the frequency of mutations in the D-4 dopamine receptors which may affect response to antipsychotic medications. Approximately 10 percent of African Americans appear to have a point mutation that results in a D-4 receptor that does not bind clozapine or dopamine.[76] The clinical significance remains uncertain.

Lithium:

As noted previously, there is a tendency to misdiagnose bipolar disorder as schizophrenia in African American patients.[13,61] **Therefore, there is concern that lithium is underprescribed to African American bipolar patients.**[58]

There have been several studies demonstrating that the RBC/serum lithium ratio is higher in African Americans than in Caucasians.[77-79] This appears to be related to a defect in lithium-sodium countertransport, which is linked to an increased risk of hypertension in African Americans. Although Strickland et al.[79] have linked the higher RBC lithium concentrations to an increase in side-effects among African Americans prescribed lithium, others have not found any increase in lithium side-effects.[80]

There have also been some studies of lithium pharmacokinetics in African Americans which have demonstrated a slightly longer elimination half-life than in Caucasians,[77] although other studies failed to find any significant differences. Given the usual practice of basing dosage adjustments on serum or plasma lithium levels, the clinical significance of this difference in half-life is uncertain.

Antidepressants:

One of the major issues in discussing the use of antidepressants in African Americans is one of underutilization. Compared to Caucasians, African Americans who are depressed use outpatient mental health services less frequently, and instead rely more on informal social supports, prayer, and folk remedies.[54-56] In addition, depression may not be accurately diagnosed by the clinician because of ethnic differences in presenting complaints.[56,58,62,81] As a result, it is estimated that only half of depressed African Americans receive appropriate treatment.[82]

It has been suggested that African Americans may require lower doses and may be more prone to develop toxic side-effects when prescribed antidepressants.[48,58] This may be due in part to pharmacokinetic differences, as the studies of CYP2D6 activity cited above suggest that a significant proportion of African Americans would be expected to metabolize both tricyclic antidepressants (TCAs) and selective serotonin reuptake inhibitors (SSRIs) less efficiently than Caucasians.[33] This has been confirmed by two studies which demonstrated higher plasma concentrations of the TCAs and their active metabolites in

African American patients than in Caucasian patients taking the same doses of medications (after correcting for body weight).[83,84] Similar pharmacokinetic studies with SSRIs are lacking.

There may also be pharmacodynamic differences between African Americans and Caucasians. For example, Raskin et al.[85] noted that African Americans showed a more rapid response to imipramine (Tofranil) than Caucasians. Similarly, Livingston et al.[86] found African Americans treated with TCAs to be at increased risk of developing delirium. Taken together, these findings suggest that antidepressants may certainly be of benefit to depressed African Americans (being at least as effective as in Caucasians), but that African Americans may be at increased risk of side-effects, which is only partly explained by pharmacokinetic differences.[48]

Benzodiazepines:

Several studies have found that African Americans are less likely to be prescribed benzodiazepines than Caucasians.[87–89] Some of this is due to the failure of African Americans to seek treatment of anxiety disorders,[90] but some may also be due to a reluctance of physicians to prescribe these medications to African Americans because of concerns about abuse.

There have been few studies of benzodiazepine pharmacokinetics in African Americans. One of the studies considered adinazolam, a triazolo-benzodiazepine that is still investigational. This study found an increased clearance of adinazolam, but a decreased clearance of its metabolite, N-demethyladinazolam.[91] Given the higher prevalence (15%–25%) of African Americans with little or no CYP 2C19 activity,[32] one would expect diazepam to have, on average, a longer half-life in African Americans. However, this has not been confirmed.

There is also evidence of pharmacodynamic differences regarding benzodiazepines, with African Americans reportedly being more sensitive. This was found in the study of adinazolam,[91] as well as studies using commonly prescribed benzodiazepines.[48,92]

Asians

Asians represent one of the fastest growing ethnic minority groups in the United States. According to the 1990 census, the Asian population in the U.S. grew by 385% from 1971 to 1990. Currently, 7.2 million Asian Americans comprise over 3 percent of the total U.S. population. Asian Americans are a very diverse ethnic, cultural, and linguistic group; they are comprised of immigrants from many different Asian countries, as well as those born in the United States. In 1990, 64% of the Asians in the U.S. were foreign born, and 15% did not speak English well.[93]

Mental illness is frequently viewed as embarrassing or stigmatizing by Asian patients and their families. Asians tend to delay psychiatric care until they are seriously disturbed. When Asians do get into the mental health treatment system, presenting psychiatric conditions have often become severe, chronic, and likely need psychopharmacotherapy.[94] As Asians tend to underutilize or avoid psychiatric care, the general public and some health professionals may perceive Asians as a well-adjusted "model minority" and as having little or no need for psychiatric services. Consequently, there is a lack of culturally and linguistically competent clinicians and treatment facilities for Asian patients.

Culturally determined health beliefs and practices can profoundly influence the psychiatric assessment and psychopharmacotherapy.[95] Cultural influences on the symptoms manifested by **Asian patients may mislead clinicians who are unfamiliar with Asian culture and health beliefs.**[96] **For example, Asian patients often present with somatic rather than psychological complaints and seek help from primary care physicians.** Even in the presence of modern Western medical services, **Asians are frequently influenced by indigenous or alternative remedies; folk or traditional medicine may be tried first for treatment of a psychiatric disorder. This must be assessed and monitored in order to avoid adverse drug interactions between traditional Asian herbal medicines and Western psychotropics.** Other issues include the assessment of efficacy and toxicity of medication compliance, and placebo effects. Several studies have reported that compliance with psychopharmacotheraphy may be more problematic among non-Western than among Western populations. Often, Western medicines are believed to be more potent and, therefore, more likely to cause side-effects than non-Western therapies, as well as there being different interpretations and perceptions of side-effects.[18,97]

Antipsychotics:

Several retrospective surveys and reports have suggested that Asian patients typically require lower dosages of neuroleptics than American or European patients,[98–100] although other studies have failed to confirm this.[101,102]

In several studies of plasma concentrations of neuroleptics, Asians have been found to have higher concentrations than Caucasians. Potkin et al.[103] and Lin et al.[104,105] have found that Asian patients had plasma haloperidol levels that were higher than those of Caucasian Americans. These authors suggested that the pharmacokinetic differences could explain, at least partially, why Asians may require lower doses of haloperidol than Caucasians do to produce similar clinical effects. Although Lin et al.[104] found that both American-born and Asian-born Asians have similar pharmacokinetic profiles, the ethnic differences are more likely due to genetics than to environmental factors.

In a study of haloperidol and its metabolite, reduced haloperidol, Jann et al.[106] reported that reduced haloperidol levels of their Chinese patients were only about one third of their age-matched non-Chinese patients. **The lower reduced haloperidol/haloperidol ratio in Chinese patients, caused either by a slower rate of reduction of haloperidol or a more active oxidation process converting reduced haloperidol back to haloperidol, could significantly affect the clearance of haloperidol and result in higher levels of plasma haloperidol.**

In two studies, Asians prescribed haloperidol were found to have a greater incidence of extrapyramidal side effects than Caucasians and African Americans.[105,107] In regard to tardive dyskinesia (TD), Kane and Smith[108] reported an average prevalence rate of 20% based on 56 studies published between 1959 to 1979 which involved a total of 34,555 patients. The reported prevalence rate of TD in the three studies conducted in different locations in Asia (Japan, Hong Kong, and Shanghai) ranged from less than 10%–20.6%.[109–111] Pi et al.[112,113] conducted an extensive study of TD in Asians involving 982 hospitalized psychiatric patients in China, Hong Kong, Korea, and Japan. In this population, the overall prevalence of TD was 17%, very similar to that reported in non-Asians. However, the prevalence among the Chinese studied in Beijing was only 8.2%. In a similar study of an Asian-

American outpatient population, the prevalence of TD was 15.7%, with 6.1% having moderate TD, and the remainder having mild TD.[114] As pointed out in a recent review, there are significant limitations in the TD studies, including: inadequate and different criteria for the diagnosis of TD; problems with inter-rater reliability using the Abnormal Involuntary Movement Scale (AIMS); cross-sectional design; and difficulties in measuring proposed predictors such as neuroleptic exposure and CPZ equivalents. **Such limitations make it difficult to compare results and confirm that differences in TD truly exist between Asians and non-Asians.**[113]

Finally, there have been recent studies of the atypical antipsychotic clozapine in Asians. Matsuda et al. found that Korean-American patients showed a greater improvement than Caucasians while receiving lower mean doses of clozapine.[115] The Korean, American patients had lower mean clozapine concentrations than the Caucasians, yet they were more likely to experience anticholinergic and other side effects. No cases of agranulocytosis were reported in the Korean American patients, and the incidence in Asians is not known. However, ethnicity has been a risk factor for clozapine-induced agranulocytosis in Ashkenazi Jews, Finns, and Native Americans, related to HLA types.[116-118]

Lithium:

Several retrospective surveys and reports, but not all, have suggested that Asian patients may respond to a lower therapeutic dose range and plasma levels of lithium (0.3–0.9 mEq/L) than those commonly used to treat non-Asian populations.[99,101,119] **However, no differences in lithium pharmacokinetics between ethnic groups have been reported.**[119,120]

Antidepressants:

It is interesting that much of the study of inter-ethnic differences in the pharmacokinetics and pharmacodynamics of psychotropic medications has involved TCAs and their differences between Asians and Caucasians.[121] There are anecdotal reports indicating that Asians require lower doses of tricyclic antidepressants,[99] although other studies of prescribing patterns have failed to confirm this.[101] It has also been suggested that Asians show a therapeutic response at lower blood levels of TCAs.[122]

The TCA clomipramine (Anafranil) is metabolized by CYP 2D6 and CYP 2C19 (see Tables 14.1 and 14.3). Given the high percentage of Asians who are CYP 2D6 "slow metabolizers" (33%–50%)[32,44] and CYP 2C19 "poor metabolizers" (20%, see Table 14.4), **it would be expected that a greater percentage of Asians than Caucasians would metabolize clomipramine slowly.** Pharmacokinetic studies of clomipramine confirmed that Asian Indian or Pakistani subjects had significantly higher mean plasma levels of clomipramine and appeared to be more sensitive to adverse drug effects than English subjects.[123,124] However, Shimoda et al.[125] did not find poor metabolizers of clomipramine among Japanese psychiatric patients with major depressive disorder.

Desipramine (Norpramin) is also metabolized by CYP 2D6 (see Table 14.1). It would therefore be expected to be metabolized slowly by a greater percentage of Asians than Caucasians. Rudorfer et al.[126] studied the pharmacokinetics of a single oral dose of desipramine in Chinese and Caucasian male and female normal volunteers. The Chinese subjects had significantly greater area under the curve (AUC) for both the desipramine and its major metabolite, hydroxy-desipramine. **A trimodal distribution of the desipramine clearance rates was found; all of the Chinese subjects were slow or intermediate metabolizers, and all of the Caucasian subjects were intermediate or fast metabolizers. The authors suggested that Asians who were slow metabolizers were at risk of toxicity from standard doses of tricyclic antidepressants.** No plasma protein binding differences were found between the two groups. These same investigators studied the kinetics of debrisoquin (a CYP 2D6 substrate), and were not able to demonstrate a relationship between the metabolism of the two drugs, i.e., debrisoquin was cleared rapidly by every subject, including those who had shown slow clearance in the desipramine study.[127] These results are perhaps not surprising, given what we now know of CYP 2D6 activity; relatively few Asians are CYP 2D6 poor metabolizers, but a high percentage of the Asian "extensive metabolizers" have a form of the enzyme that is less active than the form found in Caucasians.[32,44] The slower clearance of desipramine was most likely due to the "slow metabolizer" form of the enzyme, rather than the "poor metabolizer" form.

Pi et al.[128] compared the pharmacokinetics of TCAs in healthy Asian and Caucasian volunteers and found no significant differences between the two groups in terms of several kinetic parameters, except that the Asians reached peak serum concentrations faster than Caucasians. Subsequently, Pi et al.[129] undertook a more rigorously designed study (including controlling for body weight) involving 18 Asian and 19 Caucasian age-matched healthy volunteers. Contrary to the previous study, the Asians reached peak plasma desipramine concentrations later than Caucasians. The data also suggested the existence of a trimodal distribution of desipramine clearance in both Asians and Caucasians, with Asians having slightly fewer fast metabolizers. No significant difference in the desipramine saliva/plasma ratio between Asian and Caucasian volunteers was found.[130]

In a pharmacokinetic study of single doses of nortriptyline (Pamelor), Japanese subjects reached higher peak plasma concentrations and had a significantly higher mean AUC than American subjects. The investigators interpreted this finding as a greater bioavailability of nortriptyline in the Japanese.[131]

As noted in a recent critical review on transcultural psychopharmacology of TCAs,[121] there are clinical reports suggesting that differences may exist between Asian and non-Asian populations in the pharmacokinetics and pharmacodynamics of the drugs. Although controlled studies have not consistently supported this view, the evidence that drug disposition may differ among ethnic groups has gained support. Whether these differences are due to pharmacokinetics vs. pharmacodynamics, genetics vs. environmental factors, or shortcomings of study design are not definitively known at this time. However, recent studies of CYP polymorphism support the possibility of genetic differences.

Monoamine oxidase inhibitors (MAOIs) are uncommonly prescribed to Asians,[101] as some common Chinese foods, including fermented bean curd, soy sauce, and fermented soya bean, contain relatively high amounts of pressor amines (ranging from 0.02 to 43 mcg of tyramine per g of food).[132] Since the vast majority of Asians are fast acetylators,[133] the metabolism of phenelzine may be increased in Asians, resulting in higher dosage requirements than in Caucasians.

SSRIs are now widely prescribed for the treatment of depression and other psychiatric disorders. The frequency of their usage has already surpassed all other classes of antidepressants. Unfortunately, there has been little systematic study of possible pharmacodynamic or pharmaco-kinetic differences between Asian and Caucasian populations prescribed SSRIs.[134] This is an area where further research is greatly needed.

Benzodiazepines:

In a survey involving medical schools in Asian countries, it was reported that the dosages of chlordiazepoxide (Librium), diazepam, lorazepam (Ativan), and oxazepam (Serax) used to treat acute anxiety were actually somewhat higher than those recommended in the United States, although maintenance doses were similar.[101]

Studies of diazepam pharmacokinetics have found lower volumes of distribution and higher concentration of diazepam and its metabolite, desmethyldiazepam, in Asians than in Caucasians.[135,136] In one study, these pharmacokinetic differences became statistically insignificant after controlling for ethnic differences in skin fold thickness and the actual/ideal body weight ratio, suggesting that ethnic differences might be due to differences in the percentage of body fat.[136]

Lin et al[137] examined plasma alprazolam concentrations and acute behavioral effects in American-born Asian, foreign-born Asian, and Caucasian healthy male volunteer subjects. **Both Asian groups had higher areas under the curve (AUC), higher peak plasma concentrations, and lower total plasma clearances than the Caucasian group. There was no significant difference between the two Asian groups in any of the parameters examined. Pharmacodynamically, the only significant difference was that foreign-born Asians experienced more sedation compared to both Caucasian and American-born Asian subjects.**

Ajir et al[138] reported that Asians manifested higher maximal serum concentration (Cmax), higher AUC, and lower clearance (CL) of both adinazolam and its major active metabolite than their Caucasian and African-American counterparts. With oral administration, Asians also manifested higher Cmax for both adinazolam and its metabolite. **These findings support that Asian patients require smaller doses of adinazolam than Caucasian patients do to achieve similar levels of adinazolam and its metabolite.**

Latinos

Although Latinos have seldom been a focus of psychopharmacologic research, they are an increasingly important ethnic group to study. The Latino population was estimated at over 21 million in the 1990 Census, but this is probably an underestimation because of undercounting of undocumented immigrants.[6] Over 60% of Latinos live in the Southwest, and an additional 25% live in urban areas of New York, Florida, Illinois, and New Jersey.[6] In New Mexico, California, and Texas, over a quarter of the population is Latino; in Greater Los Angeles, they make up nearly 40% of the population.[6,139]

As with African Americans and Asians, issues related to help-seeking behavior, access to care, and the diagnostic and treatment biases of clinicians have had a major impact on the pharmacologic treatment of mental disorders in Latinos.[140] Adding to the difficulty in studying these issues, Latinos are an extremely diverse group, differing in their health behaviors due to differences in national origin, educational and economic level, and degree of acculturation.[6,141]

There is considerable evidence that Latinos underutilize mental health services.[140,142–145] One reason for this is the high proportion of Latinos (nearly 40%) who lack health insurance.[142,146] A second factor is reliance on non-mental health providers for treatment. Compared to non-Latino whites, **Latinos are more inclined to view mental and physical health as intertwined and to express mental conditions in terms of physical symptoms.**[141,145,147–149] **Resultingly, Latinos are more likely to seek** help from non-psychiatric physicians.[150] In addition, they may seek help from a variety of folk healers, including espiritistas,[140,145] curanderos,[144,149,151] or santeros.[12,141] Prayer and herbal remedies may also be used.[141,151]

For Latinos with Spanish as their primary language, interpreters pose an additional barrier to receiving appropriate services. Interpreters may distort or omit significant symptoms.[152] With bilingual patients, different impressions of the severity of illness can be obtained depending on whether the patient is interviewed in Spanish or English.[144,145]

Antipsychotics:

As with African Americans, **there is some evidence that schizophrenia may be overdiagnosed in Latinos.**[153,154] Factors contributing to this include: the misdiagnosis of folk beliefs about illness causation such as the "evil eye" (mal de ojo) or witchcraft (mal puesto) as psychosis;[11,155] and the overinterpretation of symptoms, such as hallucinations.[155,156]

Recent studies have suggested that **Latino patients with schizophrenia may require daily doses of antipsychotic medications that are 30 percent less than those required by non-Latino Caucasian patients,**[157,158] **although this was not found in a previous survey.**[159] **Recent findings have also suggested that Latinos may require lower doses of clozapine and risperidone.**[160] Any such differences are most likely pharmacodynamic rather than pharmacokinetic, as Latinos do not appear to differ from Caucasians in CYP 2D6 activity.[53] Unfortunately, Latinos have not been separately studied in most pharmacokinetic studies of antipsychotics. However, it does appear that the relationship between plasma haloperidol concentrations and oral dose is similar in Latinos and in non-Latino Caucasians.[70]

The risk of tardive dyskinesia in Latinos has not been studied. However, Sramek et al.,[72] **in a study of hospitalized patients, found no difference in tardive dyskinesia prevalence between African American, Latino, and Caucasian patients.**

Antidepressants:

Rates of depression appear to be similar in Latino populations and non-Latino Caucasian populations.[140] **However, Latinos who are depressed are more likely to focus on somatic complaints.**[161] As noted above, Latinos may be more inclined to seek care outside the mental health system for these complaints, and there is a danger of misdiagnosing a patient's folk beliefs about etiology as being delusional.

Several studies have found Latinos to respond to lower doses of antidepressant medications. For example, Marcos and Cancro[162] found that Latina women (predominantly Puerto Rican) responded to doses of tricyclic antidepressants that were only half those prescribed to Caucasian women. However, **significantly more of the Latinos complained of side effects.** Similarly, Escobar and Tuason[163] found that Colombian patients receiving imipramine complained of more anticholinergic side effects than Caucasians or African Americans in the U.S.

The increased sensitivity to tricyclic antidepressants is most likely

pharmacodynamic. There do not appear to be differences in CYP 2D6 activity[53] Unfortunately, there has been only one study of tricyclic antidepressant pharmacokinetics in Latinos, and that study by Gaviria et al.1[64] found no difference in nortriptyline pharmacokinetics between Latinos and non-Latino Caucasians.

Lithium:

As noted above, there is some evidence that Latino patients with bipolar disorder may be misdiagnosed as having schizophrenia.[154] There do not appear to have been any studies that addressed differences in pharmacokinetics or dosage requirements between Latinos and other ethnic groups. However, **Latinos may be, in some part, of African ancestry, and it is possible that some subsets of Latinos may display the elevated RBC/plasma lithium ratio described by Strickland et al. in African Americans.**[77,79]

Benzodiazepines:

There has been little study of benzodiazepine use in Latinos. Given the tendency of less-acculturated Mexican Americans to expect medication for immediate relief of symptoms,[97,144] it might be expected that benzodiazepines would be widely prescribed for anxiety-related complaints. Counterbalancing this is the attitude among both Mexican Americans and Puerto Ricans that psychotropic medications are addictive and should not be taken for prolonged periods.[97]

The only study of this appears to have been a survey of Latino patients treated by Latino physicians in New York State which was conducted after a triplicate prescription program for benzodiazepines was instituted.[165] Although it is not clear how representative the sample was, 88% of these adult Latino patients were taking benzodiazepines: 67% for anxiety and 42% for insomnia. This is an extremely high prevalence of benzodiazepine use and needs to be confirmed with further studies.

Recommendations and Conclusion

There are now data from systematic and scientifically-designed studies of neuroleptics, lithium, antidepressants, and benzodiazepines which probe the underlying mechanisms and clinical significance of pharmacogenetic, pharmacokinetic, and pharmacodynamic differences from a cross-cultural perspective. However, many questions regarding the cross-cultural aspects of psychotropic medications remain unanswered due to study design limitations. We must be cautious as to how we interpret the findings, and avoid drawing definitive conclusions based upon a limited number of studies, many of which have methodological problems. In order to understand ethnicity and culture as significant influences on psychopharmacology, future studies must overcome the many limitations of previously published studies, including: definition of ethnic populations, small sample size, factors affecting pharmacokinetic parameters, and pharmacodynamic considerations.[52,113,121,134] Also, it is necessary to apply standardized methods, to examine more representative subject populations, and to collect data on factors such as: gender, age, lean and actual body weight, birthplace, residence, alcohol/nicotine/caffeine intake patterns, concomitant medical illness and/or medications, diet, menopausal status, menstrual cycle effects, diagnosis, and severity of psychiatric disorders.

Newer psychotropic medications including "atypical" neuroleptics and SSRIs may be beneficial for all ethnic groups, since they possess equal or greater therapeutic effects and less side-effects than traditional psychotropic medications. However, the impact of ethnicity and culture on these newer medications needs to be studied. Since the diversity in CYP isozymes affects the metabolism of many psychotropic medications, further studies of the genetic differences (polymorphism) of CYP isozymes need to be carried out. Also, the possibility of pharmacodynamic differences (e.g., differences in response to the same tissue concentration of the drug and different receptor sensitivity) requires considerably more study.

Finally, clinicians who treat ethnically and culturally diverse patient populations with mental disorders should design their therapeutic regimen to be "culturally appropriate," especially in regard to the maximization of therapeutic effects and the minimization of unwanted side effects when psychotropic medications are prescribed.

References

1. Carnevale AP, Stone SC. *The American Mosaic*. New York: McGraw-Hill; 1995.

2. Gaw AC, ed. *Culture, Ethnicity, and Mental Illness*. Washington, DC: American Psychiatric Press; 1993.

3. Alarcon RD, ed. Cultural Psychiatry. *Psychiatric Clinics of North America*. 1995(Sept.); 18(3):433–679.

4. Harwood A. Introduction. In: Harwood A, ed. *Ethnicity and Medical Care*. Cambridge, MA: Harvard University Press; 1981:1–36.

5. Senior PA, Bhopal R. Ethnicity as a variable in epidemiological research. *BMJ*. 1994;309:327–330.

6. Aguirre-Molina M, Molina C. Latino populations: who are they? In: Molina CW, Aguirre-Molina M, eds. *Latino Health in the U.S.: a Growing Challenge*. Washington, DC: American Public Health Association; 1994:3–22.

7. Harrison GA. Human genetics. In: Harrison GA, Weiner JS, Tanner JM, Barnicot NA, eds. *Human Biology*. 2nd Ed. Oxford: Oxford University Press, 1977:95–178.

8. Thompson MW, McInnes RR, Willard HF. *Thompson & Thompson Genetics in Medicine*. 5th ed. Philadelphia: W.B. Saunders; 1991.

9. Barnicot NA. Biological variation in modern populations. In: Harrison GA, Weiner JS, Tanner JM, Barnicot NA, eds. *Human Biology*. 2nd ed. Oxford: Oxford University Press; 1977:179–298.

10. Gray GE, Baron D, Herman J. Importance of medical anthropology to clinical psychiatry. *Am J Psychiatry*. 1985;142:275.

11. Alonso L, Jeffrey WD. Mental illness complicated by the Santeria belief in spirit possession. *Hosp Community Psychiatry*. 1988;39:1188–1191.

12. Lawson WB. Racial and ethnic factors in psychiatric research. *Hosp Community Psychiatry*. 1986;37:50–54.

13. Bell CC, Mehta AH. The misdiagnosis of black patients with manic-depressive illness. *J Natl Med Assoc*. 1980;72:141–145.

14. Segal SP, Bola JR, Watson MA. Race, quality of care, and antipsychotic prescribing practices in psychiatric emergency services. *Psychiatr Serv*. 1996;47:282–286.

15. Hennekens CH, Buring JE. *Epidemiology in Medicine*. Boston: Little, Brown & Co.; 1987.

16. Frank JD, Frank JB. *Persuasion and Healing: A Comparative Study of Psychotherapy*. 3rd ed. Baltimore: Johns Hopkins University Press; 1991.

17. Moerman D. Anthropology of symbolic healing. *Currents in Anthropology*. 1979;20:59–80.

18. Lee S. Side effects of chronic lithium therapy in Hong Kong Chinese: an ethnopsychiatric perspective. *Cult Med Psychiatry*. 1993;17:301–320.

19. Rosenthal R, Jacobson L. *Pygmalion in the Classroom*. New York: Holt, Rinehart & Winston; 1968.

20. Grahame-Smith DG, Aronson JK. *Oxford Textbook of Clinical Pharmacology and Drug Therapy*. Oxford: Oxford University Press; 1992.

21. Roe DA. Diet, nutrition and drug reactions. In: Shils ME, Olson JA, Shike M, eds. *Modern Nutrition in Health and Disease*. 8th ed. Philadelphia: Lea & Febiger; 1994:1399–1416.

22. Anderson KE, Kappas A. Dietary regulation of cytochrome P450. *Annul Rev Nutr*. 1991;11:141–167.

23. Branch RA, Salih SY, Homeida M. Racial differences in drug metabolizing ability: a study with antipyrine in the Sudan. *Clin Pharmacol Ther*. 1978;24:283–286.

24. Desai NK, Sheth UK, Mucklow JC, et al. Antipyrine clearance in Indian Villiagers. *Br J Clin Pharmacol.* 1980;9:387–394.

25. Janicak PG, Davis JM, Preskorn SH, Ayd FJ. *Principles and Practice of Psychopharmacotherapy.* Baltimore: Williams & Wilkins; 1993.

26. Baumann P, Eap C. *Alpha-Acid Glycoprotein Genetics, Biochemistry, Physiological Functions and Pharmacology.* New York: Alan R. Liss; 1988.

27. Fujuma Y, Kashimura S, Umetsu K, et al. Alpha 2-HS-glycoprotein in the Kyushu district of Japan: description of three new rare variants. *Hum Hered.* 1990;40:49–51.

28. Lin KM, Poland RE, Silver B. Overview: the interface between psychobiology and ethnicity. In: Lin K-M, Poland RE, Nakasaki G, eds. *Psychopharmacology and Psychobiology of Ethnicity.* Washington, DC: American Psychiatric Press; 1993:11–36.

29. Juneja R, Weitkamp L, Straitil A. Further studies of the plasma, alpha1-glycoprotein polymorphism: two new alleles and allele frequencies in Caucasians and in American Blacks. *Hum Hered.* 1988;38:267–272.

30. Zhou HH, Adedoyin A, Wilkinson GR. Differences in plasma binding of drugs between Caucasians and Chinese subjects. *Clin Pharmacol Ther.* 1990;48:10–17.

31. Bjorntorp P. Obesity. *Lancet.* 1997;350:423–426.

32. Sjoqvist F, Borga O, Dahl M-L, Orme MLE. Fundamentals of clinical pharmacology. In: Speight TM, Holford NHG, eds. *Avery's Drug Treatment.* 4th ed. Auckland: Adis International; 1997:1–73.

33. Kalow W. Pharmacogenetics: its biologic roots and the medical challenge. *Clin Pharmacol Ther.* 1993;54:235–241.

34. Agarwal DP, Goedde HW. *Alcohol Metabolism, Alcohol Intolerance and Alcoholism: Biochemical and Pharmacogenetic Approaches.* Berlin: Springer-Verlag; 1990.

35. Kalow W. Pharmacogenetics: past and future. *Life Sci.* 1990;47:1385–1397.

36. Weber WW. *The Acetylator Genes and Drug Responses.* New York: Oxford University Press; 1987.

37. Mucklow JC, Fraser HS, Bulpitt CJ, et al. Environmental factors affecting paracetamol metabolism in London factory and office workers. *Br J Clin Pharmacol.* 1980;10:67–74.

38. Richelson E. *Pharmacokinetic drug interactions of new antidepressants: a review of the effects on the metabolism of other drugs.* Mayo Clin Proc. 1997;72:835–847.

39. Gonzalez FJ. Human cytochromes P450: problem and prospects. *Trends Pharmacol Sci Rev.* 1992;13:346–352.

40. Gonzalez FJ. The molecular biology of cytochrome P450s. *Pharmacol Sci Rev.* 1989;40:243–288.

41. Kalow W. Interethnic variation of drug metabolism. *Trends Pharmacol Sci Rev.* 1991;12:102–107.

42. Edeki T. Clinical importance of genetic polymorphism of drug oxidation. *Mt Sinai J Med.* 1996;63:291–300.

43. Kroemer HK, Eichelbaum M. It's the genes, stupid: molecular basis and clinical consequences of genetic cytochrome P450 2D6 polymorphism. *Life Sci.* 1995;56:2285–2298.

44. Smith MW, Mendoza RP. Ethnicity and pharmacogenetics. *Mt Sinai J Med.* 1996;63:285–290.

45. Horai Y, Nakano M, Ishizaki T, et al. Metoprolol and mephenytoin oxidation polymorphism in Far Eastern Oriental subjects: Japanese versus mainland Chinese. *Clin Pharmacol Ther.* 1989;46:198–207.

46. Kupfer A, Preisig R. Pharmacogenetics of mephenytoin: a new drug hydroxylation polymorphism in man. *Eur J Clin Pharmacol.* 1984;26:753–759.

47. Meyer UA. Molecular genetics and the future of pharmacogenetics. *Pharmacol Ther.* 1990;46:349–355.

48. Strickland TL, Stein R, Lin K-M, Risby E, Fong R. The pharmacologic treatment of anxiety and depression in African Americans: considerations for the general practitioner. *Arch Fam Med.* 1997;6:371–375.

49. Coutts RT. Polymorphism in the metabolism of drugs, including antidepressant drugs: comments on phenotyping. *J Psychiatry Neurosci.* 1994;19:30–44.

50. Zhou HH, Koshakji RP, Siberstein DJ, Wilkinson GR, Wood AJ. Altered sensitivity to and clearance of propranolol in men of Chinese descent as compared with American Whites. *N Engl J Med.* 1989;320:565–570.

51. Kalow W. Race and therapeutic drug response. *N Eng J Med.* 1989;320:588–589.

52. Pi EH. Transcultural psychopharmacology: present and future. *Psychiatry and Clinical Neurosciences.* 1998; (in press).

53. Lin K-M, Anderson D, Poland RE. Ethnicity and psychopharmacology: bridging the gap. *Psychiatr Clin N Am.* 1995;18:635–647.

54. Sussman LK, Robins LN, Earls F. Treatment seeking for depression by black and white Americans. *Soc Sci Med.* 1987;24:187–196.

55. Neighbors HW, Jackson JS, eds. *Mental Health in Black America.* Thousand Oaks, CA: SAGE Publications; 1996.

56. Griffith EEH, Baker FM. Psychiatric care of African Americans. In: Gaw AC, ed. *Culture, Ethnicity, and Mental Illness.* Washington, DC: American Psychiatric Press; 1993:147–173.

57. Jackson JJ. Urban black Americans. In: Harwood A, ed. *Ethnicity and Medical Care.* Cambridge, MA: Harvard University Press; 1981:37–129.

58. Lawson WB. The art and science of the psychopharmacotherapy of African Americans. *Mt Sinai J Med.* 1996;63:301–305.

59. Foulks EF, Pena JM. Ethnicity and psychotherapy: a component in the treatment of cocaine addiction in African Americans. *Psychiatric Clin N Am.* 1995;18:607–620.

60. Bell CC. *Pimping the African-American community.* Psychiatric Services. 1996;47:1025.

61. Bell CC, Mehta H. Misdiagnosis of black patients with manic-depressive illness: second in a series. *J Natl Med Assoc.* 1981;73:101–107.

62. Raskin A, Crook TH, Herman KD. Psychiatric history and symptom differences in black and white depressed outpatients. *J Consult Clin Psychol.* 1975;43:73–80.

63. Bell CC, Thompson JP, Lewis D, et al. Misdiagnosis of alcohol related organic brain syndromes: implications for treatment. In: Brisbane FLL, Womble M, eds. *Treatment of Black Alcoholics.* New York: Haworth Press; 1985:45–65.

64. Flaherty JA, Meagher R. Measuring racial bias in inpatient treatment. *Am J Psychiatry.* 1980;137:679–682.

65. Chung H, Mahler JC, Kakuna T. Racial differences in treatment of psychiatric inpatients. *Psychiatric Services.* 1995;46:586–591.

66. Price N, Glazer W, Morgenstern H. Race and the use of fluphenazine decanoate. *Am J Psychiatry.* 1985;142:1491–1492.

67. Strickland TL, Ranganath V, Lin K-M, et al. Pharmacologic considerations in the treatment of black populations. *Psychopharm Bull.* 1991;27:441–448.

68. Midha KK, Hawes EM, Hubbard JW, et al. Variation in the single dose pharmacokinetics of fluphenazine in psychiatric patients. *Psychopharmacology (Berlin).* 1988;96:206–211.

69. Midha KK, Hawes EM, Hubbard JW, et al. A pharmacokinetic study of trifluoperazine in two ethnic populations. *Psychopharmacology (Berlin).* 1988;95:333–338.

70. Jann MW, Lam YWF, Chang W-H. Haloperidol and reduced haloperidol plasma concentrations in different ethnic populations and interindividual variabilities in haloperidol metabolism. In: Lin K-M, Poland RE, Nakasaki G, eds. *Psychopharmacology and Psychobiology of Ethnicity.* Washington, DC: American Psychiatric Press; 1993:133–152.

71. Inaba T, Someya T, Shibasaki M, Tang S-W, Takahashi S. Influence of ethnicity on reduced haloperidol concentrations in blood. In: Lin K-M, Poland RE, Nekasaki G, eds. *Psychopharmacology and Psychobiology of Ethnicity.* Washington, DC: American Psychiatric Press; 1993:123–132.

72. Sramek J, Roy S, Ahrens T, et al. Prevalence of tardive dyskinesia among three ethnic groups of chronic psychiatric patients. *Hosp Community Psychiatry.* 1991;42:590–592.

73. Glazer WM, Morgenstern H, Doucette J. Race and tardive dyskinesia among outpatients at a CMHC. *Hosp Community Psychiatry.* 1994;45:38–42.

74. Mogenstern H, Glazer WM. Identifying risk factors for tardive dyskinesia among long-term outpatients maintained with neuroleptic medications: results of the Yale Tardive Dyskinesia Study. *Arch Gen Psychiatry.* 1993;50:723–733.

75. Jeste DV, Caligiuri MP, Paulsen JS. Risk of tardive dyskinesia in older patients: a prospective longitudinal study of 266 patients. *Arch Gen Psychiatry.* 1995;52:756–765.

76. Liu ISC, Seeman P, Sanyal S, et al. Dopamine D4 receptor variant in Africans, D4(valine194glycine) is insensitive to dopamine and clozapine: report of a homozygous individual. *Am J Med Genetics.* 1996;61:277–282.

77. Strickland TL, Lawson W, Lin K-M, Fu P. Interethnic variation in response to lithium therapy among African-American and Asian-American populations. In: Lin K-M, Poland RE, Nakasaki G, eds. *Psychopharmacology and Psychobiology of Ethnicity.* Washington DC: American Psychiatric Press; 1993:107–122.

78. Okapu S, Fraxer A, Mendels J. A pilot study of racial differences in erythrocyte lithium transport. *Am J Psychiatry.* 1980;137:120–121.

79. Strickland TL, Lin K-M, Fu P, Anderson D, Zheng Y. Comparison of lithium ratio between African-American and Caucasian bipolar patients. *Biol Psychiatry.* 1995;37:325–330.

80. Shelley RK. Are there ethnic differences in lithium pharmacokinetics and side effects? *Int J Clin Psychopharmacol.* 1987;2:337–342.

81. Adebimpe VR, Hedlund JI, Cho DW, et al. Symptomatology of depression in black and white patients. *J Natl Med Assoc.* 1982;74:185–196.

82. Sussman LK, Robins LN, Earls F. Treatment seeking for depression by black and white Americans. *Soc Sci Med.* 1987;24:187–196.

83. Rudorder MV, Robins E. Amitriptyline overdose: clinical effects on tricyclic antidepressant plasma levels. *J Clin Psychiatry.* 1982;43:457–460.

84. Ziegler VE, Biggs TE. Tricyclic plasma levels-effect of age, race, sex, and smoking. JAMA. 1977;238:2167–2169.

85. Raskin A, Thomas H, Crook MA. Antidepressants in black and white inpatients. *Arch Gen Psychiatry.* 1975;32:643–649.

86. Livingston RL, Zucker DK, Isenberg K, Wetzel RD. Tricyclic antidepressants and delirium. *J Clin Psychiatry.* 1983;44:173–176.

87. Olfson M, Pincus HA. Use of benzodiazepines in the community. *Arch Internal Med.* 1994;154:1235–1240.

88. Swartz M, Landerman R, George LK, et al. Benzodiazepine anti-anxiety agents: relevance and correlates of use in a southern community. *Am J Public Health.* 1991;81:592–596.

89. Zisselman MH, Rovner BW, Kelly KG, Woods C. Benzodiazepine utilization in a university hospital. *Am J Med Quality.* 1994;9:138–141.

90. Paradis CM, Hatch M, Friedman S. Anxiety disorders in African Americans: an update. *J Natl Med Assoc.* 1994;86:609–612.

91. Fleishaker JC, Phillips JP. Adinazolam pharmacokinetics and behavioral effects following administration of 20–60 mg oral doses of its mesylate salt in health volunteers. *Psychopharmacol.* 1989;99:34–39.

92. Henry BW, Overall JE, Markette J. Comparison of major drug therapies for alleviation of anxiety and depression. *Dis Nerv Syst.* 1971;23:655–667.

93. *1990 Summary Tape File 1C.* Washington, DC: United States Bureau of the Census; 1990.

94. Lin KM, Innui TS, Kleinman A, Womack W. Sociocultural determinants of the help-seeking behavior of patients with mental illness. *J Nerv Ment Dis.* 1982;170:78–85.

95. Kleinman A. *Patients and Healers in the Context of Culture: An Exploration of the Borderland Between Anthropology, Medicine, and Psychiatry.* Berkeley: University of California Press; 1980.

96. Lin K-M, Poland RE, Chang S, Chang W-H. Psychopharmacology for the Chinese: cross-ethnic perspectives. In: Lin TY, Tseng WS, Yeh EK, eds. *Chinese Societies and Mental Health.* Hong Kong: Oxford University Press; 1995:308–314.

97. Smith M, Lin K-M, Mendoza R. "Nonbiological" issues affecting psychopharmacology: cultural considerations. In: Lin K-M, Poland RE, Nakasaki G, eds. *Psychopharmacology and Psychobiology of Ethnicity.* Washington, DC: American Psychiatric Press; 1993:37–60.

98. Murph HBM. Ethnic variations in drug responses. *Transcultural Psychiatric Research Review.* 1969;6:6–23.

99. Yamamoto J, Fung D, Lo S, et al. Psychopharmacology for Asian Americans and Pacific Islanders. *Psychopharmacol Bull.* 1979;15:29–31.

100. Lin KM, Finder EJ. Neuroleptic dosages in Asians. *Am J Psychiatry.* 1983;140:490–491.

101. Pi EH, Jain A, Simpson GM. Review and survey of different prescribing practices in Asia. In: Shagass C, Josiassen RC, Bridger WH, et al., eds. *Biological Psychiatry*. New York: Elsevier Publisher; 1986:1536–1538.

102. Sramek JJ, Sayles MA, Simpson GM. Neuroleptic dosage for Asians: failure to replicate. *Am J Psychiatry*. 1986;143:535–536.

103. Potkin SB, Shen Y, Pardes H, et al. Haloperidol concentrations elevated in Chinese patients. *Psychiatric Research*. 1984;12:167–172.

104. Lin KM, Poland RE, Lau JK, et al. Haloperidol and prolactin concentrations in Asians and Caucasians. *J Clin Psychopharmacology*. 1988;8:195–201.

105. Lin KM, Poland RE, Nuccio I, et al. A longitudinal assessment of haloperidol doses and serum concentrations in Asian and Caucasian schizophrenic patients. *Am J Psychiatry*. 1989;146:1307–1311.

106. Jann MW, Chang WH, Davis CM, et al. Haloperidol and reduced haloperidol plasma levels in Chinese vs. Non-Chinese psychiatric patients. *Psychiatry Res*. 1989;30:45–52.

107. Binder RL, Levy R. Extrapyramidal reactions in Asians. *Am J Psychiatry*. 1981;138:1243–1244.

108. Kane JM, Smith JM. Tardive dyskinesia: prevalence and risk factors, 1959 to 1979. *Arch Gen Psychiatry*. 1982;39:473–481.

109. Binder RL, Kazamatsuri H, Nishimura T, et al. Tardive dyskinesia and neuroleptic-induced parkinsonism in Japan. *Am J Psychiatry*. 1987;144:1494–1496.

110. Chiu H, Shum P, Lau J, et al. Prevalence of tardive dyskinesia, tardive dystonia and respiratory dyskinesia among Chinese psychiatric patients in Hong Kong. *Am J Psychiatry*. 1992;149:1081–1085.

111. Ko GN, Zhang LD, Yan WW, et al. The Shanghai 800: prevalence of tardive dyskinesia in a Chinese psychiatric hospital. *Am J Psychiatry*. 1989;146:387–389.

112. Pi EH, Gutierrez MA, Gray GE. Cross-cultural studies in tardive dyskinesia. *Am J Psychiatry*. 1993;150:991.

113. Pi EH, Gutierrez MA, Gray GE. Tardive dyskinesia: cross-cultural perspectives. In: Lin KM, Poland RE, Nakasaki G, eds. *Psychopharmacology and psychobiology of ethnicity*. Washington, DC: American Psychiatric Press; 1993:153–169.

114. Pi EH, Kusuda M, Gray GE, et al. Cross-cultural psychopharmacology: neuroleptic-induced movement disorders. In: Keyzer H, Eckert GM, Forrest IS, et al., eds. *Thiazines and Structurally Related Compounds*. Malabar, FL: Krieger Publishing Co.; 1992:399–408.

115. Matsuda KT, Cho MC, Lin KM, et al. Clozapine dosage, serum levels, efficacy, and side-effect profiles: a comparison of Korean-American and Caucasian patients. *Psychopharmacol Bull*. 1996;32:253–257.

116. Lieberman J, Yunis J, Egea E. HLA-B38, DR4, DQW3 and clozapine-induced agranulocytosis in Jewish patients with schizophrenia. *Arch Gen Psychiatry*. 1990;47:945–948.

117. Amsler HA, Teerenhovi L, Barth E, Harjula K, Vuopio P. Agranulocytosis in patients treated with clozapine: a study of the Finnish epidemic. *Acta Psychiatr Scand*. 1977;56:241–248.

118. Pfister GM, Hanson DR, Roerig JL, et al. Clozapine-induced agranulocytosis in a Native American: HLA typing and further support for an immune-mediated mechanism. *J Clin Psychiatry*. 1992;53:242–244.

119. Yang YY. Prophylactic efficacy of lithium and its effective plasma levels in Chinese bipolar patients. *Acta Psychiatr Scand*. 1985;71:171–175.

120. Takahashi R. Lithium treatment in affective disorders: therapeutic plasma level. *Psychopharmacol Bull*. 1979;15:32–35.

121. Pi EH, Wang AL, Gray GE. Asian/non-Asian transcultural tricyclic antidepressant psychopharmacology: a review. *Prog Neuropsychopharmacol Biol Psychiatry*. 1993;17: 691–702.

122. Yamashita I, Asano Y. Tricyclic antidepressants: therapeutic plasma level. *Psychopharmacol Bull*. 1979;15:40–44.

123. Allen JJ, Rack PH, Vaddadi KS. Differences in the effects of clomipramine on English and Asian volunteers: preliminary report on a pilot study. *Postgrad Med J*. 1977;53(Suppl 4):79–86.

124. Lewis P, Rack PH, Vaddadi KS, et al. Ethnic differences in drug response. *Postgrad Med J*. 1980;56(Suppl 1):46–49.

125. Shimoda K. Noguchi T, Ozeki Y, et al. Metabolism of clomipramine in a Japanese psychiatric population: hydroxylation, desmethylation, and glucuronidation. *Neuropsycho-pharmacology*. 1995;12:323–333.

126. Rudorfer MV, Lane EA, Chang WH, et al. Desipramine pharmacokinetics in Chinese and Caucasian volunteers. *Br J Clin Pharmacology*. 1984;17:433–440.

127. Rudorfer MV, Lane EA, Potter WZ. Interethnic dissociation between debrisoquine and desipramine hydroxylation. *J Clin Pharmacology*. 1985;5:89–92.

128. Pi EH, Simpson GM, Cooper TB. Pharmacokinetics of desipramine in Caucasian and Asian volunteers. *Am J Psychiatry*. 1986;143:1174–1176.

129. Pi EH, Tran-Johnson TK, Walker NR, et al. Pharmacokinetics of desipramine in Asian and Caucasian volunteers. *Psychopharmacol Bull*. 1989;25:483–487.

130. Pi EH, Tran-Johnson T, Gray GE, et al. Saliva and plasma desipramine levels in Asian and Caucasian volunteers. *Psychopharmacol Bull*. 1991;27:281–284.

131. Kishimoto A, Hollister LE. Nortriptyline kinetics in Japanese and Americans. *J Clin Psychopharmacology*. 1984;4:171–172.

132. Sung SK, Lee CM, Young JD, et al. High levels of tyramine in some Chinese foodstuffs. *Human Psychopharmacology*. 1986;1:103–107.

133. Whitford GM. Acetylator phenotype in relation to monoamine oxidase inhibitor antidepressant drug therapy. *International Pharmacopsychiatry*. 1978;31:126–132.

134. Sramek JJ, Pi EH. Ethnicity and antidepressant response. *Mt Sinai J Med*. 1996;63: 320–325.

135. Ghoneim MM, Korttila MK, Chian CK, et al. Diazepam effects and kinetics in Caucasians and Orientals. *Clin Pharmacology and Therapeutics*. 1981;29:749–756.

136. Kumana CR, Lauder IJ, Chan M, Ko W, Lin HF. Differences in diazepam pharmacokinetics in Chinese and White Caucasians: relation to body lipid stores. *Eur J Clin Pharmacol*. 1987;32:211–215.

137. Lin KM, Lau J, Smith R, et al. Comparison of alprazolam plasma levels and behavioral effects in normal Asian and Caucasian male volunteers. *Psychopharmacology*. 1988;96:365–369.

138. Ajir K, Smith M, Lin KM, et al. The pharmacokinetics and pharmacodynamics of adinazolam:multi-ethnic comparisons. *Psychopharmacology*. 1997;129:265–270.

139. Sabagh G, Bozorgmehr M. Population change: immigration and ethnic transformation. In: Waldinger R, Bozorgmehr M, eds. *Ethnic Los Angeles*. New York: Russell Sage Foundation; 1996:79–107.

140. Trevino FM, Rendon MI. Mental illness/mental health issues. In: Molina CW, Aguirre-Molina M, eds. *Latino Health in the U.S.: A Growing Challenge*. Washington, DC: American Public Health Association; 1994:447–475.

141. Molina C, Zambrana RE, Aguirre-Molina MA. The influence of culture, class, and environment on health care. In: Molina CW, Aguirre-Molina M, eds. *Latino Health in the U.S.: A Growing Challenge*. Washington, DC: American Public Health Association; 1994:23–43.

142. Ruiz P, Venegas-Samuels K, Alarcon RD. The economics of pain: mental health care costs among minorities. *Psychiatric Clin N Am*. 1995;18:659–670.

143. Hough RL, Landsverk JA, Karno M, et al. Utilization of health and mental health services by Los Angeles Mexican Americans and non-Hispanic whites. *Arch Gen Psychiatry*. 1987;44:702–709.

144. Martinez C. Psychiatric care of Mexican Americans. In: Gaw AC, ed. *Culture, Ethnicity, and Mental Illness*. Washington, DC: American Psychiatric Press; 1993:431–466.

145. Canino IA, Canino GJ. Psychiatric care of Puerto Ricans. In: Gaw AC, ed. *Culture, Ethnicity, and Mental Illness*. Washington, DC: American Psychiatric Press; 1993:467-499.

146. Giachello ALM. Issues of access and use. In: Molina CW, Aguirre-Molina M, eds. *Latino Health in the U.S.: A Growing Challenge*. Washington, DC: American Public Health Association; 1994:83–111.

147. Fabrega H, Rubel A, Wallace C. Working class Mexican psychiatric outpatients. *Arch Gen Psychiatry*. 1967;16:704–712.

148. Escobar JI, Burnam MA, Karno M, et al. Somatization in the community. *Arch Gen Psychiatry*. 1987;44:713–718.

149. Maduro R. Curanderismo and Latino views of disease and curing. *West J Med*. 1983;139:868–874.

150. Karno M, Ross RN, Caper RA. Mental health roles of physicians in a Mexican American community. *Community Ment Health J*. 1969;5:62–69.

151. Kay MA. Health and illness in a Mexican American barrio. In: Spicer EH, ed. *Ethnic Medicine in the Southwest*. Tucson, AZ: University of Arizona Press; 1977:99–166.

152. Marcos LR. Effects of interpreters on the evaluation of psychopathology in non-English-speaking patients. *Am J Psychiatry*. 1979;136:171–174.

153. Lawson WB, Herrera JM, Costa J. The dexamethasone suppression test as an adjunct in diagnosing depression. *J Assoc Acad Minor Phys*. 1992;3:17–19.

154. Mukherjee MD, Shukla S, Woodle J, Rosen AM, Olarte S. Misdiagnosis of schizophrenia bipolar patients: a multiethnic comparison. *Am J Psychiatry*. 1983;140:1571–1574.

155. Mull DS, Wilcox JA, Briones DF. Pseudo-psychosis in lower-class Mexican American patients. *Psychline*. 1997;2(2):30–35.

156. Phillipus MJ. Successful and unsuccessful approaches to mental health services for an urban Hispanic American population. *Am J Public Health*. 1971;61:820–830.

157. Ruiz S, Chu P, Sramek J, Rotavi E, Herrera J. Neuroleptic dosing in Asian and Hispanic outpatients with schizophrenia. *Mt Sinai J Med*. 1996;63:306–309.

158. Collazo Y, Tam R, Sramek J, Herrera J. Neuroleptic dosing in Hispanic and Asian inpatients with schizophrenia. *Mt Sinai J Med*. 1996;63:310–313.

159. Adams GL, Dworkin RJ, Rosenberg SD. Diagnosis and pharmacotherapy issues in the care of Hispanics in the public sector. *Am J Psychiatry*. 1984;141:970–974.

160. Ramirez LF. Ethnicity and psychopharmacology in Latin America. *Mt Sinai J Med*. 1996;63:330–331.

161. Mezzich JE, Raab ES. Depressive symptomatology across the Americas. *Arch Gen Psychiatry*. 1980;37:818–823.

162. Marcos LR, Cancro R. Pharmacotherapy of Hispanic depressed patients: clinical observations. *Am J Psychother*. 1982;36:505–513.

163. Escobar JI, Tuason VB. Antidepressant agents: a cross-cultural study. *Psychopharmacol Bull*. 1980;16:49–52.

164. Gaviria M, Gil AA, Javaid JI. Nortriptyline kinetics in Hispanic and Anglo subjects. *J Clin Psychopharmacol*. 1986;6:227–231.

165. Rodriguez RF. The impact of the New York triplicate prescription program on the Hispanic community. *NY State J Med*. 1991;91(Suppl 11):24S–27S

Name Index

Name Index

Name Index

Name Index

Name Index

Subject Index

Subject Index